Jul. Cooper.

PHYSIOTHERAPY
IN SOME SURGICAL CONDITIONS

by the same author

★

**A TEXTBOOK OF MEDICAL CONDITIONS
FOR PHYSIOTHERAPISTS**

PHYSIOTHERAPY
IN SOME
SURGICAL CONDITIONS

by

JOAN E. CASH

B.A., F.C.S.P., Dip.T.P.

*A revised edition and
with additional chapters
by specialist contributors*

FABER AND FABER LIMITED

3 Queen Square

London

First published in 1955
by Faber and Faber Limited
Second impression 1955
Second edition 1958
Third edition 1966
Reprinted 1967
Reprinted with minor revisions 1968
Fourth edition 1971
Printed in Great Britain by
Western Printing Services Limited, Bristol

ISBN 0 571 04669 X

FOREWORD TO FIRST EDITION

With the rapid advances that have taken place during the past ten years in anaesthesia, blood transfusion services, chemotherapy, including antibiotics, together with a better understanding of the response of the body to trauma, all surgical procedures have been rendered freer from danger or complication. At the same time, enormous progress has been made by the newer specialities of neurosurgery, plastic surgery and thoracic surgery, the latter more recently embracing several common lesions of the heart. Therapeutically, therefore, surgery has more to offer today than ever before, and physiotherapy has contributed greatly to these exciting developments. It has evolved special pre- and post-operative treatments and exercises, not only for these new procedures, but also for the more orthodox type of operation, and in these latter has minimized the risks of post-operative chest complications and venous thrombosis.

Miss Cash is working in full co-operation with the surgeons at a hospital where all these growing points of surgery are represented and practised, and where, every day, much new knowledge is being gained. It is right and proper, then, that she should record in book form the points of her wide experience and new ideas. Her former book *A Textbook of Medical Conditions for Physiotherapists* dealt mainly with medical ward problems: the present volume is particularly for use in connection with surgical treatment. It is authoritative and right up-to-date, and contains sections on the breast, lungs, heart, abdomen, peripheral vascular disease, kidneys, etc. It will, therefore, fill a much wanted need, and should be as popular as her other book.

F. A. R. STAMMERS

5

PREFACE TO FIRST EDITION

The object of this book is to try to show why physiotherapy is of value in some of the diseases and injuries treated by the surgeon. In most surgical conditions, the purpose of physiotherapy is to assist in the prevention or treatment of complications; for this reason it is the complications rather than the diseases which have been discussed. It was felt that with an understanding of these, much of the work which is so often considered routine would become more interesting and would be carried out far more effectively.

The author has not included a section on congenital or acquired deformities or such orthopaedic procedures as arthroplasty and arthrodesis, as she originally intended to do, because it appeared that a separate book would be needed to cover this work and in addition methods are changing so rapidly that much would be out of date before it could be published.

J. E. C.

PREFACE TO THIRD EDITION

When beginning to prepare a third edition of this textbook it became clear that I would not be able to bring it up-to-date satisfactorily since no one person could make a sufficiently full study of the advances which have taken place in recent years in all the different fields of physiotherapy. The sections on general surgery, neuro-logical and thoracic surgery have, therefore, been completely rewritten by physiotherapists who have specialized in these fields. Mr. Brian Day, F.R.C.S. kindly undertook the supervision of the material for the new edition and also added new matter himself especially in the chapters on recent injuries. Mrs. Sylvia Cunningham originally proposed the names of the various contributors and initiated the contributors' work.

I would like to express my grateful thanks to Mr. Day and to the other contributors, Miss Hamilton, Miss Newton, Miss Shotton, Miss Sutcliffe and Miss Symons, for all the care and interest they have taken. Particularly, I wish to thank Miss P. Jean Cunningham. She had the difficult task of collaborating with people willing to rewrite the various sections and then reconciling the different points of view of the original author and the new contributors. I am very grateful to her. Without her hard work this third edition could never have been produced.

December 1965   J.E.C.

PREFACE TO FOURTH EDITION

Additions and alterations have been made throughout the book for the new edition and the chapter on amputations and that on the pericardium and heart have been completely revised.

J.E.C.

ACKNOWLEDGEMENTS

Miss Cash would like to thank Mr. R. Hudson Evans, M.R.C.S., L.R.C.P., and Mr. C. C. D. Martin, M.B., B.Ch., F.R.C.S.I., of the Artificial Limb and Appliance Centre, Birmingham, and Mr. H. J. B. Day, M.R.C.S., L.R.C.P., of the Artificial Limb and Appliance Centre, Manchester, for their help in the preparation of the chapter on Amputations. She would also like to thank Mr. P. S. London, M.B.E., F.R.C.S., and Mr. R. B. Brookes, F.C.S.P., of the Birmingham Accident Hospital, for their help in the chapter, Recent Injuries, and Miss S. Kelly, M.C.S.P., Superintendent Physiotherapist, Queen Elizabeth Hospital, Birmingham, for her help in the chapter, Surgery of the Ear, Nose and Throat.

Miss Cash would also like to thank Miss D. Caney, M.C.S.P., Dip.T.P., Principal, School of Physiotherapy, Queen Elizabeth Hospital, Birmingham, for her help and advice. Especial thanks are due to Miss P. Jean Cunningham, Editor of Nursing and Medical Books, Faber and Faber Ltd., for unfailing encouragement and guidance.

The following would like to express their thanks:

Mrs. S. A. Hyde would like to thank Miss D. E. Hamilton, Superintendent Physiotherapist, Addenbrookes Hospital, Cambridge, for her help, and Miss J. L. Morris, the Superintendent of the Department of Physiotherapy, Hammersmith Hospital, for her unfailing encouragement and help throughout this work, and for producing the illustrations. She also wishes to thank the cardiac surgical team for their help in the preparation of her chapter. She is particularly indebted to Professor H. H. Bentall, Mr. W. P. Cleland, F.R.C.S., and Dr. M. K. Sykes, D.A.

Mrs. M. C. Balfour, who wrote the chapters on Surgical Neurology, would like to thank Professor Gillingham, Mr. Harris and all other members of the Staff of the Surgical Neurology Department of the Western General Hospital, Edinburgh, for their invaluable help and encouragement.

Miss B. Shotton, Principal, School of Physiotherapy, Bristol Royal

Acknowledgements

Infirmary, who wrote the chapter on General Abdominal Surgery and Gynaecological Surgery, would like to thank Mr. W. Melville Capper, F.R.C.S., Consultant Surgeon, Bristol Royal Hospital, Mrs. B. R. Barkway, M.C.S.P., and Mrs. E. Green, M.C.S.P., Physiotherapy Department, Bristol Royal Infirmary and Miss M. Powell, M.C.S.P., Physiotherapy Department, Frenchay Hospital.

Miss B. Sutcliffe, Superintendent Physiotherapist, Physical Medicine Department, Westminster Hospital, who wrote the chapter on Peripheral Nerve Injuries, would like to thank Butterworth and Co. (Publishers) Ltd., for permission to reproduce photographs from Wing-Commander C. B. Wynn Parry's *Rehabilitation of the Hand*.

Miss A. Symons, Superintendent Physiotherapist, The Churchill Hospital, Headington, Oxford, who wrote the chapters on Thoracic Surgery, would like to thank all who have helped her but especially Mr. C. Grimshaw, F.R.C.S., Thoracic Surgeon, The Churchill Hospital.

CONTENTS

Contents

ILLUSTRATIONS

PLATES

Illustrations

FIGURES

Figures

Chapter I

WOUNDS

by B. CHATWIN, M.C.S.P.,
revised by J. E. CASH, F.C.S.P.

A wound is a loss of continuity of soft tissue caused by force. Very little force is needed if it is applied by a sharp instrument; everyone is familiar with the easy way in which a penknife can enter the tissues to do considerable damage. More force is required if the instrument is blunt, or if damage is caused by knocking against hard objects, or by a heavy fall. In this case, the skin may not be broken, but the underlying tissues are torn and blood vessels may be ruptured. It follows, therefore, that wounds fall into two main divisions; those in which the skin is damaged and the underlying tissues exposed, and those in which the skin remains intact. The latter type of wound is called a contusion and has been dealt with fully elsewhere (see Chapter XIV).

OPEN WOUNDS

These are also termed penetrating wounds as it is inevitable that some, at least, of the deeper structures will be affected. In size, the wound may be quite small and superficial, or it may cover a considerable area. The incision may have been a clean cut as would occur in a surgical operation, or, be caused by some severe accident producing a ragged laceration, with possibly considerable loss of skin and underlying tissues. If the wound is extensive or penetrates deeply, other structures such as nerves, blood vessels or tendons may be involved. A small puncture wound is sometimes misleading as it appears small on the surface but may have caused considerable damage to underlying structures which may not be apparent at first. An incision made during an operation is likely to be a clean wound, as the operation will have been performed under aseptic conditions. It is possible, however, that it may become invaded by organisms, particularly if the patient is suffering from some condition in which they are present, as in a mastoiditis. The wound is then said to be infected. Other wounds are very likely to be infected either at the time of the accident, or by subsequent contact with the patient's clothes.

HEALING OF WOUNDS

To understand the healing of wounds it is necessary to be familiar with the series of events in the development and repair of inflammation (see page 278). Special consideration must be given to these processes, however, as the damaged structures are in contact with the air, and as there is involvement of the skin.

In the case of clean, incised wounds, where there is no loss of tissue and the edges are closely in apposition, healing will occur by first intention. The sharp instrument causing the break in continuity acts as an irritant, and the immediate result is a vasodilatation at the edges of the wound. The narrow gap is filled by a small number of leucocytes and by tissue fluid. This exudate clots so that the edges become stuck together with fibrinous material. In the neighbouring tissue, the connective tissue cells multiply and grow out straight across the fibrin to make connection with others from the opposite side. This is immediately followed by a laying down of fibres by the fibroblasts, through a process not yet fully understood. These fibres bind the edges of the wound together. At the same time changes are occurring in the endothelium. Tiny capillary buds are thrown out. These join others and once joined they hollow out to form a lumen through which blood flows from the parent vessels. This tiny quantity of cells and blood vessels closing the gap is known as granulation tissue and may develop within twelve hours of the injury. During the subsequent few days, the fibres contract and pull the edges of the wound firmly together. By means of a multiplication of epithelial cells, the epithelium grows over the surface. The wound is thus usually completely healed in three or four days, leaving little obvious evidence of recent injury.

In the case of open wounds with tissue loss, simple pulling together of the edges by fibres will be insufficient and more tissue must be formed. This new tissue is granulation tissue. At first the gap is filled by inflammatory exudate and blood clot. Into this, new capillary loops and fibroblasts grow up from the base of the wound, forming a layer of raised red dots known as granulations. Among these granulations will be a considerable number of leucocytes from the new blood vessels and macrophages from the surrounding tissues, their purpose being to resist the invasion of the open surface by micro-organisms. Gradually the wound is filled by granulations from below upwards and the new cells filling up the gap lay down fibres. In time these fibres contract. Eventually, provided the surface remains free from bacteria, epithelium will grow over it from the edges. This epithelium differs from the normal skin, because at first it only consists of a layer or two of cells so that it is thin and transparent. It thickens quickly but never returns to normal because the appendages of the skin do not regenerate, and the skin covering the surface will have no hairs, sweat or sebaceous glands.

As the gap is wider than in the case of clean, incised wounds, more cells are present, more fibres are formed and more contraction therefore takes place. As contraction continues, the cells are flattened and the blood vessels gradually obliterated; thus, in the course of three or four weeks, the granulation tissue changes to vascular fibrous tissue and from vascular tissue to avascular scar tissue. It is evident that the more destruction and loss of tissue there is, the more scar tissue will eventually be formed. This may become a serious disadvantage because contracture of the scar may lead to loss of pliability of the tissues and even to deformity. Should a wound become infected and considerable suppuration occur, much destruction of tissue occurs, and thus considerable quantities of scar tissue will result.

In infected wounds organisms will have invaded the part, necrosis of tissue will have occurred and the surface of the wound becomes covered with a layer of thick pus containing dead tissue cells and organisms. This is known as a 'slough' and is usually adherent to the floor of the wound, sometimes having long tentacles of fibres extending more deeply into the tissues. A wound of this nature is termed an 'ulcer'. This dead area acts as a continued irritant so that inflammatory reaction occurs in the tissues lying beneath it. The exudate so formed loosens the dead cells and tentacles so that they are gradually lifted from the surface and can be removed, often coming away on the dressing. When this has occurred the wound has become clean, but, as there has been destruction of tissue, healing must be carried out by the formation of granulation tissue.

If a wound appears to be clean but fails to heal, it is said to be 'sluggish'. There is no pus or slough, but, in spite of this, no granulation tissue is laid down. This is usually due to a faulty circulation and decreased fibrinous exudate. The cells of the tissues will also be in a poor condition and fail to multiply. The actual cause may be that there is insufficient irritant to produce the required inflammatory reaction, or it may be due to some underlying defect, such as venous congestion, in the circulation of the part. No healing is possible under these conditions and the open area is very likely to become infected, particularly if the patient has been doing the dressings himself over a long period.

FACTORS DETERMINING HEALING

It is obvious that certain conditions must be present for healing to take place and that the type of healing which occurs will depend upon the state of the wound and surrounding tissues. Healing will occur by first intention if the edges of the wound are in apposition. If the wound is gaping, the surgeon can assist the healing by drawing the edges together with sutures. This is the procedure with operation incisions and with many clean-cut lacerations, but, in the latter case, suturing can only be done during the first eight hours as, after that time, the wound has, in all probability, become infected. Healing will also depend on the care taken of the newly forming granulation tissue. The little vascular loops can be broken down easily and bleeding, which delays the healing process, will occur. Two points are therefore important: first, that no strain should be put on a recently sutured wound although a little movement is good as it stimulates healing; second, that great care should be taken not to damage granulation tissue when changing the dressings. Healing will only occur where there is no infection, and strict aseptic precautions must be taken when changing the dressings. A good blood supply is also an important factor, partly to ensure sufficient fibrinous exudate to glue the edges together, and also to provide nutrition to the living cells so that they can multiply and lay down new tissue. As this multiplication plays a large part in the formation of new tissue, a healthy state of tissue cells in the surrounding area is essential. The general condition of the patient is also important, as it is essential that the blood should contain its full supply of corpuscles and antibodies, and that its chemical composition should be normal so that fibrin can be formed and new cells laid down.

Physiotherapy in the Healing of Wounds

A clean, incised wound, which will heal by first intention, does not require physical treatment as it will heal without assistance and is best left alone. Where there has been considerable loss of tissue, physical treatment can be of help to stimulate the formation of granulation tissue, and it is these wounds which will be seen in the physiotherapy department. Since the main object in the treatment of wounds is to gain rapid healing and therefore minimal scar tissue formation, everything should be done to achieve this end. It has already been seen that vascularity is an important point, thus any physical means which stimulate the circulation may be used. In order to estimate the treatment which should be given, it is necessary to make a careful examination of the whole area.

EXAMINATION OF A WOUND

If possible the physiotherapist who is carrying out the treatment should *remove the soiled dressing*, as it is an important factor in estimating the condition of the wound. It may be soaked in pus, denoting the presence of a deeper infection, or wet with a clear fluid, showing increased exudate. If it is coated with a thickish, yellow substance it is probable that slough has come away and observation of the wound shows it to be cleaner than at the last attendance. Attention should then be given to the *floor of the wound*. Its colour should be noticed, whether it is yellowish-grey, showing the presence of a slough, or covered with red dots, denoting granulation tissue. A pale pink colour with no red dots, indicates that the wound is sluggish and not healing. Often the wound will be at different stages over its area and careful note should be taken of the yellow, infected areas which need cleaning and the parts which are granulating well and will need little or no treatment. Special attention should be paid to any parts that are deeper than the rest. The *edges* should be carefully inspected. Well-defined, clear-cut edges denote a spreading wound, particularly if they appear inflamed. If the walls are shelving, it is healing well. In a sluggish or indolent wound, the edges often have bulbous oedematous margins and may overhang the floor by as much as a quarter of an inch (see Plate I). This may be discovered by applying gentle pressure on the skin near the edge then moving slightly backwards and forwards, when the edge will be seen to move over the floor of the wound. The *base* is the zone of tissue surrounding the wound and should not be neglected. It may be indurated and feel hard to the touch, owing to the sclerosis of connective tissue. This occurs if the decrease in circulation has been long-standing, as is so often seen in so-called varicose ulcers. On the other hand the skin may be thin and scaly, or have open eczematous weeping areas showing it to be in a very poor condition. Gentle pressure should be applied an inch or two away from the area to estimate the amount of oedema which is present. Lastly the *limb* should be examined as a whole; the general condition and the circulation of the limb are important. The mobility of all joints and strength of muscles should be tested, as decrease in functional ability may be an important contributing factor to delay in healing.

Having examined the wound, it is important to *keep a record* not only of its appearance but also of its exact size and shape. This can be done by placing over it a piece of sterile Cellophane paper and tracing round the edges on the paper with a pen. If two pieces of Cellophane are placed one over the other, the one underneath which has been in contact with the wound can be thrown away and the top piece of paper dated, and kept in an envelope for future reference. During the course of treatment, successive tracings on separate pieces of paper can then be placed over each other and held to the light so that the parts which have healed or extended can be determined (see Fig. 1). It is important to place some mark indicating

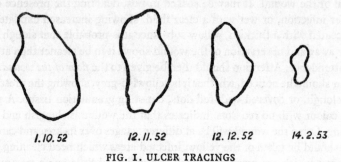

1. 10. 52   *12. 11. 52*   *12. 12. 52*   *14. 2. 53*

FIG. I. ULCER TRACINGS

the position in which the paper was held over the wound so that the paper can be held in exactly the same position when comparison is made. A graph of the area in square centimetres may be charted. A special instrument, the planimeter, can be obtained for this purpose. The needle should be moved along the ink lines of the tracing and the area read on the scale of the apparatus. Another method for discovering the area is to place the tracing over graph paper marked in millimetres and make a rough count of the number of squares it covers.

TREATMENT OF A GRANULATING WOUND

The increase in circulation may be brought about by the use of *ultra-violet and infra-red rays*. The value of these rays lies in the fact that, as both are absorbed in the skin or subcutaneous tissue, the effect will be to increase the superficial circulation and so alter the blood supply to the actual tissues round the wound itself. The infra-red rays penetrate deeper than the ultra-violet, but their effect can only last for several hours at the most, while, although the ultra-violet rays are absorbed in the superficial layers of the skin, the reaction will take several days to disappear. The usual practice is to give a dose of ultra-violet rays and then treat with infra-red until the ultra-violet reaction has died down making it possible to repeat the dose. The equivalent of a second or third degree erythema should be used. The second degree acts as sufficient stimulant to a wound that is granulating, while the stronger dose is required if it appears to be indolent. An area of skin around can also be treated, as this will spread the effect on the circulation to the surrounding tissues. It is advisable to use the Kromayer lamp at a distance of from two to six inches, so that the air will filter out the shorter rays which are destructive and might damage the new tissue which has been laid down. An alternative procedure is to use the blue uviol filter which will have the same effect. If the skin is inflamed or eczematous, it is wise not to expose it, as treatment will still further increase the inflammatory changes and may produce a blister.

Following treatment, a dry dressing may be applied, or Vaseline petroleum jelly gauze or some other lubricant may be used, if there is any likelihood of the dressing sticking to the wound. Sometimes the surgeon may order a stimulating lotion such as gentian violet or red lotion. As these are sensitizers to ultra-violet rays, this should be borne in mind when estimating the dosage for successive treatments.

The reaction to this application of ultra-violet rays may be judged by observation of the dressing at the next attendance (increased exudate is a sign of increased vasodilatation) and by noticing the colour of the skin which has been irradiated, although if it is in a poor condition there is often very little change to see. It is possible to give regular doses with ultra-violet rays, each reaction taking several days to disappear. Between these doses, the patient attends for dressings and can be given a treatment of mild warmth with the infra-red lamp. Care should be taken to remove all ointments from the area before treatment as these may add to the effect of the infra-red rays and produce a burn.

Granulation tissue should be laid down on the floor and edges so that the cavity is gradually filled up, and eventually reaches the level of healthy tissue. During treatment a careful watch should be kept that this is occurring; for, if any part of the cavity becomes sealed off by new tissue, it is likely to become infected and arrest healing. Particular attention should be paid to any overhanging edges and everything possible should be done to stimulate the formation of granulation tissue beneath them. The deeper parts of any ulcer should always be treated first, before any attention is given to the remainder. Sometimes parts may over-granulate, forming mushroom-like blobs of granulation tissue. As the amount of scar tissue formed depends upon the quantity of granulation tissue, these blobs should be destroyed by touching them with some caustic substance, such as copper sulphate, and so preventing formation of more scar tissue than necessary.

While concentrating on the wound itself, it is important that the general condition of the part should not be neglected. It is almost certain that the function will be impaired, owing to the fact that the patient will not be using the part normally. Exercises should be given to maintain the range of movement and muscle strength, but should be carefully controlled so that there is no undue stretching of newly-formed tissue. Massage should also be given if any oedema is present. After the wound has healed, if there has been prolonged splintage, it may be necessary to improve the condition of the skin which has been covered with plaster, by giving massage with oil. Any joints which have become stiff should be given exercises, which should be preceded by the application of some form of heat such as infra-red rays, hot water baths or paraffin wax, but if wax is used care should be taken not to cover the area of the wound with wax until it is quite healed. Should excessive scarring occur or adhesions bind the wound to the underlying tissues, it may be necessary to give treatment to stretch and free the scar. This has been described elsewhere (see page 39).

TREATMENT OF AN INFECTED WOUND

In this case it is most probable that there will be a slough adherent to the floor of the wound, and this can be removed by obtaining a very severe reaction with ultra-violet rays. A strong dose is essential for this purpose and should be obtained with the Kromayer lamp, placed so close to the wound that it is just not touching it. In this way, no rays will be absorbed in the air, and all of them will be used to obtain the desired circulatory reaction. If the wound is large it is possible to irradiate the whole area at once by using the Alpine Sun lamp at a distance of twelve or eighteen inches. In addition, the shorter abiotic rays will be absorbed in the slough itself and will destroy a certain number of bacteria, but, unless the slough is very thin, the effect on the bacteria as a whole is likely to be negligible. As the slough absorbs so many rays, few will actually reach the tissues beneath and it is necessary to give a much stronger dose than usual in order to produce sufficient reaction in the tissues lying beneath. It is not possible to treat any of the surrounding skin as this strong dose would produce a blister; therefore, it is necessary for the skin to be screened right up to the edges of the wound, by spreading on the surface some ointment, which is opaque to the ultra-violet rays, such as Vaseline petroleum jelly or zinc.

If the slough is very thick, or consists of hardened gangrenous tissue, no ultra-violet rays will be able to penetrate to the bed, but a dose to the surrounding skin may produce sufficient vascular changes beneath the slough to be effective. A second or third degree dose should be given.

The effect of this treatment is to increase the blood supply and the ability to fight the infection. It is also of value in that it will produce sufficient exudate to cause increased pressure from within and so force the slough away from its bed. This will free it, so that it can eventually be removed. If treatment has been effective, the dressing will be coated with thickened, yellowish pus and the floor of the wound will look pink and clean.

If a wound is infected and has no slough, there may be only a thin film of pus lying on the floor. In this case treatment by *zinc ionization* is sometimes found useful. A solution of zinc sulphate is used under the positive pole and the zinc ions, having a positive charge, will be driven into the tissues. When these ions enter the tissues, they unite with the proteins of the tissue cells to form a solid zinc albuminate. On removal of the pad after treatment this can be seen as a thin greyish film covering the whole floor of the wound. Zinc is mildly antiseptic and, in this way, the actual tissues on the surface have been converted into an antiseptic covering. While this remains in place, granulation tissue can be formed beneath so that the cavity can gradually fill up from the bottom. The effect of a treatment lasts for about one week, after which it should be repeated.

In order to ensure that the zinc covers the floor, the cavity should be carefully packed with sterile gauze until it is level with the surface. This gauze should be soaked in the solution. It is advisable to cover the floor first with a single layer of gauze which can be left in place after the treatment, as, if it were removed, it would bring with it a certain proportion of the zinc albuminate covering which has been formed. When the surface is even, a pad and electrode can be placed over the whole in the usual way. Most of the current will enter the tissues through the wound, as it has no skin to offer high resistance. It should be remembered, therefore, that the size of the active pad is virtually the size of the non-skin area. To ensure that this is the case, the resistance of the skin may be still further increased by covering it with Vaseline petroleum jelly and non-absorbent wool before placing the pad over it. Some authorities state that it is possible to give a very much higher current over a non-skin area and an average of six milli-amperes per square inch can be taken as a maximum, but, in practice, much less is usually tolerated by the patient.

While the treatment of all infected wounds is the same, there are two special types which will be dealt with more fully, as they are the most likely to be seen. The one is the gravitational ulcer, while the other is the pressure sore such as might occur during a prolonged period of rest.

GRAVITATIONAL ULCER (See Plate II)

This is the term used for ulceration of the lower third of the leg just proximal to the malleoli. It is usually due to venous obstruction resulting from thrombosis of the deep veins of the calf spreading to the popliteal vein. In the process of organization and canalization of the thrombus the valves of the veins are destroyed and the effectiveness of the 'leg muscle pump' correspondingly reduced. Capillary pressure rises and oedema results.

The ulceration commonly begins on the medial side of the leg because here the skin and subcutaneous tissues are drained directly by a communicating vein into the posterior tibial veins. If valves are destroyed reflux of blood from the deep veins will occur and these tissues will be particularly affected by venous congestion. As pressure rises in the capillaries interchange of gases is impaired, nutritional changes occur and the skin resistance is lowered. Red blood cells escape into the tissues, pigments are liberated and act as irritants. Itching and scratching are often followed by infection and this leads to fibrosis and shrinking of the oedematous tissues. This sometimes causes the development of a 'waist' just above the malleoli with oedema distal and proximal. The skin over the area becomes either papery thin or dry and scaly and the area is pigmented, hard and sometimes eczema is present. Eventually, either spontaneously or as a result of minor injury, the skin breaks down and a spreading ulcer develops. Secondary infection then readily occurs.

In addition to the ulcer the general condition of the leg is impaired due to the venous obstruction and consequent oedema. Fluid collecting in the foot and around the ankle gradually organizes, the capsules of the joints shrink and joints become stiff. The leg feels heavy and is sometimes tender and painful, the patient walks with a limp and limits his activities. The foot may be held in the most comfortable position and an equinus deformity sometimes develops.

TREATMENT

Treatment is directed towards the prevention of thrombosis and, if it has developed, to the prevention of chronic oedema (see Chap. XX). If an ulcer has developed the main object of treatment is to get rid of the oedema and unless this is done healing is impossible. The patient is carefully examined to exclude any factors which might be causing raised intravenous pressure, such as a large ovarian cyst. Any factors causing delay in healing, such as vitamin C deficiency, are dealt with and a diet sheet is provided if the patient is overweight.

Bed rest with the foot of the bed raised and a cage over the legs may be ordered for a short period to reduce oedema, or if the ulcer is very painful or spreading, but it is not normally desirable as it predisposes towards further thrombosis.

The most effective treatment is firm elastic support combined with exercises and walking. This method reduces oedema because it compresses the veins and activates the 'leg-muscle pump'. As the calf muscles contract they exert pressure on the veins since the supporting bandage prevents outward expansion of the muscle belly.

given with the **legs** elevated and in sitting on the side of the
egs have been **bandaged**. Correct walking is taught and the
ged to walk as **much** as possible. While exercises are given
range in all **joints** of the foot and ankle, the most important
tarflexion and **dorsiflexion** of the ankle because of its effect
eins and lymphatics. Great stress is laid on regular home
exercises.

ulcer is assisted **not** only by the use of ultra-violet therapy
tening the indurated area around. Finger kneadings starting
ry of the area **should** be done using sterile lanolin. The
dually work **inwards** towards the edge and actually on the
er. If the ulcer is **adherent** it may be gently pressed from side
the fingers **and** thumb.

assage steps **must** be taken not to break down surrounding
is dry and **scaly** and tending to crack it usually responds
e with lanolin. **If** it is papery thin, massage in the area must
one at all or **very** gently and with extreme care.

rays will be **used** both to combat infection and stimulate
he methods already described. (See p. 24.)

PRESSURE SORES

es can be divided into superficial and deep sores. Super-
in in the skin. **These** break down leaving a shallow, painful
res begin in the **subcutaneous** tissues. Muscle and fat have
to pressure **than** skin and destruction may occur in these
covering them **shows** only erythema. Eventually the skin
nd the deeper **necrosed** tissues are exposed. Both types of
pressure. **This** drives the blood out of the vessels and de-
ue of nutrition. In a patient with normal sensation the
discomfort and he alters his position to relieve this, but if
f sensation or he is unconscious or too ill to move pressure
ieved.

rs may precipitate sores: ill-fitting splints, friction from
persistent soaking of the skin resulting from incontinence
condition in venous obstruction may all lead to skin break-
sites for pressure sores are the heels, malleoli, great trochan-
nd sacrum. In **the** latter case, if a patient is nursed in a
osition he tends to slide down and this causes a shearing
acral area, rupturing deeper tissues and small blood vessels
tly leading to a deep pressure sore.

28

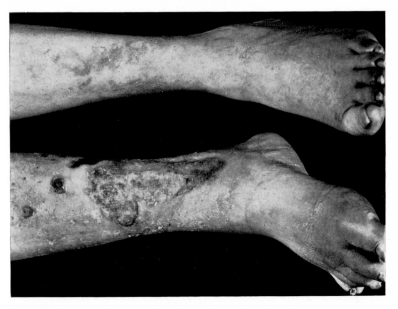

II. Gravitational ulcer: left healed;
right unhealed (*see* p. 25)

I. Bedsore over the sacrum
(*see* p. 21)

overhanging
edge

granulation
tissue

slough

healed area

The compression bandage may b...
bandage applied once or twice a week...
the patient is taught to apply befor...
necessary again during the day. In tl...
legs elevated to reduce swelling befor...
is applied over any necessary dress...
sometimes applied over the ulcer, es...

It is essential that the patient shou...
stretching in the bandage many time...
should walk. This encourages altern...
deep veins and strengthens the musc...

Direct treatment of the ulcer is s...
applications are used. Excision of t...
veins and grafting of the excised are...

Physiotherapy

This has the main object of reduci...
ing again. To achieve this object th...
thened and full range of movement...
also be given to the healing of the ul...
local ultra-violet light and by softer...
the ulcer.

Reduction and control of oedema is b...
under pressure, massage, elevation...
therapist's job to teach the patient...
Particular points to note are: the b...
the proximal limit of the oedema; i...
gets up or after a period of rest with...
not too tight and should become les...
be smooth with no wrinkles. As s...
elasticity a new one must be supplie...

Faradism under pressure and m...
vated. Massage consists mainly of...
begins by stimulating the circulatio...
tous region. Gradually the affecte...
proximal part and when the oeder...
immediately distal is dealt with and...
attention is usually needed to the h...
caneus and around the malleoli.

Exercises...
bed when th...
patient enco...
to increase t...
exercise is p...
on the deep...
practice of t...

Healing of tl...
but also by s...
at the peripl...
fingers will g...
edge of the u...
to side betwe...

In giving...
skin. If the s...
well to massa...
either not be...

Ultra-viole...
healing using...

Pressure s...
ficial sores b...
ulcer. Deep s...
less resistanc...
while the ski...
breaks down...
sore are due...
prives the ti...
pressure caus...
there is loss...
will not be r...

Other fac...
rucked sheet...
and poor ski...
down. Likely...
ters, elbows...
propped-up...
force on the...
and consequ...

Pressure Sores

TREATMENT

Pressure sores should not be allowed to develop. They can usually be prevented by ensuring that unconscious patients or those suffering from loss of sensation do not suffer from prolonged pressure. If the patient is confined to bed and unable to help himself he must be turned every two to three hours night and day. If he is up sitting in a chair he has to be taught to relieve pressure by lifting himself up by his arms—at first every ten minutes and later at regular intervals. Care is also taken to see that splints do not rub, sheets are smooth, the patient does not slide down in the bed and the skin is kept dry. The skin is washed and dried once or twice daily, but rubbing with oil or spirit seems to make little difference.

Once a sore has developed all pressure must be taken off it until it has healed. This will involve the use of special packs and mattresses. The actual sore is treated by excision of any slough, antibiotics in solution to clear up infection and wet sterile saline dressings, covered with a dry dressing and sealed off with porous Elastoplast.

Physiotherapy can help in the prevention and in the treatment of sores. When treating any patient liable to develop pressure sores the physiotherapist should examine the skin carefully and if it shows any erythema, and if the physician is willing, mild heat in the form of infra-red rays should be given several times daily to stimulate the circulation. If a sore is present a course of ultra-violet and infra-red rays will help to control infection and stimulate healing. This should follow the lines indicated on page 24. Short-wave diathermy has been tried and might prove as or more effective for deep infected pressure sores.

Pressure Sores

TREATMENT

...

Chapter II

LOCAL INFECTIONS

by B. CHATWIN, M.C.S.P.,
revised by J. E. CASH, F.C.S.P.

A local infection is present when suppuration occurs in an area of
inflammation. A very severe irritation will produce the usual
inflammatory reaction but will also cause destruction of cells and,
therefore, pus formation. The reaction will be greatest at the point of irritation and it is here that necrosis of tissue occurs. It will be remembered that
an increase in the number of polymorphonuclear leucocytes is one of the
inflammatory changes, and this is an important factor in suppuration as
these leucocytes produce an enzyme which digests the dead cells. For this
reason they are known as pus cells. In the process of digestion, tissue
becomes liquefied and an opaque, yellowish fluid is formed. This is termed
pus. It contains serum, cells and the remaining debris of partially destroyed
tissue cells. At the margins, where pus comes in contact with living cells, a
milder irritation occurs, resulting in the formation of granulation tissue
which encloses the area, localizing the infection. The condition now present
is known as an abscess.

As more and more pus is formed, so the pressure within the abscess
increases, and the wall gives way at its weakest point so that the pus tends
to spread. It will move through the tissues along the path of least resistance,
to reach, either the surface of the skin, or a cavity within the body where it
can be discharged. The exact path taken by the pus is thus determined by
the structures in the region. There is a tendency for fluid to pass down
tendon and muscle sheaths. For example, an abscess formed in the lumbar
vertebrae will track down the sheath of the psoas muscle and eventually
reach the surface high up in the thigh, over the site of the insertion of the
muscle. The pus from an abscess in the hand, however, will not have far to
travel but will open on the skin of the palm. The track formed by the pus is
called a sinus and it may extend for a considerable distance. Its wall, like

those of the abscess, will be fibrous tissue. If an abscess tracks in two directions and discharges on to the surface and also into a body cavity simultaneously, it is termed a fistula.

As soon as the pus has been evacuated from the abscess, healing can begin. This will be by means of the formation of granulation tissue. This must spread from the floor of the abscess cavity up the sinus, eventually to reach the surface, where epithelium will grow over it from the surrounding healthy skin.

If the abscess is in the superficial tissues, it is possible to watch its development. At first the usual signs of inflammation will be present and the area will look red and swollen, and be hot and painful. As the changes continue, it will be noticed that there is a smaller area in the centre where these signs are intensified. If the abscess lies in the skin or just beneath, it may be possible to see the yellow head, where pus has collected, showing through the layers of the skin. If it is not superficial, a dusky redness may show over the site of the abscess. It is often possible to feel a fluctuating fluid, if gentle pressure is applied, although this may not be possible if the capsule is thick. In this case, the area will feel tense and indurated.

While the infection is present, organisms will be absorbed in the lymph stream and carried to the lymph glands which drain the area. It is, therefore, probable that these glands will become inflamed and be hardened and painful. If the lymph vessels themselves are affected, they will also become inflamed, and a lymphangitis occurs with red streaks showing on the limb in the lines of lymphatic drainage. If the organisms are absorbed into the blood stream, they will be carried round the body, spreading the infection to other tissues or producing a general septicaemia. This is most likely to occur in the earlier stages, before the infection has been localized by the surrounding capsule.

A local infection may occur in any of the body structures and the principles of treatment are the same for all. There are, however, certain sites which are more liable to become infected than others, and such infections are more likely to be seen in the physiotherapy department. These will be dealt with separately.

BOILS AND CARBUNCLES

BOILS

A boil is a staphylococcal infection of the skin involving a sebaceous gland and hair follicle, with subsequent suppuration and local gangrene. It is frequently found on the back of the neck where the collar rubs the skin. It will also occur in the buttock, groin or axilla, but may be found anywhere in the body where there are hair follicles. The boil starts with the usual inflammatory changes occurring in a localized area of skin. Sometimes the reaction of the tissues is sufficient to produce resolution and the symptoms gradually disappear without suppuration having occurred. More often this is not the case. Cells are destroyed and an abscess develops producing a prominent rounded swelling which may be the size of a marble or even larger, and is extremely painful. As pus increases in quantity and nears the surface, a yellow area appears in the centre where the skin will break down, forming an opening for evacuation of pus.

Not all the dead tissue is necessarily liquefied in the formation of the abscess and there is usually a semi-solid slough also, which is often called the core. This must separate before healing can begin. After separation has occurred there remains a small cavity with overhanging edges and a floor of granulation tissue, which should heal rapidly. The length of time taken for a boil to develop will depend upon its severity, a usual average being from three to five days. Healing may be expected to be complete in three to five days after the slough has been removed.

CARBUNCLES

A carbuncle shows all the characteristics of a boil but is very much larger and deeper, involving the subcutaneous tissue as well as many hair follicles. Spread of infection occurs because the pus, instead of moving directly to the surface, passes into the connective tissue beneath the skin and spreads outwards in all directions, reaching the surface in many places, so that the centre of the area of infection is covered with small openings through which pus is exuding. For some days the pus will be evacuated through the many openings, but gradually necrosis of the superficial tissues occurs and the whole of the central area becomes open, showing beneath it a whitish-yellow slough. When this separates, it will be found to be a solid mass of dead tissue with long stringy tentacles extending outwards into the surrounding tissue. A large cavity remains with ragged, overhanging edges and granulation tissue beginning to show on the floor.

Because of its size and depth it will take some time to heal. The inflammation around the carbuncle will also take some time to disappear, and redness and swelling tend to remain for some days after the core has separated.

Treatment by Physiotherapy

Boils. The patient is usually given a course of antibiotics. During this time, the application of dry heat will help. This is because heating will accelerate the inflammatory reaction and so shorten the time taken for the infection to develop, or possibly bring about resolution without pus formation. Dry heat is preferred to wet heat as the latter softens the tissues, lowers their resistance and therefore aids the spread of infection. It is therefore quite common to find both chemical and physical methods of treatment being used concurrently. The short-wave diathermy current is the most useful form of heat, because it is possible to produce effects in the deeper tissues rather than in the boil itself. Also the method of application is very much more convenient than that of other currents, as the electrodes do not need to be in contact with the part. The principle underlying the treatment is to give very small doses of heating which are so slight that the heat produced is only just perceptible to the patient, or possibly not even appreciated at all. In this way the normal reaction of the tissues can be accelerated and increased blood supply will be available to combat the infection, without at the same time heating the tissues and also the organisms. If more heating were given, not only would the reaction be too great, but the organisms themselves would become heated and, according to van't Hoff's law, their activity would be increased. These very small doses may be achieved by giving the patient a low current and by limiting the duration of the treatment to a few minutes. They should be repeated at least twice daily, or more often if possible, so that the effect on the circulation can be maintained without producing a rise in temperature of the part.

The patient should begin to have this treatment as soon as the condition is diagnosed. If it is given at this very early stage, it is often possible to bring about resolution of the inflammation without abscess formation and the symptoms will disappear in a day or two. If this does not occur, the increased circulation will provide more leucocytes so that the necrosed tissue is digested more rapidly and the time taken for abscess formation will be considerably lessened. As the short-wave diathermy current has a deep effect, the vasodilatation will be correspondingly deep. This will mean an increase in tension in the structures beneath the abscess and it will force the pus towards the surface more quickly, hastening its evacuation and bringing relief from pain to the patient.

The technique used for giving treatment should be carefully studied, in order that the maximum effects are produced in the tissues beneath the boil and not on the surface. The usual through and through method of placing the electrodes is most suitable as it is likely to produce a through heating effect; but, if the boil is very prominent, a wider air space than normal is necessary to prevent the field from concentrating over the boil (see Fig. 2a).

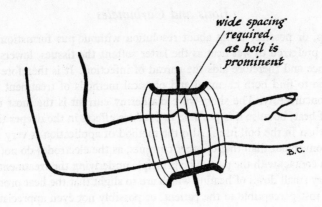

wide spacing
required,
as boil is
prominent

(a) Direct through-and-through method

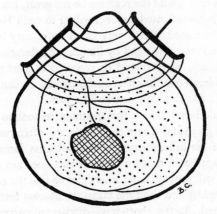

(b) Lateral through-and-through method

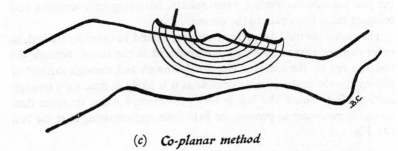

(c) Co-planar method

FIG. 2. METHODS OF PLACING SHORT-WAVE ELECTRODES IN THE
TREATMENT OF BOILS

Also, after the abscess has formed, the presence of a collection of fluid pus may cause the field to concentrate on the abscess within the tissues. To deal with either of these difficulties, it may be necessary to avoid placing the electrodes over the boil itself. On the back of the neck, or in a limb, this can be effected by placing the electrodes on each side of the part and so giving a lateral through and through application (see Fig. 2b).

The co-planar method is an alternative in which the electrodes are placed parallel to the surface of the part on each side of the boil. In this case, providing they are sufficiently far apart from each other, the field will dip down into the tissues beneath the boil (see Fig. 2c).

Treatment should be continued until after the slough is removed. The dosage can be gradually increased by lengthening the duration of each treatment as the acute condition subsides, but should not exceed more than ten minutes. After a few days, the slough will separate and one further treatment is necessary to ensure that there is no remaining infection in the deeper structures. Treatment should then be changed and the ultra-violet rays should be used to promote healing. One or possibly two stimulating doses will usually be sufficient and these should be given on the lines laid down for the treatment of a granulating wound.

It is possible that the skin surrounding the boil may become infected by the pus as it discharges. When this occurs, a crop of small boils develops, scattered over quite a large area of skin in the vicinity. These may be treated by a counter-irritant dose of ultra-violet rays given to the whole area. Quite a severe reaction may be obtained only being restricted if the area treated is very large. A course of general light baths with ultra-violet rays may be given, together with the local treatment, in order to improve the general condition of the patient and so increase the resistance to infection.

Carbuncle. The treatment of a carbuncle is identical with that of a boil. Progression of treatment will, however, be at a slower rate owing to the fact that it takes very much longer for each stage of the carbuncle to develop. During treatment the patient should be carefully watched owing to the danger of septic absorption, and any increase in the severity of the symptoms or rise in temperature should be reported to the surgeon in charge of the case.

INFECTIONS OF THE HAND

Infections of the hand are very liable to occur, owing to the fact that the hand, usually with the skin unprotected, is in constant use in everyday life. The original cause of infection is probably a small puncture of the skin, so slight that it is ignored at the time. Scratches from thorns, pin pricks, wooden splinters, are all common causes; while a factory worker may encounter a metal splinter while operating his machine. The infection is caused by the staphylococcus entering the tissues through the wound. This is extremely likely to occur if the damage is done while the patient is at work and the hands are dirty. Alternatively the invasion by the organism may not occur for several days and may be the result of failure to keep the scratch properly covered while carrying out the normal daily duties.

An irritation is caused by the presence of bacteria in the tissues and inflammatory changes develop rapidly. The fingers and possibly the whole hand, particularly the dorsum where the tissues are lax, become very swollen and intensely painful with a characteristic throbbing pain, which may keep the patient awake at night. Owing to the pain the hand is held stiffly and this serves to increase the amount of exudate, causing a marked degree of swelling and the likelihood of gross adhesion formation.

As the irritation is often severe there may be considerable necrosis of tissue and a large amount of pus may be formed; and, since the infection is often deep-seated, it may take considerable time to track towards the surface. This will affect the progress of the condition in two ways. First it will mean that the time taken for drainage will be prolonged, and secondly that there will be considerable loss of tissue, causing permanent scarring and disability. In addition, a severe infection may spread from the connective tissue to specific tissue such as tendons or bones. An infection of a tendon may cause the tendon itself to slough, making voluntary movement impossible in the joint which it controls. If the bone is involved, an osteomyelitis develops, necrosis of bone tissue occurs and spicules of dead bone may need to be removed before healing can begin.

The gravity of the condition must not be ignored, as the complicated structures of the hand will suffer through a period of immobility. The organization of inflammatory exudate may cause adhesions to bind tendons and joints, producing permanent disability. This condition is sometimes spoken of as a 'frozen hand' and may seriously affect the whole future of the patient and prevent him from returning to his normal work and independence. Not all infections, however, produce these far-reaching results and it is possible for only a small, local area to be involved.

The actual site of the infection will depend upon the site of the scratch, but there are certain parts more commonly affected than others and these produce definite clinical pictures.

PULP INFECTIONS OF THE FINGER

The tips of the fingers are very prone to scratches and cuts and consequently are likely to become infected. The pulp lies on the front and sides of the terminal phalanx and is divided into compartments by fibrous bands which radiate outwards from the phalanx to the skin. These fibrous bands tend to restrict the infection to one of these compartments, so that only a small part of the finger-tip will become involved. If the condition progresses, the fibrous bands may break down and pus may spread through the whole of the pulp. The condition may vary, therefore, from a very small, local infection in one place with a 'pinhead' of pus, to a marked inflammation of the whole of the pulp. As the space is small, a small quantity of pus will cause a marked increase in pressure, and pain and tension will occur within a few hours. The whole of the distal segment of the finger may become swollen and painful and be held rigidly. Infection may spread down the finger to the middle and proximal segments and even into the palm of the hand.

PARONYCHIA

An infection of the nail-bed is termed paronychia and is caused by splitting of the cuticle, possibly by careless manicuring. A small, painful spot of redness appears at one corner and may spread to form a red, swollen, painful rim. Pus collects under the nail, which will then need piercing or removing before drainage can occur. Paronychia is seen both in the acute and chronic forms. The chronic type tends to prove intractable as it is such a low-grade infection that there is insufficient reaction to promote healing. However it will often respond well to a succession of third-degree doses given round the nail-bed with the Kromayer lamp using an average-sized applicator rod. Short-wave diathermy is another treatment which can be given using mild thermal doses.

PALMAR SPACE INFECTION

Infection of the palm may be due to puncture of the skin in that area; but it is more often the result of the spread of infection from the fingers. In the latter case, the infection may gradually creep along the finger until it reaches the palm, or the organisms may be carried to the palmar space in the lymphatic drainage. Fascial bands in the connective tissue divide the palm into three distinct compartments so that the infection is likely to be limited to one of these. The little, ring and middle finger will infect the middle palmar space, while the thumb and index finger will do the same for the thenar palmar space.

There will be pain over the whole of the hand which will be held rigidly. Tenderness will be present and will increase in intensity over the area of infection. Swelling is not likely to become very apparent in the middle palmar space, owing to the tough covering of palmar fascia, but is marked over the thenar eminence, and often spreads into the dorsum of the hand.

TENDON SHEATH INFECTION

If the sheath of the tendon becomes infected, the name of acute suppurative tenosynovitis is given to the condition. It may occur as a result of laceration in which the sheath itself has become damaged. Pus will form within the sheath, distending it and causing a very painful condition, especially on movement of the finger concerned. The real danger of the condition lies in the fact that the tendon itself may become necrosed and a portion of it slough away producing permanent disability.

INFECTION FROM CRUSHING

In a severe accident to the hand, when laceration occurs, probably at the time of injury, organisms may enter the tissues through the wound. This type of injury is commonly caused by allowing the hand to be caught and crushed while operating a heavy press, and infection is likely owing to the conditions under which the accident occurred. In this case all the structures of the hand will be damaged and, in addition to the changes produced by the infection, there will be those caused by the severe crushing. The skin is usually lacerated; there is often severe contusion of soft structures including blood vessels and sometimes nerves; metacarpals and phalanges may be fractured and one or more fingers may have been partially or completely amputated, either at the time of the accident or later owing to the amount of injury they have sustained. The infection is likely to be widespread and is a complication which will retard the progress of recovery and restoration of function. Extensive damage to soft tissues leads to marked inflammatory changes with gross oedema, which are liable to produce much adhesion formation and stiffness. Damage to blood vessels may result in thrombosis and oedema, or even gangrene. Damage to nerves will cause weakness or paralysis of muscles and diminished or loss of sensation. This is particularly serious in the hand, as without sensation, function is impaired. Severe scarring following laceration will also be the cause of limitation of movement. The function may be altered by loss of part, or the whole, of one or more fingers, but the surgeon, when operating, will endeavour to leave the patient at least part of the thumb and middle or index fingers so that the pincer movement of the hand is still present.

Treatment by Physiotherapy

Treatment of an infection of the hand is carried out on the same lines as those laid down for the treatment of a boil: namely, repeated applications of very mild heat which is sufficient to increase the blood supply, but insufficient to raise the temperature of the part. The site of infection makes no difference to the technique employed, as the whole of the hand should be treated in all cases even though only one finger may be affected. Local application of short-wave diathermy can be made, using a through and through technique with electrodes large enough to include the hand and fingers in the field. Some authorities prefer to use the cable electrode, applied in several turns round the hand and with the usual thickness of towelling placed between the cable and the hand. This produces a maximum effect in the fluid tissues but has the disadvantage of covering the incision through which pus is draining, so that it cannot be watched during treatment. Also, as the hand is covered from the air, it cannot lose heat from the surface and there is a tendency to produce overheating. A more general effect on the circulation can be obtained by extending the turns of the cable up as far as the axilla, so that the whole arm is included in the treatment as well as the hand. This method is sometimes used alternately with the local through and through application. The dosage should be restricted, so that almost no sensation of heat is experienced, and, as with a boil, several treatments of short duration can be given each day.

As the infection is in the deeper structures, it is usually necessary for the surgeon to make an incision in order that pus can drain freely. For this reason the physiotherapist should keep a careful watch on the condition during the early stages and report the presence of fluctuating fluid. It should also be remembered that pus is draining, and the wound should be carefully dried before each treatment and covered with a dry dressing. During treatment there is likely to be increased discharge which may necessitate an additional swabbing during the treatment. The dosage should only be increased when the signs of the acute condition are disappearing and pus is draining freely.

It may take several days, after draining has begun, to clear the infection completely and the course should be continued until there is evidence that there is no remaining infection. This can be determined by the fact that there is no further pus or exudate on the dressings, no pain on any special spot and decreased redness. When this stage is reached, doses of ultra-violet rays may be given to stimulate healing, using the same technique as suggested for the treatment of a granulating wound (see Chapter I).

During and after the period when short-wave diathermy is given, it is necessary to prevent stiffness. It is probable that a plaster splint will have been applied to immobilize the part and provide rest. With the surgeon's permission this should be removed and one active movement given daily to each joint in as wide a range as possible within the limit of pain. This will serve to maintain movement during the period when the infection is active. If one finger only is affected, stiffness in the other joints of the hand should be prevented by giving active exercises whenever possible.

After healing has occurred, the patient is often left with a stiff oedematous hand sometimes with sensory diminution or loss and consequently with exceedingly poor function. Stiffness is usually largely due to the organization of the inflammatory exudate and resulting fibrous tissue formation, to loss of elasticity and to shrinkage of the capsules of the joint, to the mechanical difficulty of moving a swollen area and to weakness and atrophy of extrinsic and intrinsic muscles. It may also, in part at least, be due to fear. The oedema is the result of the excessive extravasation of fluid, resulting from vascular damage and to the interference with tissue drainage, if lymphatic and blood vessels are ruptured and thrombosed. It is partly also the result of diminished function. Physical treatment then aims at the establishment of better drainage and the relief of oedema; at softening and stretching fibrous thickenings and increasing the pliability of the capsule and other soft tissues; at strengthening the musculature of the hand, training sensation if nerves have been involved, and, most important of all, at re-education of the normal use of the hand.

Establishment of tissue drainage and relief of oedema may be obtained by means of some form of heat applied proximally to the area of oedema, or by means of faradism under pressure carried out with the hand and forearm elevated above the level of the axilla. Massage will follow the faradism and should also be done with the limb in elevation. Effleurage and kneading to the area proximal to the oedema will be given to stimulate the flow of blood and lymph. Deep squeezing kneading on the hand will be interspersed with short strokes of effleurage done slowly and deeply. Finger kneadings to the interosseous spaces, the thenar and hypothenar eminences and effleurage and kneading to the digits will also be given.

When the oedema is softened and reduced by the previous measures, active finger, thumb and wrist movements are practised. These should be done slowly and vigorously for their pumping effect.

Softening and stretching fibrous thickenings, increasing pliability and freeing scar tissue. These may be obtained by the use of paraffin wax, ultra-sound, accessory movements and active exercises. Ultra-sound is particularly useful when the hand shows thickened, hard, fibrotic areas. It is successful in softening the area and improving the elasticity of the tissues. Wax is preferable when scars are adherent or tending to contract and crack. It may be followed by massage with lanolin. Accessory movements loosen the capsules and any folds which have adhered to each other or to underlying bone. Voluntary movements will then be easier to perform.

If the scars formed in the healing of open wounds are adherent or tending to contract, they may be softened by the use of histamine ionization and loosened by suitable massage. If they are extensive, hard and seem liable to crack, massage is ideally preceded by the use of paraffin wax, and lanoline may be used as a lubricant. Ultrasonic therapy is another form of treatment which can be given because of its beneficial effect in softening fibrous tissue.

Strengthening the musculature may be obtained by the constant use of active exercise with the maximum resistance the muscles can work against whilst completing the full range of contraction. Both extrinsic and intrinsic muscles should be exercised in this way.

Training sensation. This is important when nerves have been damaged. Without the ability to recognize textures, sizes and shapes, to feel differences in temperature and painful stimuli, the value of the hand is severely reduced. Careful training on the lines indicated for median nerve injuries must be carried out. (See page 273.)

Re-education of the normal use of the hand is vitally important, because there are so many finely co-ordinated movements. Each patient, according to his own occupation, develops his own type of movement. The best exercise is the practice of the movements involved in his particular type of work or movements as nearly similar to these as possible.

LYMPHADENITIS

Lymphadenitis, or adenitis as it is sometimes called, is an inflammation of the lymphatic glands and may be acute or chronic. The condition is caused by some primary infection elsewhere in the body, the glands becoming infected through the lymphatic drainage. The glands which drain the site of infection will be those to become infected. Thus infections of the hand and arm will cause adenitis of the glands of the axilla; sepsis of the teeth, tonsils or mouth will involve the cervical glands. Infections of the foot and leg will lead to an infection in the glands of the groin.

Another cause of adenitis is the tubercle bacillus. In this case the organism settles in a gland, providing the irritation which causes the inflammation. The inflammatory changes and subsequent abscess are produced in the gland itself and the sinus will be found extending from the gland to the surface of the skin. As this may be some distance and the sinus may be narrow, drainage is not as simple as in other infections and healing will not occur until after all pus and dead tissue have been evacuated. Sometimes the surgeon will remove the infected gland itself.

Treatment by Physiotherapy

For staphylococcal infections the short-wave diathermy current may be used to produce mild heating. Treatment should begin at once and continue until all signs of the infection have disappeared. The dosage and technique of application are similar to those used for a boil. If a sinus is present it is necessary to ensure that all pus is allowed to drain away from the bottom. The surgeon does this by inserting a piece of rubber into the sinus to form a drain down which the fluid can pass. The drain will be seen protruding from the opening and may be fastened to the dressing by means of a safety-pin. If treatment is given special care should be taken not to disturb the position of the drain but to remove the safety-pin before giving short-wave diathermy. The use of ultra-violet rays to stimulate healing should also be modified owing to the length of the sinus. It is important to ensure that the granulation tissue is first laid down at the base of the sinus and the rod applicator may be introduced into the sinus so that the rays will be absorbed in the place where healing should begin. It may, however, not be possible to reach the bottom, in which case counter-irritant doses given to the skin in the region of the opening of the sinus will produce an increased circulation to stimulate healing.

If the infection is tubercular in origin, the application of heat is contra-indicated, but treatment may be given with ultra-violet rays. If it is possible to introduce the sinus rod, a very strong dose should be administered in the hopes of producing a sufficiently severe reaction to destroy the organism. This should be repeated until the discharge ceases, after which dosage should be decreased in order to stimulate healing. If the use of the sinus rod is not practicable, counter-irritant doses should be given to the skin over the glands as suggested previously.

Chapter III

BURNS

THE SKIN AND ITS FUNCTIONS

To obtain a clear understanding of the problems presented by burns, certain points about the structure and function of the skin should be borne in mind.

It will be remembered that there are three layers of skin; the epidermis, the dermis and the subcutaneous tissue. The epidermis is stratified epithelial tissue; and therefore it shows several layers of cells, the deepest of which are columnar and capable of multiplication. Growth of new skin takes place from this layer. The dermis consists of fibrous and elastic

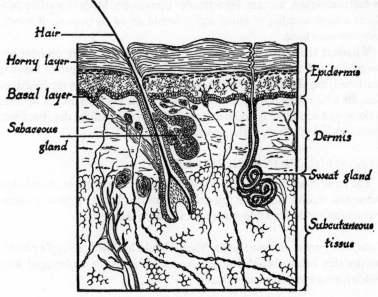

FIG. 3. THE STRUCTURE OF THE SKIN

43

tissue in which are found blood and lymph vessels, nerves, touch corpuscles, hair follicles, and sweat and sebaceous glands. This layer has an upper papillary zone, mainly built up of very sensitive and vascular eminences, named the papillae. It has also a lower, denser, reticular zone resting on the subcutaneous tissue, which is a looser connective tissue containing considerable quantities of fat. Many of the hair follicles and sweat glands extend into this layer (see Fig. 3).

The skin has many functions. One of its most important is its power to act as a barrier, on the one hand against the entry of bacteria, and on the other against the loss from the body of protein and fluid. If there should be extensive loss of skin in a severe burn, infection is very likely to occur, while loss of fluid is liable to affect the general condition of the patient very severely.

BURNS

A burn is caused by excessive heat applied to the tissues. Many burns occur in the home, either as a result of clothing catching fire, contact with a hot object, or from faulty electrical equipment, or from steam or very hot water. These latter burns are known as scalds. Industrial burns, often caused by molten metal, corrosive substances, friction or electrical currents of high amperage, account for a smaller percentage. Modern warfare produces a large number of burns and it would do so particularly if atomic weapons were used.

Whatever the cause, the damage is the same. The tissue proteins are coagulated and actual necrosis may take place. A varying depth of tissue is destroyed, the severity depending on the temperature and on the length of time for which the excessive heat is applied. If the full thickness of the skin is destroyed and there is no infection, the burnt skin will be dry, hard and black, this being known as the slough.

CLASSIFICATION AND HEALING

The most usual classification is into first degree or partial-thickness skin burns and second degree or full-thickness burns. Partial-thickness burns may be further divided into superficial and deep skin loss.

Superficial partial-thickness burns. These should heal with a supple elastic, healthy skin because epithelial cells are available in the undamaged hair follicles, sebaceous and sweat glands.

Deep partial-thickness burns. These heal less well and the skin will be of poor quality because only the deepest parts of the sweat glands remain to provide epithelial cells.

Full-thickness burns. These present a different problem since no epithelial cells remain. If infection does not occur, granulations develop beneath the slough and gradually loosen it until it eventually separates leaving a raw area covered with red granulations. Epithelial cells grow in over the surface, but if the area is wide their rate of growth becomes slower as they get further from the edges and it takes considerable time to cover the wound. Meanwhile more granulation tissue is forming in the depth of the area and the deeper layers are being converted into scar tissue. The scar tissue contracts strongly and is responsible for the deformities so often seen in severe burns.

To assist prognosis classification is sometimes made according to the total area of skin burnt. Muir states that, in assessing burns, if the total area of the superficial part of the burn, as a percentage of body area, is divided by four and the total percentage of full-thickness burn added, 35 per cent is the point at which the chance of survival is equal to the chance of death. Other factors such as age, site of burn, general condition of the patient and infection have also to be taken into consideration in making the prognosis.

THE EFFECTS OF THE BURN

Burns, other than those causing erythema only, have far-reaching effects. Shock, anaemia and infection are all liable to occur.

Shock. The immediate effect of excessive heat on undestroyed vessels is a vasoconstriction, but this is rapidly followed by a widespread dilatation and an increase in the permeability of the vessel wall. These changes result in an increased formation of tissue fluid with a high protein content. The fluid seeps between the layers of the epidermis, causing blistering, and passes into the deeper tissues, bringing about oedema. Again, since much plasma protein escapes into the tissue spaces, the osmotic pressure of the blood falls and fluid is not attracted back into the vessels. This loss of fluid into the tissues, into the blister and onto the surface, means a decrease in the volume of circulating blood, which, if not too great, can be compensated for partly by a constriction of the skin and splanchnic vessels. If the fluid loss continues severe vaso-constriction occurs resulting in inadequate blood supply to the viscera, damaging the kidneys and preventing absorption of water from the alimentary tract. This is harmful compensation. Eventually a state may be reached in which inadequate fluid is present in the circulatory system and circulatory failure, uncompensated shock, is present and death may result.

Anaemia. Not only is there a fluid loss, but also there is a marked fall in red blood corpuscles, partly due to stagnation in the dilated capillaries, and partly due to their damage or destruction as they pass through the burnt area. The presence of anaemia will have a considerable bearing on the patient's prospect of recovery as well as on the rate of healing.

Infection. One of the greatest dangers of burns is infection. The burnt area, having been sterilized by the heat, immediately after the trauma is free from bacteria; but it is very liable to become infected, since the protective function of the skin has been lost and the necrotic tissue is an ideal breeding ground for bacteria. Bacteria may reach the area from the air, from clothing, from the hands of those handling the patient or from the dressings. Once in the wound they will multiply rapidly. Continuous infection implies greater tissue destruction, constant absorption of toxic substances, floating off of grafts and lowered resistance and vitality of the area as well as deterioration in the patient's general condition. All these facts may mean delay in healing and this leads to the danger of scarring, contracture and deformity.

OBJECTS OF TREATMENT

The first object of treatment is the preservation of life by preventing circulatory failure.

The second object is the control of infection. If the burn is seen within the first few hours, infection may be prevented; if the patient does not come for treatment until after a longer period, the burn may already be infected and this infection must then be treated and controlled.

The third consideration, which has a close bearing on the first and second, is the general condition of the patient, his resistance, nutrition, recuperative powers and morale. The general condition deteriorates if continuous pain is experienced, if there is extensive fluid or protein loss and if infection occurs and is persistent. All these factors have therefore to be considered.

The fourth consideration is to obtain quick healing. The more rapid the healing the less the likelihood of infection, the less loss of fluid and protein and the less formation of scar tissue and contraction.

Prevention of uncompensated shock. On admission to a casualty department or Burns Unit, a case of burns is seen immediately by a senior member of the unit. A careful estimation is made of the size and depth of the burn and the amount of fluid lost. Since fluid loss is likely to continue for twenty-four hours or more, it is essential to make up what has been lost and to continue giving fluid as long as necessary, often for two to three days. This is done by the immediate administration of reconstituted human plasma or one of its substitutes. At some time during or after this period, blood may be given instead of plasma, to make up for the destroyed red blood corpuscles.

During this time no active treatment of the burn is undertaken except for the application of an adequate cover, thick enough to prevent infection.

Prevention or control of infection. A burn admitted within six hours of the accident should be clean because the heat destroys the bacteria; but if not very carefully treated it will rapidly become infected. In the case of burns not seen until after six to eight hours have elapsed, colonization with bacteria is almost certain. Swabs are usually taken to establish the presence and nature of bacteria and chemotherapy is then instituted. Attention to the burn in both cases is usually undertaken by a special dressing team in a special air-conditioned room where it is unlikely that the burn will become infected from the air. Under sedation the burn is gently cleaned and the wound is then treated by exposure or by dressings. In the first method the wound is left uncovered. The surface rapidly dries and a crust is formed under which healing occurs. Infection is not common with this method because the conditions of dryness, coolness and exposure to air are inimical to the growth of bacteria.

In the second method the wound is dressed with an inner non-adherent layer to which antiseptics may be applied and an outer porous firm layer. The dressing is usually left for three days, being covered with extra bandage if fluid seeps through. It is then changed and left for seven to ten days. By the third week partial-thickness burns should be healing. Any area of full-thickness burn will now be dealt with by wet dressings to encourage the slough to separate. When granulations look healthy the wound will be covered with a skin graft.

If the burn can be recognized as a full-thickness burn at once then the slough may be excised and an immediate skin graft performed. Often it is difficult to be certain of the degree of the burn, partial- and full-thickness destruction being present at the same time.

Improvement of the patient's general condition. The anaemic condition is treated by transfusions of whole blood. Severe protein loss leading to

Burns

debility, increased liability to pressure sores and emaciation is counter-acted by a high-protein and high-calorie diet together with iron and vitamin therapy. General muscle wasting may be lessened by suitable physiotherapy.

Rapid healing. This depends partly on the depth of the burn, but also on the prevention of infection, avoidance of oedema and improvement of the patient's general condition.

PHYSIOTHERAPY IN RELATION TO BURNS

Nearly all patients suffering from burns receive physical treatment once shock is overcome. The treatment comprises measures aiming at the general well-being of the patient and those dealing with the local condition.

GENERAL TREATMENT

The general condition of the patient is liable to deteriorate because fear, pain, fluid and protein loss, toxic absorption and confinement to bed, all lead to loss of appetite and weight, poor general muscle tone, slowing of circulation and lowered morale. With the modern treatment of burns none of these should be really severe but they may all be present in a minor degree.

Physical treatment should, therefore, comprise light general exercise excluding any immobilized area, breathing exercises and as early ambulation as the surgeon considers suitable. In hospitals in which burns are treated in special units, this work is best done by the group method since far more competition and enjoyment is obtained and morale is consequently maintained or improved.

A special point should be made of breathing exercises, especially in the elderly, those who by nature of their burns are confined to bed and those in whom the affected area includes the upper respiratory passages, neck, face or chest. If flame or hot smoke have been inhaled the mucous membrane of the respiratory tract will become oedematous and considerable respiratory distress results. Tracheostomy is then usually necessary and the physiotherapist will be needed to give breathing exercises, coughing and help with intermittent suction to remove secretions. Breathing exercises are also particularly important if the chest is covered with bandages which must not be removed.

In many patients attention to posture is vitally important. A very careful check of the position in bed, explanation to the patient of the importance of correct posture and progressive strengthening exercises for all postural muscles are all essential.

LOCAL TREATMENT

The main object of the physical treatment of the affected area is the prevention of contractures and the restoration of full function or of as full a function as the condition will allow. This return of function depends on the absence of deformity, the maintenance or restoration of the full range of movement in the joints, the maintenance of good tone and bulk of the muscles and the obtaining of a healthy, supple, elastic skin. In addition, one of the greatest factors in obtaining full function is the mental condition of the patient in relation to his injury.

Prevention of contracture is particularly necessary in cases of burns with deep partial-thickness or complete-thickness skin loss, because, unless early skin grafting is possible, much fibrous tissue tends to form in the process of healing. In addition there is the danger of organization of fluid if the post-traumatic oedema is not controlled. Again, skin grafts on the flexor surfaces of limbs have a great tendency to contract from the time they have 'taken' to about twelve weeks after the operation. As fibrous tissue contracts, movement may become severely limited, not only because of the scar contracture, but also because of gradual adaptive shortening of the capsule and other peri-articular structures of the joints. This danger is minimized by the use of splints and active exercises.

Thin plaster splints are often used over dressings either with or without grafts. When the dressings are discarded, removable plasters or light metal splints are applied. These need constant supervision by the physiotherapist to ensure that they are correctly applied and are fulfilling their function. Particular care is needed in certain regions, such as the neck and chin, axilla, flexor surfaces of elbows, wrists, hips and knees. For example, burns of the neck and chin and axilla, if unchecked, may result in gross flexion of the neck and adduction and medial rotation of the arm. In these patients the use of pillows and sandbags and a constant check on the position of the part are essential. It is wise to gain the co-operation of the nursing staff and the interest and co-operation of the patient in such difficulties.

Active exercise is also vital in preventing deformity. If dressings are encased in plaster, rhythmic muscle contractions are essential. As soon as the plaster has been removed active exercises are begun. These are best done many times a day; five minutes out of every hour is not too often. One of the most comfortable ways of obtaining active work is in a bath, and, where full-length baths are available and the surgeon permits, full-body baths are ideal, especially for children. In the special bathroom the outer dressings are removed and the patient is lifted into the bath. The water used is maintained slightly above body temperature and to it salt or Lux may be added according to instructions. Small children do well in Lux baths because they enjoy playing with the bubbles and they will often do movements which they would otherwise avoid. The soapy water has an excellent effect on the areas of skin grafts or unhealed areas waiting for grafting. In addition, dressings float off easily and unhealed areas can be gently cleaned without pain. At the end of the treatment the patient is lifted, if necessary, on to a trolley covered with a sterile sheet and fresh dressings are applied, or the areas may be left exposed.

Active work should be carried out in as full a range as possible and progressed every day. Quite early, functional activities should be added. Remedial occupational therapy is desirable.

Whether all this work is effective or not, depends upon whether the patient's interest and co-operation are obtained. Children with extensive burns, who may need many operations, are often inclined to be spoilt and become difficult to manage and unwilling to work. Much therefore depends on the ability of the physiotherapist to handle the patient well, to be firm though kind and to make the work interesting.

One point must be noted. In cases in which skin grafting has been performed, passive movements and massage, so often employed in the past, should definitely not be used to stretch or to prevent deformities, since these hasten the tendency towards contractures. After about twelve weeks they can be employed if desired, but they must be avoided before this time.

Maintenance of a full range of movement is essential. Without physical treatment joints tend to become stiff, because oedema often occurs, due to the damage to blood and lymphatic vessels and to circulatory stasis resulting from lack of use. Oedema may also be the later result of decreased tone in muscles and vascular walls. Then, when the limb becomes dependent for the first time, vasodilatation occurs followed by excessive exudation of tissue fluid.

Oedema, due to the injury, may be avoided by the use of a firm crêpe bandage which the physiotherapist may need to reapply in the course of her treatment. It may also be avoided by the suspension of the limb in such a position as will obtain the assistance of gravity in draining the area. Splints applied over the dressings may make such suspension possible.

Oedema, which arises from the injury or from decreased tone, may also be avoided by the use of active exercises and gradual resumption of the dependent position. For example, many metal burns of the feet occur in industrial injuries. These are nearly always full-thickness skin loss and they are usually seen and treated immediately after the accident. The usual procedure is to excise and then cover with a full-thickness skin graft. The leg is then encased in a below-knee plaster for six or seven days. During this time static contractions of muscles within the plaster and active exercise of free joints are given, to avoid circulatory stasis and loss of tone. At the end of this period the plaster is removed and, if the graft has taken, active exercises are continued and progressed in bed for a further two days. The next day the leg is allowed to hang over the side of the bed for repeated periods of five to ten minutes to become used to the dependent position. The following day the patient sits out of bed for two periods of one hour. Progression is then made to walking. Thus haemorrhages beneath the grafts, oedema and stiffness of foot and ankle are avoided.

It is important to realize that, in the case of grafts, the part should not be dependent before eight or nine days, because otherwise haemorrhage may occur beneath the graft which then fails to 'take'.

Another reason for the development of stiff joints may be the difficult and uncomfortable position a healthy part may be asked to maintain in the case of tubular pedicle grafting. Stiffness and discomfort may be avoided by active exercises of joints not immobilized, static contractions of muscles and the application of short-wave therapy through the plaster for immobilized joints.

Condition of muscles is maintained and atrophy minimized by the use of early and progressive exercises, observing the same precautions as in the previous procedures. Care must be taken not to disturb skin grafts, or break down capillaries, or death of the graft may occur.

Condition of the skin needs special attention. In the case of healing without a graft, the new skin is thin and delicate and will not tolerate physical treatment; but, as it becomes thicker and loses its transparent, bluish appearance, the recovery of elasticity and suppleness will be much assisted by wax baths and the gentle application of lanolin or one of the similar preparations. If wax is used it must be applied at a low temperature because the sensation is markedly reduced or absent and the delicate skin blisters readily. An attempt is often made to raise the temperature of the wax by one degree each day, until a temperature rather higher than that normally used is being tolerated.

In cases where grafts have been applied, gentle massage with lanolin over the graft and its edges may help to smooth the skin and loosen it from underlying tissue, but it should not be used longer than necessary. In the later stages any signs of contracture are best treated by wax baths and active exercises.

BURNS OF HAND

These always present a special problem because the hand invariably becomes oedematous and contractures and stiff joints are particularly serious. Usually as soon as the burn is dressed the hand is splinted and elevated. In the very early days active movements seem to increase the oedema but as soon as the burn is healed intensive physiotherapy is necessary. Burns of the dorsum of the hand tend to get into the position of extension of the metacarpo-phalangeal joints and flexion of the inter-phalangeal joints. Stiffness in this position makes a good grip impossible. Careful splinting is therefore necessary and movements usually begin when epithelialization is complete.

Burns of the palm of the hand caused by grasping a hot object often result in full-thickness skin destruction. If possible this is treated by excision of the slough and immediate grafting. The graft tends to shrink and therefore in children the hand is splinted for three months and in adults until the graft is healed, when the splint is removed during the day for normal use and exercises but re-applied at night. In children's burns the splint is removed for short periods daily when the graft has taken and active movements are practised with particular attention to extension of the fingers and abduction of the thumb.

SKIN GRAFTS

A skin graft implies the transference of whole-thickness or partial-thickness skin from a donor area, often the thigh, to a clean, recently burnt area, or one which has begun to granulate. Its purpose is to provide a cover to lessen fluid loss and protect against infection or to speed up the process of epithelialization. If such a graft lives, a much more pliable scar results than would occur with spontaneous healing. A skin graft may be a free graft, that is one in which a section of donor skin is completely freed from its bed and transplanted to a new site; or it may be a skin flap in which one or both ends of the donor skin are temporarily left intact so that its circulation is maintained.

Free grafts may be split skin grafts or full thickness skin grafts. Split skin or Thiersch grafts are sheets of skin, cut with a Blair knife or Paget's dermatome, or with an electric dermatome, and the exact thickness can be varied according to the area to be grafted. These sheets are laid over the area with their edges slightly overlapping. They are pressed firmly into place and are usually retained, for a period of about fourteen days, by layers of Tulle Gras covered thickly by wool and bandage. To prevent movement of the part, which might disturb growing capillaries, thin plaster splints are often applied over the dressings and bandages. Full thickness skin grafts or Wolfe grafts consist of whole-thickness skin from which the fat has been removed. A single strip is laid over the burnt area and its edges are sutured to the freshly prepared edges of this area. Usually the donor area is covered with a Thiersch graft.

Flap grafts may be fixed-base grafts or tubular grafts. Both make use of whole-thickness skin with its adipose tissue and blood vessels. In a fixed-base pedicle a flap of skin is raised leaving one end undisturbed. The free end is sutured to the area needing skin. After about fourteen days the graft will have obtained a blood supply from the raw area as well as from its base and the base may now be detached and sutured to the recipient area.

In a tubular pedicle two parallel incisions are made and the skin between is freed from its bed. The free edges are sutured so that a tube is formed attached at both ends. A Thiersch graft is applied to the area from which the tube has been raised or the donor area is sutured. By about fourteen days later, a good blood supply and venous and lymphatic drainage should be established in the tube. One end can then be safely detached and moved to the required area. Ten or fourteen days later the other end is divided and moved, the tube being 'unsewn' and the skin smoothed out over the area. In this way whole-thickness skin can be moved a considerable distance as, for example, from abdomen to forearm and forearm to forehead, by a series of operations.

One of the problems in any type of graft is the maintenance of the circulation. In free skin grafts, firm pressure helps to ensure that capillaries will grow from the burnt area into the grafted skin; while, in skin flaps, leaving one end attached to the donor area ensures the circulation, but, in spite of this, viability is not always maintained and then grafts fail to 'take'. One of the essential precautions is to avoid disturbing the graft, since movement may rupture the growing capillaries. For this reason plaster splints are often used, especially in the case of tubular grafts in which, in order to transfer the skin a considerable distance, joints may be fixed in awkward positions. Splints are also of great value to avoid kinking of the pedicle and so diminishing its blood supply.

SPECIAL POINTS IN PHYSICAL TREATMENT IF SKIN GRAFTS HAVE BEEN APPLIED

Heat, ultrasound, massage and movements may all be used during or after skin grafting operations.

Heat should not be given directly to a graft because the graft is insensitive for many months, but it is of value given to the area to help movements if joints have become stiff, provided the graft itself is covered. It is useful if applied to the muscle groups of a limb which has to be maintained in an abnormal position during the period of transference of a flap graft. By heat the cramp and discomfort can often be relieved.

Ultrasound. This is particularly valuable when a pedical graft has been freed from the donor area. It is used for its micro-massage effect, improving local circulation, stimulating cell metabolism and reducing any oedema. It decreases the formation of fibrous tissue under the graft. These effects are likely to increase the chances of a successful graft.

Massage may be used to smooth out a split-skin or full-thickness skin graft and to loosen it from underlying tissue. It must not be given until the graft has 'taken' and is thickening, usually between two and four weeks. It is then given, lightly and without pressure, by the fingers for a few minutes and is only continued with for as long a period as is necessary. Great care must be taken or the graft may blister. Massage is also occasionally ordered for a tubular graft to assist its drainage. It is then given very lightly with the finger-tips. In the same way as heat it is useful to the joints and muscle groups during the various stages of transference of flap grafts.

Movements are not given to the area until the graft has firmly taken but they are of value to neighbouring joints, if they cannot disturb the graft, because they will stimulate the circulation and lessen the danger of stiff joints. After the graft has become firmly anchored active movements are valuable to lessen the danger of contracture, since grafts seem to have a tendency to contract up to about twelve weeks from the time of operation.

Chapter IV

THE PART PLAYED BY PHYSIOTHERAPY IN THE TREATMENT OF COMPLICATIONS COMMON TO ALL OPERATIONS

COMPLICATIONS

No matter how simple and straightforward an operation, or how physically fit the patient who undergoes it, there are always certain risks which cannot be avoided, though preventative measures may lessen their possibility. Of these the most dangerous to life is thrombosis because it can give rise to pulmonary or cerebral embolism. Next in importance are chest complications. Whenever a general anaesthetic is necessary and morphia has to be administered, there is the possibility of trouble, though naturally thoracic surgery is most likely to be associated with chest complications. Another complication is post-operative haemorrhage. This may take place within twenty-four hours of the operation or any time after the third day. Immediate haemorrhage is the result of the rise of the blood pressure which occurs as the post-operative shock begins to subside. Late or secondary haemorrhage tends to occur if sepsis intervenes. The septic process may invade blood vessels and destroy their walls, or may delay healing so that catgut sutures are absorbed before vessels are completely healed. Some impairment of muscle function with resultant muscle imbalance may arise, particularly if extensive division of muscles is necessary. This may lead to deformities and, if care is not taken, in rare cases to stiff joints. Finally, wounds may fail to heal. Resuturing may have to be carried out and the excessive fibrous tissue which results will lead to weakening of the area and possibly to incisional herniae.

THROMBOSIS AND EMBOLISM

Thrombosis may occur following any operation, though it is probably most common after operations on the pelvis. It tends to occur at any time

55

between the first and twenty-first post-operative day. It is important to realize that there are two distinct types of thrombosis. In one type the vein, often the long saphenous, becomes inflamed and consequently the blood within it rapidly clots. This type is known as a thrombo-phlebitis. In the second variety thrombosis precedes inflammation. This is known as a phlebo-thrombosis. Of the two types the second is by far the more serious because it arises silently, giving rise to no symptoms, and the first evidence that it has occurred may be a pulmonary or cerebral embolism.

THROMBO-PHLEBITIS

The probable cause of this is damage to the vein wall. In operative surgery the most likely cause is the insertion of an intravenous drip. The vein is irritated and becomes inflamed and the blood rapidly clots. The clot becomes adherent to the vein wall, and, since the vein is temporarily obliterated by the clot, embolism, though possible, is unlikely. In many cases the inflammation spreads to the surrounding tissues, and a cellulitis is evident. As the vein is nearly always a superficial one, there will be redness in the region of the vein, and the area will be painful and exquisitely tender to touch and may show considerable oedema. Usually the patient's temperature will rise, largely as a result of the absorption of toxic products produced by the disintegration of the clotted blood. The inflammatory condition gradually resolves, if the irritant is removed, and in many cases the clot is absorbed by the action of phagocytic cells. The vein becomes once more patent. Sometimes, however, organization of the clotted blood takes place by growth into it from the vessel wall of fibroblasts and capillary loops, and the vein becomes changed into a fibrous cord. This is of little significance, since there is a very extensive venous collateral circulation and adequate venous drainage will be established by other veins.

It will be realized that the presence of thrombo-phlebitis is not dangerous to life though it may be very uncomfortable for the patient. Treatment is therefore directed to aiding resolution of the cellulitis and to relieving discomfort. If the cause is an intravenous drip, it will, for obvious reasons, be removed and only inserted elsewhere if necessary.

Physiotherapy

Physiotherapy can help to fulfil the objects of treatment mainly by the application of heat to the area of cellulitis. Both short-wave diathermy and inductothermy prove most effective; inflammation rapidly subsides and pain and tenderness disappear. Usually no other treatment is necessary. If movements were being given at the time of onset they should be continued.

PHLEBO-THROMBOSIS

This type of thrombosis tends to start in the veins of the foot and calf, sometimes spreading to the larger popliteal, femoral and iliac veins. The cause is still not fully understood, but there are a number of possible explanations.

In the first place it is known that following surgery there is a rise in the number of platelets and amount of fibrinogen in the blood. The greater the handling of the tissues and the longer the operation the greater will be the platelet and fibrinogen content of the blood and the more likelihood of thrombosis.

A second very important factor is the altered speed of blood flow. If the flow is slow there is a tendency for platelets to fall out of the stream and in addition thrombo-plastic substances are not so readily carried away. Following surgery flow tends to be slowed. Post-operative sedation, abdominal distension, faulty posture with hips and knees bent, diminished muscle contractions, reduced respiratory excursion will all affect the venous return.

A third factor is minor intimal damage. This may happen during the operation and until the patient recovers consciousness and begins to move about. The deep muscle relaxation, if the legs are resting flat on the table or bed, causes excessive pressure on the veins producing ischaemia and damage to the vein walls.

When these various factors are present, platelets adhere to the site of damage. There is a release of thromboplastic substances and fibrin is formed. Red and white cells are caught up in the fibrin network. The speed at which the thrombus builds up depends on the rate of blood flow. If the flow is slow the thromboplastic substances are not carried away and more fibrin is formed, the thrombus developing quickly and sometimes extending for a considerable distance along the vein as a 'tail' floating freely within the vein. Gradually the thrombus becomes canalized by the growth into it of endothelial cells. It is also organized by the penetration of cells from the deeper part of the vein wall. The latter process is speeded up by the fact that the presence of the developing thrombus irritates and sets up inflammation of the wall. Occasionally this inflammation spreads to the surrounding tissue involving the adjacent artery and causing arterial spasm.

Early diagnosis of the condition is vital because of the danger of break off of the thrombus before it becomes adherent, or of the 'tail', leading to embolism. The earliest signs are tenderness on palpation of the calf, a slight rise in temperature and pulse rate and sometimes pain in the calf muscles on dorsiflexion of the foot with the knee straight. After a few days signs of venous obstruction may appear. Oedema develops in the foot and round the ankle, masking the extensor tendons and filling out the hollows and the superficial veins appear fuller. If the vein wall is inflamed there may be pain and cramp in the calf and tenderness over the vein.

If the thrombosis extends into the femoral or iliac veins the whole leg becomes oedematous and sometimes it is pale and cold, possibly the result of arterial spasm.

TREATMENT

Attempts are made to avoid thrombosis by protection of the deep veins during the period of surgery and unconsciousness. The ankles are supported on sandbags so that pressure is taken off the calves and the legs are elevated until the patient is moving actively.

A careful watch is kept for early signs and the physiotherapist is expected to check for tenderness in the calf and discomfort on dorsiflexion of the foot. Measurements should be taken daily to detect any oedema. If these signs are present the surgeon will immediately institute anti-coagulant therapy. As soon as the patient is sufficiently conscious to co-operate breathing exercises are started. These should, if possible, be taught pre-operatively. Diaphragmatic and lateral costal breathing are particularly stressed. Vigorous toe and foot exercises are also begun with special emphasis on foot dorsiflexion and plantarflexion. Progression is usually quickly made to knee, hip and trunk exercises, depending on the particular operation. The patient is encouraged to relax and to move freely round the bed and, if the surgeon permits, is got up on the first day and starts walking that day or the next.

If thrombosis is established anti-coagulants are continued, the leg is rested with the foot of the bed raised and active exercises are discontinued for three days though breathing exercises and active work for the un-affected limb are continued. The patient is allowed up again when his temperature and pulse have been normal for two or three days but he must now wear an elastic bandage until such time as the leg no longer tends to swell when standing.

If the thrombosis extends to the femoral vein swelling is unlikely ever to subside completely. Physiotherapy is then given with the object of reducing oedema, preventing organization, and strengthening the leg-muscle pump. It will follow the lines described for gravitational ulcer (see page 25).

EMBOLISM

Embolism may be another serious complication, the two common sites being the pulmonary and the cerebral vessels. Pulmonary embolism most commonly follows a phlebo-thrombosis. Part of the thrombus may become detached from the vein wall or part of the 'tail' may break off. The embolus then passes in the blood stream, through the heart into the pulmonary circulation. Embolism may be due to one large embolus or multiple small emboli.

If large, the thrombus may 'stick' at the bifurcation of the pulmonary artery, roll up into a ball and completely obstruct all blood entry into the lungs. The patient will then die within a matter of seconds. If rather smaller, the clot may block one of the two vessels and one lung will fail to receive blood. If the patient is young and fit, he may survive with one lung out of action. The embolus may of course be much smaller, or there may be multiple small emboli, blocking only small branches, and the patient who is suddenly stricken with pain in the chest and spitting of blood will recover, but will be left with a small infarct which will gradually be converted into scar tissue.

Cerebral embolism appears to be particularly liable to occur after a mitral valvotomy, oesophagectomy, pneumonectomy, and radical mastectomy. The signs and symptoms vary with the size of the vessel blocked and the site of the embolus. There may therefore be a transient loss of consciousness with rapid and full recovery, or, on the other hand, the patient, if he survives, may be left with a hemiplegia.

Physiotherapy in Embolism

A severe pulmonary embolism is likely to prove fatal, but in the case of small or multiple emboli when physiotherapy is already being given for the particular operation, physiotherapy will continue, but if the patient is getting up he will probably now be confined to bed for seven days. It is most important, however, that the circulation should be stimulated and the legs exercised, and full activity in bed together with breathing exercises should be stressed.

More treatment is needed if the patient recovers from a cerebral embolism but is left with disabilities such as a hemiplegia. Physiotherapy is then required for the weakness or loss of voluntary movement. This treatment will be conducted on the usual lines for the condition except that progress may be delayed as a result of the original condition. If, for example, the cerebral embolism has followed a mitral valvotomy, the patient may not be allowed to get up to start the usual walking re-education at the third or fourth day, but may be confined to bed for seven days. Passive movements can, however, be started at once and a start may be made on active re-education. When the patient is allowed to get up and walk, the routine training in balance, getting up from a chair and sitting down, and walking as used for a hemiplegia will be begun.

CHEST COMPLICATIONS

Chest complications are liable to follow any operation, particularly those in which general or spinal anaesthetics are used. They are clearly likely to be most common in thoracic surgery since in most cases the lungs are already involved. After thoracic surgery the highest incidence is probably in abdominal operations, particularly those which require supra-umbilical incision. The two main complications are bronchitis and post-operative lung collapse. These may lead to broncho-pneumonia, bronchiectasis or lung abscess. The factors which predispose towards these complications are increased formation of secretions and decreased ability to eliminate them. The increased secretions may be due to slight irritation of the bronchial mucous membrane by the anaesthetic. Sometimes the mucus formed is stringy and viscid in type and consequently particularly difficult to eliminate. In addition, it is possible that septic material may be inhaled from the nose or throat which will set up inflammation and further secretion. Very occasionally, if a tube is not passed through the oesophagus prior to operations on the intestine, pressure on the stomach may cause gastric secretions to travel along the oesophagus and these may be inhaled into the lungs; while, if the patient is not very carefully watched, post-operative vomiting may result in inhalation of vomitus.

Normally secretions are eliminated by means of the action of the cilia lining the mucous membrane and by the cough reflex. The cilia are, however, inhibited in their movement by the anaesthetic and the cough reflex depressed by post-operative analgesics. If, in addition, the operation is thoracic or abdominal, coughing is voluntarily inhibited through fear of pain and will be made difficult if a recumbent position is used. If secretions collect they may form a plug which can block one of the bronchi or bronchioles, obstructing air entry or exit from the lobules distal to the obstruction. Air is then gradually absorbed from the alveoli of these lobules and the area collapses. One of two events may then occur: the mucus plug may become infected and inflammation may spread to the walls of the tubes setting up a broncho-pneumonia, or the bronchioles just proximal to the block may dilate and a bronchiectasis result.

The drop in vital capacity, which inevitably follows operations on the thorax or abdomen, is a further factor in predisposing towards these complications. The diaphragm is responsible for as much as sixty per cent of the normal respiratory movements, but, in the first twenty-four hours after the operation, its movement may be only twenty per cent of the normal. The result of this fact is that the lungs, particularly the bases, are not fully ventilated and the circulation is slowed, with consequent congestion. Not only is the vitality of the lung lowered, but there may be increased filtration of tissue fluid and slight oedema of the lung bases.

Collapse of part of a lung usually occurs within twenty-four to forty-eight hours of the operation and will be suspected if there is a sudden rise of temperature, pulse and respiratory rates, dyspnoea, sometimes cyanosis and diminished movement of the chest wall. Pneumonia occurs after a rather longer interval, usually three or four days. The temperature rise is more gradual, but eventually high, and there is a productive cough.

Physiotherapy

Treatment for chest complications, like that for thrombosis, is mainly preventative, though, naturally, if complications have arisen, attention will be directed towards their cure. Clearly, if the main cause of chest complications is lowered vital capacity and accumulation of secretions through decreased cough and diminished respiratory movements, the purpose of physiotherapy is to raise vital capacity, stimulate coughing and encourage full use of the lungs. In cases where elimination of mucus is difficult, it is a further object to assist in its removal so that bronchoscopy will not be necessary.

Since vital capacity is lowered, the first principle of treatment is to train the patient to use the lungs, especially the lower areas, fully. This is not easy if the patient is still hazy from the anaesthetic and in some discomfort. It is important therefore to train good breathing before the operation. Particular stress is laid on gaining good expiration and on the ability to perform diaphragmatic and lower lateral costal breathing at will. An understanding of the value of the correct breathing is essential, so that the patient will co-operate as soon as he recovers from the anaesthetic.

The second principle of treatment is based on the likelihood of secretions accumulating. The patient must be taught how to cough with the least strain and pain. He must also be taught deep breathing so that the movement of air will help to drive out mucus. These again are best taught preoperatively. Two points require stress in teaching coughing. Firstly, strain on the wound will be relieved if the patient supports the operation site with his hands and if the knees are drawn up and the trunk bent slightly towards the area of the incision. Secondly, following an inspiration, a short, sharp expiration, with strong contraction of the diaphragm, produces the easiest and most effective cough.

Sometimes, in spite of adequate coughing and practice of breathing exercises, mucus does collect and there is danger of collapse. Then a third principle applies: the mechanical assistance of elimination of mucus. This is carried out by the use of percussion on the sides and back of the chest, postural drainage and encouraging the patient to move about more freely. There is usually no reason why the patient should not be 'tipped' to aid elimination. If he is being nursed in the half-lying position, bed rest and pillows may be removed and the crook lying and crook side lying positions may be taken up, while the foot of the bed can be elevated on blocks. Breathing exercises and percussion will be given in these positions. Incidentally, movement and percussion usually help to relieve the flatulence which so often causes abdominal distension and further hampers breathing.

One of the most important points to bear in mind is that the practice of breathing exercises once daily is useless. If they are to be effective in preventing chest complications, they must be used all day long until good breathing becomes a habit. Much depends therefore on the ability of the physiotherapist to gain the patient's interest, understanding and co-operation. Frequent short visits are essential, until it is clear that the patient is sufficiently enthusiastic to work on his own.

A method now commonly in use is that of drainage by means of a tracheostomy tube. This method has the advantage of eliminating the unpleasantness of repeated bronchoscopy and the exhaustion which accompanies 'tipping' and vigorous chest percussion. It is particularly useful following operations in which chest complications are likely to occur or where, if chest complications do occur, the mucus is viscid and cannot easily be coughed up.

Pre-operative physiotherapy is exactly as before because tracheostomy may not be done but if, after the operation, a tracheostomy tube is in position, postural drainage will be omitted though breathing exercises, chest shakings and attempted coughing will be carried out to help to bring the secretions nearer the trachea. The physiotherapist will now help in the drainage of the secretions by use of a mechanical sucker. The catheter, attached through a glass connection to a bottle, is inserted into the tracheostomy tube and the motor switched on. This process may be repeated every two to three minutes.

HAEMORRHAGE

Haemorrhage may complicate any operation, but it is particularly liable to occur when surgery has been necessary in a very vascular area, such as the thyroid gland or tonsils. Blood may actually be seen staining the bandage if there is external haemorrhage. On the other hand, there may be no obvious blood if haemorrhage is internal. In either case, if bleeding is excessive or prolonged, various signs and symptoms will arise. The pulse will be feeble, the blood pressure low, and respirations fast and often of the sighing type. The skin will become cold and clammy and the complexion and mucous membranes pale. The patient will be restless, feel thirsty and complain of faintness and giddiness.

Should haemorrhage occur, physical treatment is immediately stopped and first aid treatment given until further help can be obtained. If possible the patient should be placed in the lying position and if the bleeding is external, digital pressure may be applied above the site of haemorrhage. The main measures are, however, precautionary. If there is any reason to suspect the possibility of haemorrhage, as, for example, where there is sepsis, vigorous movements between the third and fourteenth days should be avoided.

MUSCLE ATROPHY AND MUSCLE IMBALANCE

Muscles may be in poor condition, both as regards tone and bulk, before an operation is undertaken, or they may be in excellent condition, but affected by the operation. Into the first group comes the elderly patient whose muscles are weak and flabby, and the patient who has been ill for some time, possibly suffering from nutritional disturbances such as might be present in gastric or duodenal ulcer. Again there is the bronchiectatic child or adult whose musculature is poor.

In the second group, muscles may be affected both generally and locally by surgery. Most operations demand a certain amount of lessening of general activity. This is true from the menisectomy to the serious pelvic or brain operation. This inactivity is often increased by fear. The effect of muscular activity on the blood vessels is diminished, venous return is lessened, cardiac output is correspondingly reduced and the normally freely circulating oxygenated blood is available in smaller quantities for all the muscles; consequently their metabolism is reduced and their bulk and power diminished.

For several reasons muscles in the region of the operation may very easily be affected. Sometimes muscles are deliberately cut, though often this is avoided. In thoracoplasty, for example, the scalene muscles, the levator scapulae and the rhomboids are all divided. No real harm results from this if they are adequately sutured, though a small amount of scar tissue must result. This, however, will not markedly reduce the power if it is kept supple. On the other hand, some exudate and haemorrhage may occur, which, if it organizes, will later hamper the action of the muscle. Incision of muscle will therefore temporarily reduce bulk and power, though with adequate treatment this effect may be lessened and will not be long lasting.

Complications Common to all Operations

The nerve supply to the muscles may be damaged at the time of operation, though this is always avoided where possible. For example, in surgery of the cervical lymph glands, the accessory nerve is occasionally damaged and trapezius and sternomastoid may both be affected. Again, in a thyroidectomy, it is difficult to avoid the recurrent laryngeal nerve and the muscles of the larynx may then be weakened. In cholecystectomy the ninth, tenth and eleventh intercostal nerves may all be severed and marked weakness of one side of the abdominal wall will result.

In radical mastectomy, if the dissection has to be carried far back, the nerve to serratus anterior may be slightly damaged and a paresis of the serratus result. Occasionally, stretching or pressure of one or more nerves may occur. If the relaxant drugs, such as curare, are used during an operation, there is complete absence of tone in the muscles, and consequently no protection for the nerves. If a position is necessary in which pressure on a nerve might occur, there is a greater tendency for a paresis to result. Again it may be possible that the assistant holding the arm during a radical mastectomy may allow it to fall back into extension so stretching the brachial plexus and causing a partial paresis. If an Esmarch's rubber bandage around the thigh is used for a tourniquet in operations on the knee, a drop foot occasionally occurs, probably owing to ischaemia of the lateral popliteal nerve. This neurological damage means atrophy of the muscles with diminished or lost tone and reduced or absent power according to the extent of the lesion.

In some operations certain positions may be necessary which prevent active use of the muscles. For example, many surgeons fix the arm to the side for some days following a mastectomy, and the arm is fixed in adduction and medial rotation in operations for recurrent dislocations of the shoulder. This lack of movement must inevitably result in diminished metabolic processes and, therefore, in atrophy.

Pain may result in inhibition of muscle, either deliberately through fear, or as a result of reflex action. In cases of operations on joints, distension or damage of the capsule stimulates its nerve endings and reflex inhibition results. This is often seen in operations on the knee or the shoulder. In operations on the spinal cord, patients are afraid to move, especially if much pain in the back or leg has preceded the operation. The result is atrophy of the spinal muscles.

Effects of muscle atrophy. Whatever the cause, it appears that atrophy and hypotonia of muscle will occur following any surgical procedure. The most outstanding effect of this is alteration in posture, usually affecting the body as a whole. For example, atrophy and hypotonia of the spinal muscles will lead to a loss of the erect carriage of the back. If the gluteal muscles are also affected, increased pelvic tilt will be followed by spinal deformity. When the patient first gets up and begins to walk about, his general posture is likely to be poor; postural flat feet and round shoulders with poking head may be particularly noticeable. Should weakness of the trunk muscles be unilateral then muscle imbalance is particularly noticeable and may well lead to gross deformity. This is most clearly seen in thoracic operations or in cases of interference with the nerve supply of abdominal muscles. Scoliosis is a very likely result and one which should have been avoided.

Another noticeable effect of muscle atrophy is diminished power, with possibly serious results, since the muscles are the first line of defence of the joints. Inadequate muscles will result in continuous minor traumata to joint structures and a chronic synovitis may develop. This is particularly liable to happen if care is not taken following operations on the knee joint.

If the abdominal muscles are the ones to be affected, then their function is impaired and not only will posture be disturbed, but they will no longer adequately protect the abdominal viscera or maintain the intra-abdominal pressure. If intra-abdominal pressure drops, then respiration, venous return, elimination, and support of the abdominal viscera will all be disturbed. Again, scarring in abdominal muscles means a weak point and may lead to incisional hernia (see page 66).

Muscle weakness may be one of the factors leading to stiffness of joints. If the muscle has insufficient power to move the joint through its full range, then full range is never attained and adaptive contractures will result. This is not uncommonly seen following a radical mastectomy, though muscle weakness is not necessarily the only reason for its development.

Physiotherapy

Muscle atrophy can usually be avoided except in the case of nerve involvement. The principle is the practice of active contraction and, if possible, active exercises, before the operation, immediately after the operation, and for a considerable period after this. All muscle groups should be exercised as vigorously, as often, and in as wide a range as possible. If active movement is impossible, then static contractions should be used. In the case of a radical mastectomy, for example, static contractions of deltoid, biceps and triceps can be taught, even if the arm may not be moved. Where static contractions cannot be obtained, passive exercise, by the use of the faradic current, may be substituted, but it should only be used until active work can be undertaken.

UNHEALED WOUNDS AND INCISIONAL HERNIA

Surgical incisions will heal quickly and with little formation of scar tissue under suitable conditions. There must be adequate apposition of the tissues. The wound must not become infected or infection should not be already present when the operation has to be performed. There must be an adequate supply of blood containing the substances necessary for repair. Excessive strain on the site of incision, such as might result from constant coughing, must not occur, though healing is stimulated by some pull on the wound, provided that it is not excessive. It is safe to say that a wound will not break down, unless it is inadequately sutured or unless it becomes infected.

Certain factors are liable to cause considerable delay in healing and even break down of the incision. If a haematoma forms in the wound, healing will inevitably be delayed. This complication is likely to arise if the operation has been carried out on a very vascular area. Blood then tends to ooze on to the surface, often for several days, and clots to form a haematoma. Both thyroidectomy and radical mastectomy are liable to give rise to haematoma formation for this reason. Therefore, small drainage tubes are often used for the first two or three days. Extensive incisions sometimes result in delayed healing and as these are necessary in such operations as mastectomy and nephrectomy, it is difficult to avoid the complication in these particular cases.

If the wound should become infected, healing will be slow and 'bursting' of the wound is possible. It is rare today for wounds to be infected in the operating theatre, but, later, infection from the throat or hands of the dresser or from the dust-laden air of the ward, may occur. Much can be done to prevent such infection. Any person having any connection with dressing the wound should wear a suitable mask; the dressing should be done using forceps and taking care to touch nothing with the hands. There should be minimum movement of the bedclothes or other material from which dust and micro-organisms might be shaken into the air to fall on the surface of the wound.

The presence of infection in a previously clean wound may be recognized by the fact that the wound becomes painful, throbs and is very tender. The temperature of the area rises and sometimes redness and oedema may be seen around the wound; the sutures then tend to cut through the tissues and the wound to gape either in its whole length or between the sutures.

Healing is likely to be less satisfactory if the area is already infected. The presence of sepsis necessitating operation, as, for example, in the case of a gangrenous appendix, or in empyema, involves the use of drainage tubes to permit free drainage of the pus and ensure healing from the base upwards. If tubes remain in for any length of time they are apt to cause irritation of the walls of the track with consequent fibrous tissue formation; then healing becomes difficult when the tube is eventually removed. In addition, where tissues are damaged and there is sepsis, the proteolytic ferments, liberated by bacteria and phagocytic cells, tend to digest the tissues in the region of the wound and may do so for a considerable distance. This loss of tissue must be replaced by granulations which will later become converted into scar tissue. For these reasons, tubes are usually shortened quickly and removed as soon as possible, usually between three and seven days.

In the case of incisions of the abdominal wall, abdominal distension might cause bursting either of the whole wound or areas between the sutures. Persistent distension is therefore to be avoided.

If, as a result of these factors, scarring occurs in the musculature of any of the walls of the abdominal or pelvic cavities, then there is always the possibility of protrusion of the contents of the cavity through the weakened area. This condition is known as incisional hernia.

It will be seen from these facts that certain points are very important when dealing with wounds of operative surgery. The most important point is obviously to obtain quick healing without infection. To obtain this, great care is necessary in dressing the wound. If a wound becomes infected, steps should be taken to allow free drainage and stimulate healing.

Physiotherapy

Firstly, active exercises are good, since, as has already been seen, some strain on the wound stimulates the healing process. Excessive strain is of course to be avoided; therefore an abdominal operation should not be followed by outer range abdominal exercises or heavy work such as double hip and knee flexion.

Secondly, if a clean wound becomes infected, cleaning may be assisted and subsequently healing stimulated by the use of some form of dry heat. If the infection is superficial, infra-red or radiant heat are satisfactory, but if the infection is deep-seated, short-wave therapy should be used. In the first case, treatment is usually only given after the sutures have been cut and the wound allowed to gape so that free drainage is established. In either case treatment should be given at least twice daily.

Where wounds are already present and infected and operative surgery is necessary, as might easily be the case in road accidents, the wound is often covered with Vaseline petroleum jelly gauze and the affected limb encased in plaster. The plaster may then be left untouched for some weeks. Physiotherapy may indirectly aid healing by stimulating circulation through active exercises for joints not included within the plaster and by light, general exercises and breathing exercises. Exercise is also necessary to lessen atrophy of muscles and stiffness of joints, which might otherwise result.

Since the healing of wounds which are either slow to heal or which require re-suturing is characterized by the formation of much scar tissue, certain after-effects may be noticed. Firstly, the scar may be an unsightly keloid one, in which the scar is red, raised and puckered. This is a contra-indication to physiotherapy, as massage and active exercises are usually found to stimulate the production of more scar tissue. Secondly, the scar will be adherent to underlying tissue and will probably hamper movement. It may also cause discomfort, as it pulls on other tissues. Not only will it be adherent, but it may well contract and produce deformity. Therefore, as soon as the wound is firmly healed, massage with lanolin should be used. It should be carried out over the surface of the scar to keep it supple and should be done in such a way as to lift the scar to try to loosen it from the underlying tissue. For particularly hard scars, ionization with iodine or chlorine ions may be used. On suitable areas, paraffin wax treatment nearly always results in scars becoming softer and more elastic. The sooner the treatment can be started, the more successful it will be.

Occasionally a scar may be painful, probably because a superficial nerve has become caught up in the fibrous tissue. Different measures have been advocated for this complication. One principle is to soften the fibrous tissue. Pain may then be relieved. This could be attempted by salicylate or iodine ionization, but it is, in fact, probably much more successfully done by X-ray irradiation. Alternatively, the fibrous tissue may be excised and the nerve freed. Physiotherapy then has no place in the treatment.

TERMS USED TO DESCRIBE CERTAIN
SURGICAL PROCEDURES

Certain terms are commonly used to define surgical procedures. In many cases a suffix is attached to the name of the organ or part being treated, and, if the suffix is understood, further definition is unnecessary.

The suffix *ectomy* is derived from the Greek word-meaning 'a cutting out'. Hence, if the colon is removed, we use the word, colectomy, or, in the case of the stomach, gastrectomy.

The suffix *otomy* is derived from the Greek word meaning 'to cut' and, if an incision is made in order to perform a wider operation or to carry out an investigation, the suffix may be used. A craniotomy is a cutting into the skull and might readily be followed by the removal of a cerebral tumour. A thoracotomy is the making of an incision through the chest wall and may, for example, be performed for thoracoscopy or for the division of adhesions.

The suffix *ostomy* is derived from the Greek word meaning 'mouth' and indicates therefore the making of an opening. Colostomy is the formation of an opening through the abdominal wall into the colon, and a suprapubic cystostomy the forming of an artificial opening through the abdominal wall just above the pubis into the bladder.

The suffix *oscopy* originates from the Greek 'to look' and indicates an inspection of a hollow organ or body cavity by means of an instrument devised for this purpose. The word endoscopy is commonly used to describe this process and the instrument is known as the endoscope. Often the prefix is altered according to the organ or cavity to be examined in this way. Thus an examination of the more proximal parts of the bronchial tree may be carried out by a bronchoscope and is known as a bronchoscopy. Similarly the stomach may be examined by the gastroscope and the pleural cavity by thoracoscopy. It is usually possible to withdraw, by suction, material from the walls or lumen of the organ through the endoscope or to insert a knife to scrape the walls or to divide adhesions.

The suffix *ography* indicates a writing or written description. The process entails, as a rule, the filling of the organ or vessel with a radio-opaque substance, followed by X-ray photographs of the part. Thus an angiograph is a written description of the state of certain vessels seen in the above way, a cholecystography is an examination and description of the state of the gallbladder. The X-ray photograph is usually known as the 'gram'—hence cystogram, angiogram.

Plasty comes from the Greek word meaning 'to mould' and is usually a suffix indicating that a certain tissue is being repaired, remodelled or built up. Hence a hernioplasty is a repair of a hernial orifice. An arthroplasty is the remodelling of a joint, often by means of using other material than body tissue.

The word *resection* is derived from the Latin, *re* = again, and *secare* = to cut, and indicates the operation of cutting out. Thus a rib resection indicates the removal of a rib and a resection of intestine the removal of part of the gut.

Many other words may be used, but these are some of the words most frequently met with.

Chapter V

GENERAL ABDOMINAL SURGERY.
GYNAECOLOGICAL SURGERY

by B. SHOTTON, M.C.S.P.

The physiotherapist is asked to assist in the post-operative treatment of a large variety of abdominal conditions. Some of the operations commonly performed on stomach, intestines, other abdominal viscera, and on the abdominal wall itself will be considered here, and a later section will deal with operations on the genito-urinary system. Finally, operations on the abdominal aorta will be discussed briefly.

INCISIONS
(See Fig. 4.)

VERTICAL INCISIONS

True midline incisions do not bleed freely as they are made through fibrous tissue, but they may be slower to heal than other types. They are most frequently used by gynaecologists below the level of the umbilicus.

Paramedian incisions are more commonly used, supra- or sub-umbilical, about 1 inch from the midline, the rectus muscle being retracted laterally to cut through the posterior layer of the sheath.

Pararectal incisions just lateral to the rectus muscle are rarely used, since nerves to the rectus would be cut, thus grossly weakening the muscle.

OBLIQUE INCISIONS

A subcostal incision runs below the ribs. A right one would be used for gall-bladder operations, and a left one for splenectomy.

An oblique lumbar incision as for nephrectomy would commence further back at the lateral border of sacrospinalis, and pass forward parallel with the twelfth rib towards the anterior superior iliac spine.

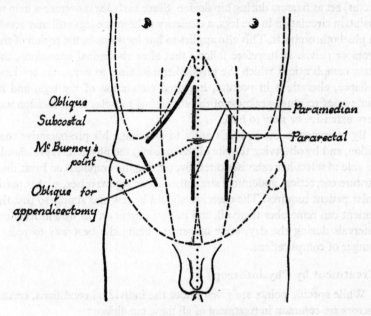

FIG. 4. ABDOMINAL INCISIONS

McBurney's incision is commonly used in appendicectomy. McBurney's point is at the junction of the medial two thirds and lateral one third of a line joining the umbilicus to the anterior superior iliac spine. The incision is at right angles to the line at this point.

TRANSVERSE INCISIONS

These are less frequently used, as they may not give good access, although they heal well.

The physiotherapist should have a knowledge of the site of incisions most commonly used for abdominal operations, since on the site several factors important to post-operative treatment depend. With a *high* incision near the diaphragm or ribs, the patient will find deep breathing painful, and this may predispose to chest complications. Full elevation of the arm may also be painful. With a *lateral* or *oblique* incision, the patient may find the movements of rotation or of side-flexion to the opposite side painful: he may therefore tend to sit with the spine side-flexed, the concavity towards the side of the wound. Again, full arm movements may be painful. With *all* incisions, but especially those towards *midline,* the patient may find any early hip and knee movements painful, as the abdominal muscles (mainly rectus) act as fixators during hip flexion. Since early leg movements help to maintain circulation in the legs, a tendency to keep the legs still may result in phlebothrombosis. This also applies to low incisions in the region of the groin or pelvis. It therefore follows that after abdominal operations, the main complications which the physiotherapist aims to overcome are lung collapse, alterations in posture, impaired circulation of the legs, and in some cases residual weakness of the abdominal muscles if the incision was very extensive or slow to heal.

By reference to the patient's notes to determine his pre-operative condition, and by observing the site of the incision, the physiotherapist should be able to select her exercises carefully, putting the emphasis on breathing, posture correction, abdominal strengthening or leg exercises, as that particular patient requires. The exercises should be few and simple so that the patient can remember them all, and perform them on his own at frequent intervals during the day, early movement being the best way to reduce danger of complications.

Treatment by Physiotherapy

While specific points are given under the individual conditions, certain factors are common in treatment of all these conditions:

PRE-OPERATIVE TREATMENT

The value of pre-operative physiotherapy is today generally accepted. The physiotherapist is able to gain the confidence of the patient, and explain the value of the exercises that he will do post-operatively. Some practical points to note are:

Postural Drainage. If there are lung secretions to be cleared, postural drainage should be used several times a day. The sputum should be measured carefully, and the surgeon informed when the amount is minimal, as the patient will then be ready for operation.

Breathing Exercises. These should be taught in as much detail as the nature of the impending operation and the co-operation of the patient allow.

Coughing. The difference between a real cough which can bring up mucus, and a mere clearing of the throat, should be stressed.

Arm Exercises. The 'prayer' position is often the best, the palms being held flat together, fingers pointing upwards: thus the more painful arm is aided by the normal arm which does not, however, do all the work of lifting. A short lever is best at first, the elbows being kept flexed until the hands are past the nose, then straightened until the upper arms are against the ears.

Leg Exercises. Toe and ankle movements are taught in full range, also static contractions of quadriceps and glutei: all these movements should be done rhythmically and repeated at frequent intervals, e.g. for five minutes in every hour. The patient can also be shown how to flex his hip and knee keeping his heel on the mattress, so that the minimum of lifting strain is put on the abdominal muscles for the first few days.

Posture correction. The patient should be taught to sit equally on both buttocks. His arms, when hanging to his sides, lie equally outside his hips. His shoulders are slightly braced and level.

POST-OPERATIVE TREATMENT

Some practical points to note are:

Bed Cradles should be used to release tight or heavy bed clothes and facilitate leg movements.

Breathing. Dressings are usually kept to a minimum to avoid restriction, Elastoplast being used to secure dressings rather than bandages. If pre-operative breathing was taught, any suitable type of breathing can now be used: but if not, then it is frequently easier to get maximum thoracic excursion and maximum air interchange by lateral costal breathing. Many patients find this simpler than localized diaphragmatic breathing, and it should be remembered that the diaphragm is actually working to help to raise the ribs. Emphasis will naturally be placed on those parts of the lungs needing specific attention. Thus with a right-sided incision, the right arm will be painful to move, and the right basal expansion must be particularly encouraged. But left basal expansion may also be limited for two reasons: first, the patient may have had a long operation, lying on that side; secondly he may lie on his left side after the operation to relieve pressure on the right. Bilateral breathing exercises are therefore probably best.

The best way to be sure that the lung tissue is expanding satisfactorily is by reference to an X-ray, or more simply by finding out from the doctor that the breath sounds are normal. An experienced physiotherapist may be able to detect collapse of lung tissue by gentle percussion. Another quick and easy method is to ask the patient to hold his breath, which he will find difficult if there is some collapse. The pulse is taken at frequent intervals. Any rapid rise in pulse rate could, and frequently does, indicate early collapse of lung. This can be detected before the patient shows a rise in temperature.

Coughing. This can be aided by firm pressure over the wound by the physiotherapist or by teaching the patient how to support the part himself. Relaxant drugs are now in frequent use during surgery. These prevent trauma to the abdominal muscles, since these can be drawn apart more easily during the operation, but normal muscle tone does not always reappear until several days after operation. This is sometimes the reason why it is difficult for the patient to produce a strong cough. Postural drainage may help to clear secretions, but the physiotherapist should be certain that there is no reason why tipping may be contra-indicated.

Leg Exercises. The test for Homan's sign should always be made, and any adverse signs reported. For the first two days after operation, it is always safe to do foot exercises and static contractions as previously described, the stress being on full range and frequency. In lower abdominal operations, the physiotherapist should consult the surgeon as to when hip and knee movements may be started. These should be commenced as described preoperatively, progressed by lifting the heel, then to straight leg raising. Double leg exercises are rarely needed or advisable. Early ambulation rapidly replaces leg exercises, many patients being allowed out of bed twenty-four to forty-eight hours after operation, and thereafter to walk easy distances of increasing length. Sitting in a chair for long periods should be discouraged, since this position causes pressure on the veins of the legs.

Posture. Two common faults should be borne in mind here:
  (a) The 'arm-chair' position of pillows into which the patient slumps should never be tolerated; the back needs firm support.
  (b) Many patients mistake a drawing-in of the abdominal wall by lifting the thorax and arching the back, for the desired static abdominal contraction. This is always best taught by making the patient flatten his lumbar hollow, at the same time drawing his pubic symphysis and his sternum closer together. Trunk movements can usually be started on the fourth day, when healing should be well progressed; in fact, they are frequently taking place before this, during movements around the bed and for toilet purposes.

WARD CLASSES

In many long wards these are impracticable, since there will be patients at different stages following different operations, sometimes under the care of different surgeons whose opinions of rate of progress may differ. Large ward classes also hold up the nursing procedures of the busy ward. It is therefore simpler in most cases to treat the patients individually, or in small groups of three or four; and the present trend towards small wards, or partitioning of large ones makes this the treatment of choice.

PROGRESSION OF EXERCISES

Some of the previous points can therefore be summarized: Whenever possible, pre-operative exercises should be given. Immediate early exercises (one to two days) can always include foot movements, static contractions of glutei and quadriceps, and posture correction. Early ambulation is encouraged. Trunk exercises can be started on the fourth day. Clips and stitches are usually removed by the seventh to tenth day.

Once out of bed and ambulant, exercises can be continued in small groups, but here the difficulty is space, many wards having no day-room available which can be utilized.

Except in specific cases, physiotherapy should no longer be needed after the tenth day. If there are no complications patients are sometimes discharged to a convalescent home while the stitches are still in, or sent home after the tenth day.

OPERATIONS ON THE STOMACH

PARTIAL GASTRECTOMY

This operation may be performed in cases of ulceration. Two standard operations on which other varieties are based will be described here:

(a) Billroth I

This is commonly performed for gastric ulceration. The proximal line of transection is across the body of the stomach, and the distal line is at the first part of the duodenum, about two-thirds of the stomach being removed. The duodenum is then anastomosed to the remaining part of the stomach.

(b) Polya Operation

This is more commonly used if the ulcer affects the proximal part of th duodenum. The proximal and distal lines of transection are as before, but here the duodenal stump is closed, and the remaining part of the stomach is anastomosed to the proximal loop of the jejunum.

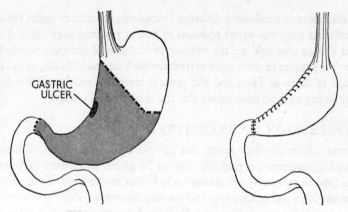

FIG. 5. BILLROTH I. PARTIAL GASTRECTOMY

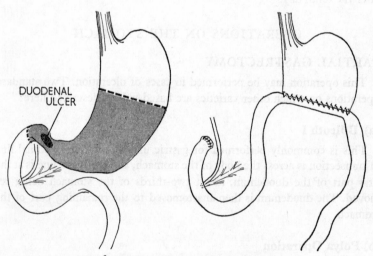

FIG. 6. POLYA TYPE. PARTIAL GASTRECTOMY

To obviate vomiting or distension, most patients have a naso-gastric tube passed for 24 to 72 hours following operation. Fluid balance is maintained by intravenous drips of glucose or saline. Small feeds of milk or weak tea are then introduced, and the diet gradually progressed. At first the patient will take only small quantities of food and will therefore need frequent feeds; but this is eventually largely overcome by dilatation of the remaining part of the stomach.

TOTAL GASTRECTOMY

This operation is performed for carcinoma of the stomach. The whole stomach is removed, and the lower end of the oesophagus is joined to the jejunum. Most of the pancreas may also be removed, but the remaining part still passes pancreatic juice into the duodenum, which is therefore anastomosed into the wall of the jejunum.

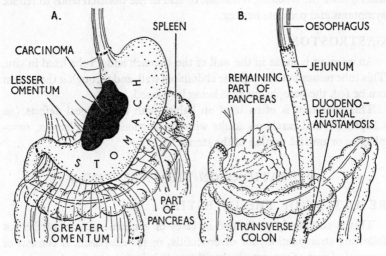

FIG. 7. TOTAL GASTRECTOMY

In cases of partial or total gastrectomy, the patient may be in a poor state of health, and unable to co-operate for long at a time. Later, care is taken to see that the patient does not become anaemic; this may happen because of the loss of normal stomach stimulus to the production of red blood cells.

Physiotherapy

Routine treatment should be given little and often noting the following points:

The base of either lung may tend to collapse. The patient can be laid flat and rolled onto either side for lung drainage if required. The presence of the naso-gastric tube and the soreness of the patient's throat make coughing difficult, thus much encouragement is needed to get him to clear his sputum.

As there will be control of fluid intake and output, the physiotherapist should be careful not to give anything by mouth unless permission is given and the amount charted. If the patient vomits during treatment, this should be reported.

VAGOTOMY

It has been shown that section of the vagus nerves to the stomach abolishes the nervous phase of gastric digestion and reduces the production of acid. This operation is therefore often used in the treatment of duodenal ulcers, since the resulting reduction of acid in the stomach tends to reduce symptoms and promote healing.

GASTROSTOMY

An opening is made in the wall of the stomach and a tube fixed in situ. This tube passes out through the abdominal wall, and through it the patient can be fed, the oesophagus thus being by-passed.

This operation is often used on babies with oesophageal defects (*see* Chapter X) and rarely on adults with obstruction of the pharynx, oesophagus, or cardiac portion of the stomach.

OPERATIONS ON THE INTESTINES

RESECTION OF THE INTESTINE

This is commonly performed in cases of gangrene of part of the gut following strangulation; for diverticulitis, or for neoplasm. It consists of removal of part of the gut, the healthy ends being anastomosed.

COLOSTOMY

This may be performed as a temporary measure in cases of diverticulitis or carcinoma. A loop of colon is brought to the surface, and is kept in position by a glass rod until it becomes fixed by adhesions to the abdominal wall.

The intestinal contents are discharged onto the surface through an opening in the wall of the colon, and the part of the colon distal to the opening is rested. Later, the affected distal part may be resected, the continuity of the colon restored by end-to-end anastomosis and the colostomy may be closed.

In cases of carcinoma of the rectum, a permanent colostomy is performed, the lower diseased part of the gut and the carcinoma being resected. For this extensive operation, approach from the abdomen and from the perineum is necessary, the operation being termed abdomino-perineal excision of rectum (A.P.E.R.).

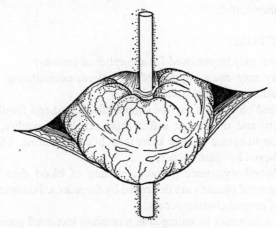

FIG. 8. COLOSTOMY

Physiotherapy

After these operations on the intestines, general breathing exercises must be given, the patient finding it difficult and painful to cough. Leg exercises are also of importance to prevent phlebo-thrombosis. Routine foot movements and static contractions of glutei and quadriceps can be given, but any hip or knee exercise which involves movement of the sutured perineum will be painful; these can probably be commenced gently within a day or two.

The patient may be embarrassed by the colostomy bag, and is self-conscious about the lack of control in emptying the bowel. In time, many patients develop the ability to control the opening of the bowel to a certain extent by tension of the abdominal muscles through which the opening has been made. Care of the colostomy bag is taught by the ward sister.

ILEOSTOMY

When the whole colon is excised in ulcerative colitis, the ileum is brought to the surface as an ileostomy.

General Abdominal Surgery

OPERATIONS ON OTHER ABDOMINAL VISCERA

APPENDICECTOMY

The 'grid-iron' incision is used, at right angles to McBurney's point, the muscles not being divided but split along the line of their fibres. Unless there are complications, the incision is very small, and recovery is usually rapid and uneventful.

SPLENECTOMY

The spleen may be removed for a number of reasons:

(a) Injury may cause rupture of the spleen, necessitating immediate operation because of haemorrhage.

(b) The red blood cells may be abnormally shaped and fragile (sphero-cytosis) and the patient suffers from acholuric jaundice, a familial disease so named because there is no bile in the urine. The jaundice is relieved by splenectomy.

(c) In thrombocytopenic purpura, clotting of blood does not occur because the platelets are destroyed by the spleen. Following splenectomy, normal clotting occurs.

(d) The spleen may be enlarged as a result of increased pressure in the portal circulation (portal hypertension).

The abdomen is usually opened by a left paramedian or a left subcostal incision.

Physiotherapy

Routine post-operative treatment can be given, with special attention to the left lung base and to leg exercises, but it must be remembered that the patient is often anaemic and may be given a number of blood transfusions. He may also be rather shocked for the first 24 to 48 hours after operation. Thrombosis may occur since the platelet content of the blood is temporarily increased after operation. Thus Homan's test is important, and the patient may be on anti-coagulant therapy.

PORTAL-CAVAL ANASTOMOSIS

This operation is performed for the relief of portal hypertension. The portal vein is divided before it enters the liver, and is implanted into the inferior vena cava. (The liver will still receive a blood supply via the hepatic vessels, from the abdominal aorta.) A right thoraco-abdominal approach is used, the diaphragm being partly divided to facilitate the procedure.

Physiotherapy

Great care will be needed to maintain the expansion of the right lung, owing to the opening of the thoracic cavity and the great discomfort felt by the patient on the right side. A drainage tube from the pleural cavity is often used for a few days. Postural drainage of the right lower lobe is nearly always permitted and is frequently of great value.

CHOLECYSTECTOMY

When there is chronic inflammation of the gall bladder, with obstruction to the flow of bile and the formation of gall stones, the gall bladder and the cystic duct may be removed. A paramedian or an oblique sub-costal incision is used. The cystic duct is divided close to its junction with the common bile duct. The gall bladder is removed after careful separation from the liver to which it is attached by the peritoneum. A short drainage tube is often provided for 4 to 5 days, since there may be a small leak of bile from the bed of the gall bladder.

Physiotherapy

Patients are frequently obese. Special attention must be paid to the right lung base. These patients are difficult to treat since obesity makes lung expansion and early mobility difficult. Convalescence may be slow owing to loss of appetite and to lethargy.

In some cases, a T-tube is retained in the common bile duct for up to 10 days, after which the surgeon may order a cholangiogram to outline the bile ducts. In these cases, it is even more difficult to get full expansion of the right lung base. Of all cases undergoing abdominal surgery, these patients often prove the greatest problem for the physiotherapist because of persistent lung collapse.

OPERATIONS ON THE ABDOMINAL WALL

A hernia is a protrusion of a viscus through an abnormal opening in the wall of the containing cavity. The word is most often used in reference to a hernia of the intestine or omentum through the walls of the abdomen. To produce a hernia, two factors are present. Firstly, there is the area of weakness. Secondly, there is a rise of intra-abdominal pressure: this may occur gradually as a result of increasing obesity, or suddenly as a result of violent effort as in prolonged coughing, straining at stool or lifting heavy weights. The sites at which herniae occur most commonly will be considered in turn.

INGUINAL HERNIA

During foetal life, the testes descend through the abdominal wall to become contained in the scrotal sac outside the abdominal cavity. An oblique canal is thus formed in the lower part of the abdominal wall, parallel to and just above the inguinal ligament. This weak point in the wall is strengthened as a result of its oblique direction, and by the conjoint tendon which arches over it and protects the medial part of its posterior wall.

In elderly men with obesity, flabby abdominal muscles and chronic bronchitis, it is not difficult to see how a hernia can occur at this point, a 'sac' of peritoneum protruding down the canal and forming a bulge anteriorly just above the inguinal ligament.

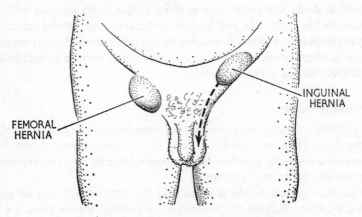

FIG. 9. FEMORAL AND INGUINAL HERNIAS

If a loop of gut protrudes with the sac, the blood supply of that part of the gut may be obliterated by the narrow neck of the sac, forming a *strangulated* hernia, a serious condition needing immediate operation.

Hernia also occurs frequently in younger men with excellent general abdominal tone, but with a congenital weakness just at the point of the inguinal canal.

Operations

If it is considered that the musculature of the inguinal canal is in good condition and the deep abdominal ring unstretched, the operation will be that of *herniotomy*, consisting merely of removal of the protruding peritoneal sac. In most cases, however, some repair of the canal is required, the operation being that of *herniorrhaphy*. The incision is one inch above and parallel to the medial three-fifths of the inguinal ligament. There are many varieties of this repair, but all are designed to occlude the gap between the conjoint muscles and the inguinal ligament. The aponeurotic fibres of the conjoint tendon may be stitched down to the inguinal ligament close to the medial side of the emerging spermatic cord. The external oblique aponeurosis is then drawn down over the front of the cord and stitched to the inguinal ligament. A *hernioplasty* involves repair of the weak area by introducing fibrous tissue to help to fill up the deficiency. This may be taken from the fascia lata, or from the aponeurosis of the external oblique muscle.

Physiotherapy

Patients are frequently allowed up within a day or two of operation, and are discharged to convalescent homes before removal of the stitches. Complications are rare unless the patient has a chronic chest condition. Discouragement of smoking both before and after operation is of great importance. Routine early breathing exercises, foot, and static contractions of quadriceps and glutei may be given, and the patient encouraged to move his hips and knees gently. If he needs to cough, he can support the incision with his hand, or can flex the hip slightly on that side. Static abdominal contractions combined with head raising should also be taught in the lying position. If the patient is sent to the gymnasium post-operatively, a graded scheme of abdominal exercises and instruction in lifting techniques would be of benefit. In many instances, however, these patients fail to reach the physiotherapy department before they return to work, and do very well without further treatment. This is probably because in younger men, as has already been stated, the general musculature is already excellent, and if they have strenuous occupations, they should already be well trained in correct lifting techniques. With elderly men, it is doubtful whether physiotherapy can do much to improve their muscles and posture at this late stage, and they may do better to wear a truss if the surgeon considers this necessary.

FEMORAL HERNIA

A similar protrusion may occur through the femoral canal, a swelling appearing in the groin just below the medial end of the inguinal ligament (see Fig. 9).

UMBILICAL HERNIA

This may be seen in babies and young children. It often disappears spontaneously as the muscles develop and grow stronger, but may need operative repair.

General Abdominal Surgery

INCISIONAL HERNIA

This may occur at the site of the scar following operation in any part of the abdominal wall.

DIAPHRAGMATIC (HIATUS) HERNIA

In some patients, the oesophageal opening in the diaphragm is lax, part of the stomach protruding upwards into the thorax. The extent of the lesion can be clearly seen on X-ray following barium swallow. The patient often presents with symptoms of palpation and heartburn, indigestion and regurgitation of bitter fluid, so leading to discomfort on lying flat.

OPERATIONS ON THE GENITO-URINARY SYSTEM

PROSTATECTOMY

After the age of fifty, it is not uncommon for the prostate gland to become enlarged. The main symptom is difficult micturition with frequency, due to pressure on the urethra. Later, retention of urine may occur, necessitating urgent operation. Intra-venous pyelogram (I.V.P.) may help to confirm diagnosis, dye being injected into a vein in the arm, and X-ray pictures of the renal tract being taken at frequent intervals afterwards to note time and density of its excretion. This condition may be treated by trans-urethral cautery and resection, by supra-pubic operation involving the bladder, or by rectro-pubic operation in which the prostate is enucleated from its capsule. Patients are usually admitted to hospital a few days before operation, so that cystoscopy may be performed and urinary function tested. It is important to keep the patient as active as possible, since enforced and sudden rest in an elderly person could result in slowing of the circulation and in phlebo-thrombosis.

Following operation, routine breathing, foot and leg exercises should be given and the patient will be allowed up within a few days. The catheter is retained for a few days until local swelling subsides, and can be used to irrigate the bladder, and to keep it empty and so promote healing. Fluid intake and output charts are again used, and the physiotherapist should help to encourage the patient to drink as much as he can.

CYSTECTOMY AND URETERO-COLIC ANASTOMOSIS

This operation is usually performed in malignant disease of the bladder, confirmed by intravenous pyelogram and by cystoscopy. After removal of the bladder, the ureters are transplanted into the sigmoid colon. By burying the terminal part of the ureters in an oblique tunnel in the bowel wall, an attempt is made to reproduce the valvular action normally present in this situation. The patient may achieve a measure of control over the flow of urine.

Physiotherapy

Since the patient is probably elderly, breathing exercises will be required, and he should be encouraged to move his feet and legs as much as possible. Early ambulation is probable.

NEPHRECTOMY

One kidney may be removed provided that the other is healthy. Reasons for removal of the kidney are tumours, infection (pyonephrosis), tuberculosis, multiple calculi, or hydronephrosis (gross enlargement of the renal pelvis at the expense of the parenchyma of the kidney). The operation is usually performed through an oblique lumbar incision. After closure, a drainage tube is left in for two to five days to prevent accumulation of exudate, which might become infected, in the dead space left by the removal of the kidney.

Physiotherapy

Breathing exercises to both lung bases should be given: to the operation side because of the large painful incision; and to the other side as the patient will have been lying on this side during the operation and probably frequently afterwards for the first few days. Arm exercises on the side of the operation should be commenced immediately. Routine leg exercises including gentle hip and knee movements must be encouraged as often as possible. Posture correction will be necessary to prevent the patient leaning towards the side of the incision. Gentle trunk exercises can be started on the fourth or fifth day when the drain has been removed, and early ambulation is encouraged.

It is important for the physiotherapist to remember that all patients who have had operations on the kidney or bladder will be on fluid intake and output charting, but plenty of fluid intake must be encouraged.

GYNAECOLOGICAL CONDITIONS

OVARIAN CYSTECTOMY

An ovarian cyst may be completely excised. Any normal ovarian tissue is retained, since there is a tendency for these cysts to be bilateral, and if one ovary is removed, the patient may return later with the only remaining ovary cystic.

General Abdominal Surgery

OOPHORECTOMY

If it is impossible to conserve the ovary, it is removed. This operation may also be performed bilaterally in the treatment of carcinoma of the breast. When oestrogen starts to be produced in quantity at the time of puberty, the breasts enlarge and mature under its influence. Since this ovarian hormone controls normal breast growth, it is not surprising that it also has an effect on abnormal tissue growths in the breast. Spread of growths to other tissues (metastasis) can often be checked temporarily by the removal of both ovaries, although it is not fully understood how the withdrawal of oestrogen produces this effect. Bilateral adrenalectomy or even removal of the pituitary gland may also be attempted.

SALPINGECTOMY

Removal of a Fallopian tube may be performed for chronic salpingitis, or following rupture of a Fallopian tube as a result of a tubal pregnancy (ectopic gestation).

MYOMECTOMY

This operation is commonly performed to remove benign growths of the uterus, namely fibroids. Since these are mostly composed of plain muscle tissue, the term 'myomectomy' is used. This condition is commonest in women between the ages of thirty and fifty who have not borne children. The body of the uterus is affected more commonly than the cervix in proportion 95 per cent to 5 per cent.

HYSTERECTOMY

(*a*) *Sub-total.* This may be performed in women over forty with extensive fibroids, and consists of removal of the body of the uterus only. This operation is less in favour than total hysterectomy, since the cervix, which

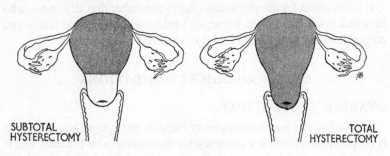

SUBTOTAL HYSTERECTOMY

TOTAL HYSTERECTOMY

FIG. IO

remains behind, is a common site of disease, and may therefore give trouble later.

(b) *Total.* This would be a preferable operation for extensive fibroids in women over forty. This operation consists of removal of the whole uterus including the cervix, and is usually performed through a midline abdominal incision. The vagina is closed in its upper part and left intact. The ovaries are retained. These patients, therefore, continue to ovulate until their natural menopausal time occurs, and do not show early menopausal changes.

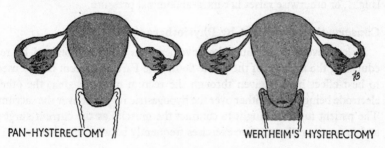

PAN-HYSTERECTOMY   WERTHEIM'S HYSTERECTOMY

FIG. 11

(c) *Total hysterectomy with bilateral salpingo-oophorectomy.* (See Fig. 11.) This may be performed for malignant disease in these organs.

PROLAPSE OF THE UTERUS

The uterus depends partly for its support on the transverse ligament which is extensive and complex in structure, but also on the adequate function of the muscles of the pelvic floor. These structures may become stretched and damaged as a result of prolonged or difficult labour. Prolapse due to lack of support may not, however, arise until after the menopause, since at that time all muscles and ligaments tend to atrophy, and an increase in obesity may cause a rise in intra-abdominal pressure, resulting in pressure on the uterus from above. Chronic bronchitis may also be a predisposing factor. The whole uterus may lie outside the body, carrying with it the vagina which will have been turned inside out.

Operation

A hysterectomy may be performed through the vagina.

PROLAPSE OF VAGINA

The vagina is severely stretched during childbirth, and some of its circular muscle fibres may be torn. This may leave weakened areas anteriorly and posteriorly. If posteriorly, the rectum may tend to protrude through the weak area into the vagina when the intra-abdominal pressure is raised as in coughing. This rectal bulge is called a *rectocele*. If anteriorly the bladder may bulge downwards and backwards into the vagina, this bulge being called a *cystocele*.

Complications. Stress incontinence may occur, the patient passing a small quantity of urine (and occasionally of faeces) when she coughs, sneezes, laughs, or otherwise raises her intra-abdominal pressure.

Conservative treatment by Physiotherapy

In less severe cases, much improvement can often be obtained by re-educating the muscles of the pelvic floor. The Faradic current can be used to best effect here if given through the rectum or the vagina, the other electrode being placed either over the hypogastric region or over the sacrum. The patient must be taught to contract the muscles as the current surges, and to continue these active exercises frequently between treatments.

Operations

These are of a variety of types, but the main object is repair of the pelvic floor, especially the levator ani muscles, which by meeting in midline form the main support for all the pelvic contents. Repair of the posterior uterine wall is known as *posterior colporrhaphy*: of the anterior wall and supports of the bladder, as *anterior colporrhaphy*. These two repairs plus amputation of the cervix and tightening of the transverse cervical ligament are known as a Manchester repair, or Fothergill's operation.

POST-OPERATIVE CARE FOLLOWING GYNAECOLOGICAL OPERATIONS

Many of these patients are given blood transfusions. The pulse and blood pressure are taken at frequent intervals in the first twenty-four hours, since a fall in blood pressure could indicate that intra-abdominal haemorrhage was taking place. A catheter may be passed if emptying of the bladder gives rise to difficulty at first. Dressings are kept to a minimum. Stitches are removed between the seventh and tenth days. Patients are usually allowed up within forty-eight hours of the operation.

Physiotherapy

For the first few days, physiotherapy can be of value in maintaining the circulation of the legs by vigorous and frequent toe and ankle exercises, also static contractions of the quadriceps and glutei. Hip and knee movements can be introduced after a couple of days. It is essential that the patient does not lie with a pillow under the knees to relieve tension on the abdominal muscles, since this could easily cause stasis in the veins of the legs. Bilateral breathing exercises are of value, also static abdominal contractions and pelvic floor exercises. These patients can often be treated satisfactorily in a ward class. After a few days when the patient is ambulant again, breathing and leg exercises can be discontinued, but the patient should continue the pelvic floor exercises until she can control these muscles easily in any position, e.g. standing, and not merely in the lying position with the legs crossed. Faradism may again be used if necessary.

Chapter VI

SURGERY OF THE BREAST

by B. SHOTTON, M.C.S.P.

Since the position of the breast and its lymphatic vessels have a very important influence on the surgery of this region and this, in its turn, affects the necessity for physiotherapy, the physiotherapist must have some knowledge of the anatomy of the breast. The average female breast extends vertically from the second to the sixth rib, and horizontally from the lateral border of the sternum to the mid-axillary line. It has one process, the axillary tail, which extends up along the lower border of the pectoralis major into the axilla. The breast lies in the superficial fascia, being separated from pectoralis major and serratus anterior by deep fascia. It is firmly connected to the skin by fibrous bands which are continuous with the fibrous framework of the breast and are known as Cooper's ligaments. The breast consists of glandular tissue; fibrous tissue, which acts as a supporting framework and divides the glandular substance into lobules; and fatty tissue between the lobules. Just below the centre of the breast is a conical eminence, the nipple, perforated by fifteen to twenty lactiferous ducts, and around this is an area of dark skin, the areola. Lymphatic vessels form a plexus in the interlobular spaces and in the walls of the ducts, while those of the more central part of the gland form a network, the sub-areola plexus, just deep to the areola. From this network, lymphatic vessels pass in various directions. Those from the greater part enter a dense network in the fascia over pectoralis major, from which vessels pass to the axillary lymph glands. Others drain into the internal mammary lymph glands, and there may be some communication with lymph vessels of the opposite breast. A few vessels from the upper part of the breast drain into the supra-clavicular lymph glands, while those from the lower and medial part anastomose with a lymphatic plexus on the upper part of the sheath of rectus abdominis, and probably communicate with lymphatic

90

vessels in the extra-peritoneal areolar tissue. Small local cysts may be removed by means of a small incision. The whole breast is sometimes removed for cysts or tumours. Neither of these operations should cause any great disability to the patient apart from occasional difficulty in regaining arm movements.

When the nature of a tumour in the breast is uncertain part may be removed and a frozen section performed. Should the growth prove to be malignant the operation will proceed and either a simple or a radical mastectomy will be carried out.

SIMPLE MASTECTOMY

This is removal of the breast through a vertical or diagonal incision, the pectoralis major muscle is left intact, but some surgeons remove the axillary lymph nodes. In the case of young people the operation may be followed, two or three weeks later, by a course of deep X-ray treatment. For older patients cytotoxic drugs are often preferred. These drugs destroy rapidly multiplying cells and so should destroy tumour cells. At the same time white blood corpuscles are also destroyed and great care has therefore to be taken against infection.

For these patients physiotherapy begins at once, the patient usually getting up on the first day. Breathing exercises, coughing, leg and trunk exercises are given. Arm movements should be full on the first day.

RADICAL MASTECTOMY

The area is exposed by an extensive incision. The following structures are removed:

1. The breast itself, together with the skin overlying the tumour, and including the nipple.

2. The entire system of lymphatic glands in the axilla, together with the channels which connect them with the breast, and the axillary fat in which these lie.

3. The sterno-costal part of pectoralis major, the whole of pectoralis minor, the upper part of the external oblique aponeurosis, and the anterior digitations of serratus anterior. If the growth is in the upper part of the breast, the whole of pectoralis major will be removed. Haemorrhage is carefully arrested, and the wound is closed, a rubber drainage tube being used for forty-eight hours. In cases where the skin cannot be approximated, a Thiersch graft may have to be used. Sterile dressings are applied and covered with thick layers of cotton wool, the upper arm being bandaged

lightly against the patient's side to maintain pressure and to prevent early movements of the shoulder. The patient is nursed in the semi-sitting position, the arm being supported by pillows.

Complications

1. The area is slow to heal, or may break down.
2. Movements of the shoulder will be limited, painful and weak.
3. There may be pulmonary complications.
4. The arm may become oedematous.
5. There may be damage to the brachial plexus.

Physiotherapy plays its part in preventing or overcoming these complications.

Physiotherapy

Breathing exercises should be practised for the first week, since the tight supporting bandages tend to restrict chest expansion. The fact that the patient is sitting up will help her to breathe more easily. While a few surgeons allow early shoulder movement, many do not allow this for the first week. If commenced too early, there is a danger of haematoma formation, and the chance that more serious exudate from the severed lymphatics will pass into the tissue spaces and form adhesions. There should be no restriction to other arm movements, however, and finger, thumb, wrist, radio-ulnar and elbow movements should be commenced immediately. These movements should be done frequently and in as large a range as possible to help to maintain circulation in the arm and thus prevent oedema. The physiotherapist should note any weakness which might indicate involvement of the brachial plexus, but this is a rare complication. Intercosto-humeral numbness around the region of the scar is common, and often worries the patient considerably. Posture should be corrected, as the patient may lean towards the side of the incision to relieve tension. After one week the dressings may be reduced and shoulder movements commenced gently. All movements should be attempted, not forgetting rotation, while the 'prayer' position is probably the method of choice for obtaining elevation. Loss of the pectoral muscles and part of serratus anterior results in these movements being grossly weakened. In many cases the patient will never regain full range movements, but it is always possible to get useful functional range in every direction, and this the physiotherapist must aim to do.

Rest for the first week gives the area a better chance of healing, but should the wound be slow to heal or break down again later, the physiotherapist may be asked to treat it. If heat is given, great care must be taken because of diminished sensation and vascularity of the area. If ultra-violet rays are used, care should be taken to see that no sensitizers are used in the dressings and that the patient is not yet receiving X-ray treatment.

Attendance as an out-patient will probably have to be continued for a number of weeks for deep X-ray treatment, and during this time the patient is encouraged to continue her exercises and to do functional activities at home. Occupational therapy would also be of value.

CHRONIC OEDEMA OF THE ARM

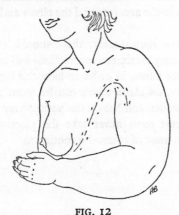

FIG. 12

In a number of cases, oedema of the arm may develop. This may be due to thrombosis of the axillary vein, or extensive fibrous tissue formation in the axilla preventing lymphatic drainage from the arm. It may also result from the wide removal of the vessels and glands draining the arm. If this occurs soon after operation, the limb is at first very tender. Later, however, it becomes white and heavy, and movements of the elbow and hand may become limited. It is at this stage that the physiotherapist may be called in.

It is advisable to *measure* the arm at a number of levels before treatment is commenced, and again afterwards. In this way, the benefit of the treatment can be assessed, and the amount of recurrence of oedema by the next attendance can also be noted.

Faradism under pressure. The patient should be lying rather than sitting, so that the arm may be elevated with the least amount of strain at the axilla. Faradism under pressure causes the muscles to contract. They cannot expand outwards owing to the firm bandage, so they press against the tissue spaces and bone, thus forcing fluid onwards. It is worth spending a little time experimenting with position of the electrodes in order to get the best contractions in the muscles. Short periods of activity with rests in between will probably be more tolerable to the patient than a prolonged session. After the Faradism, the limb is often much softer and more easy to massage; but in some cases of gross oedema, the Faradism has little effect unless preceded by massage. *Massage* should commence at the proximal end of the arm, with short, slow, deep strokes of effleurage, followed by kneading exerting firm pressure in a proximal direction, and then relaxing. As the area becomes softer, work progresses down the arm, special attention being given to the areas around the elbow and hand.

Exercises should follow immediately: these should be performed slowly and rhythmically, getting maximum contractions and maximum stretching of vessels passing over joints, in order to have the best effect on the circulation. If necessary, *an elastic sleeve* can be worn to control oedema. If the limb is very swollen and heavy, the patient may rest it in a *sling* for short periods, but rest must never take the place of active exercises. Shoulder movements must of course be continued.

Chapter VII

SURGERY OF THE EAR, NOSE
AND THROAT

THE EAR

Any part of the ear may become affected by disease, and, in order to appreciate the condition fully, it is necessary to have an understanding of the construction of the ear and the manner in which it acts as an organ of hearing and balance.

The ear consists of three parts: the outer or external ear, the middle ear, which includes the tympanic cavity, and the internal ear or labyrinth (see Fig. 13).

THE EXTERNAL EAR

This consists of the expanded portion or auricle of cartilage and skin, and a partly cartilaginous, partly bony tube, known as the external auditory meatus. The meatus is lined by skin continuous with that covering the auricle. In the subcutaneous tissue of its cartilaginous portion are glands which secrete a wax. Immediately posterior to the meatus is a thin layer of bone separating the meatus from the mastoid air cells. The function of the auricle is to collect sound waves; that of the meatus is to convey the vibrations to the drum head at the base of the tube.

THE TYMPANIC CAVITY

This is an air-containing space in the temporal bone, separated from the external ear by a thin semi-transparent structure known as the tympanic membrane or drum head. The inner wall is formed by the bony capsule of the internal ear. In this wall are two windows. The oval window opens into the vestibule, the central part of the internal ear. Fitted into this window, by means of a fibrous ring, is the foot plate of the stapes. The round window, which is closed by a membrane, lies a little behind the oval window and opens into the cochlea of the inner ear. Just above the oval window in the inner wall is part of the facial canal containing the facial nerve.

The anterior wall contains the opening of the Eustachian tube, by means of which the middle ear communicates with the naso-pharynx. This ensures that the pressure of air on both surfaces of the ear drum remains equal.

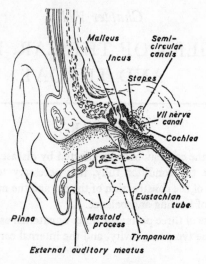

FIG. 13. THE EAR (RIGHT)

The upper part of the tympanic cavity, known as the attic, communicates posteriorly by a narrow passage, the aditus, with the mastoid antrum from which the mastoid air cells spread out into the surrounding bone. The whole air-containing structure, from the Eustachian tube to the mastoid air cells, is the middle ear cleft.

Across the tympanic cavity lies a chain of tiny bones, known as the ossicles. Their purpose is to assist in the conduction of vibrations from the tympanic membrane to the inner ear. First is the malleus, resembling a hammer, attached to the tympanic membrane. It articulates with the second, the incus, resembling an anvil, and this in its turn articulates with the stapes, or stirrup, whose foot-piece fits into the oval window.

Both the walls of the tympanic cavity and the ossicles are covered with mucous membrane. This is continuous with that of the naso-pharynx, through the Eustachian tube, and with that of the mastoid antrum and air cells, through the aditus. This means that inflammation of the nasal mucous membrane can spread, by direct continuity, to the middle ear and mastoid antrum.

The Ear

THE INTERNAL EAR OR LABYRINTH

This lies in the petrous portion of the temporal bone. It consists of two parts: the bony labyrinth, and the membranous labyrinth. The central part of the *bony labyrinth* is the vestibule immediately deep to the tympanic cavity. The anterior part is the cochlea communicating with the vestibule. The posterior part, also communicating with it, consists of three semicircular canals set at right angles to one another and representing the three planes of space. The cochlea obtains its name from its resemblance to a snail's shell. It forms a spiral tube wound round a central pillar of bone, known as the modiolus. The whole labyrinth is lined with endosteum, and contains a fluid identical to cerebro-spinal fluid, known as perilymph, in which floats the membranous labyrinth (see Fig. 14A).

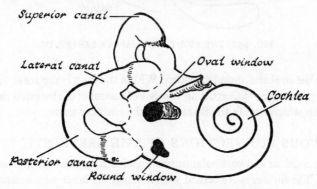

FIG. 14A. THE RIGHT BONY LABYRINTH

The membranous labyrinth is anchored at various points to the surrounding bony labyrinth. It consists of two sacs (the utricle and saccule), three semicircular canals and the duct of the cochlea. The semicircular canals open at each end into the utricle; the cochlear duct opens into the saccule and the saccule and utricle communicate. The membranous labyrinth thus forms a system of communicating sacs and ducts (see Fig. 14B). It contains endolymph, a fluid secreted in the cochlea and resembling perilymph.

The utricle and saccule are tiny membranous sacs lodged in depressions in the vestibule. Each shows a thickening in its wall known as the macula, which is the sense organ. In the macula are many flask-like hair cells, their free edges showing long tapering processes which project into the endolymph, and come in contact with tiny crystals, the otoliths. Between the hair cells ramify the fine fibrils of the vestibular nerve.

The semicircular canals open into the utricle. One end of each canal is dilated to form the ampulla, and in each of these is found an elevation similar in structure to the macula, and known as the crista.

The duct of the cochlea lies within the bony spiral tube. It is divided into three parts by membranous septa and communicates with the middle

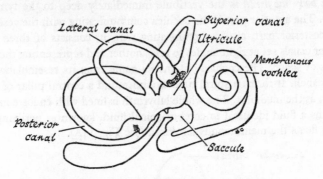

FIG. 14B. THE RIGHT MEMBRANOUS LABYRINTH

ear by the oval and round windows. Within the duct is the sense organ of hearing, the organ of Corti. This consists of a number of elongated hair cells between which ramify the filaments of the cochlear nerve.

NERVOUS CONNECTIONS OF THE LABYRINTH

The cochlear and vestibular nerves together form the eighth or auditory nerve. The former is concerned with hearing, the latter with balance.

The cells of origin of the cochlear nerve are found in the cochlear ganglion within the cochlea. Their peripheral processes terminate between the hair cells of the organ of Corti. Their central processes travel in the auditory nerve through a bony passage, the internal auditory meatus, to the pons where they relay in the cochlear nucleus. The bipolar cells of the vestibular nerve lie in the vestibular ganglion found in the internal auditory meatus. Their peripheral processes terminate between the hair cells of the cristae and maculae. Their central processes pass through the auditory nerve into the pons. Many relay in nuclei to enter the spinal cord forming the vestibulo-spinal tract, while others relay into the cerebellum.

FUNCTION OF THE LABYRINTH

The cochlear nerve, the cochlea and possibly the saccule too are concerned with hearing. Sound waves set up in the ear are collected by the auricle, transmitted by the meatus and impinge on the tympanic membrane, causing it to vibrate. These vibrations are transmitted across the tympanic cavity by the ossicles and by the air within the cavity. As the foot-piece of the stapes fits into the oval window of the vestibule, the vibrations are transmitted to the vestibule and the cochlear duct, causing movement of the fluid contained within it. The hair cells of the organ of Corti are stimulated, setting up impulses in the terminal processes of the cochlear nerve. As the stapes presses into the vestibule, the moving fluid bulges the membrane of the round window outwards, towards the tympanic cavity. If either window becomes obstructed by disease, the stapes would be unable to move, and stimulation of the organ of Corti would not occur.

The vestibular nerve, the semicircular ducts and the utricle are concerned with balance. When the head is moved, the fluid in the ducts and utricle tends to lag behind and consequently the hair cells of the cristae and maculae are stimulated. This results in the setting up of impulses in the filaments of the vestibular nerve. Again, the position of the head in space determines the direction of the pull of gravity on the otoliths. These pull on the tapering processes of the hair cells so that nerve impulses are generated. It is usually considered that alterations in the posture of the head influence the maculae, while movements of the head affect the cristae. Once the vestibular nerve is stimulated, appropriate messages are sent to muscles to maintain or restore balance and correct posture.

SYMPTOMS WHICH MAY ARISE IN DISEASES OF THE EAR

Pain, deafness, tinnitus (a sensation of noise caused by abnormal excitation of the auditory apparatus) and vertigo (giddiness) are common symptoms of ear defects. The physiotherapist will be concerned chiefly with the vertigo and should therefore have some understanding of its significance. Vertigo means an awareness of 'disordered orientation' of the body in space. The patient may feel that the surroundings are moving round him or that he is moving in relation to his surroundings, or that some part of his body or limbs is in an incorrect posture or is unsteady. Nausea and vomiting are common and there are often accompanying disturbances such as sweating, pallor or alterations in blood pressure.

Disturbance of balance may arise as a result of many factors, since correct orientation in space depends upon the reception by the vestibular nuclei, red nucleus and cerebellum, of messages from the labyrinths, eyes, skin and muscles and joints. Naturally it also depends upon the sending out of messages to the muscles of all parts of the body. Vertigo is essentially a disorder of sensation, due to the disturbance of the vestibular end organs or the afferent pathways to the brain. We are particularly concerned here with the disturbance of the vestibular nerve and ear. In this connection, excessive accumulation of wax in the external meatus, blockage of the Eustachian tube resulting in alterations in pressure in the tympanic cavity, inflammation of the middle ear, calcification of the oval window, inflammation or intermittent action of the labyrinths, head injuries or persistent movement may all cause vertigo. It should be remembered also that giddiness may be psychogenic, and, again, that it often persists when its organic cause has been relieved. Surgery involving the labyrinth will inevitably upset the mechanism by which equilibrium and stability is maintained and vertigo may be a temporary after-effect.

Aural Lesions in which Physiotherapy is of Value

Otitis media, mastoiditis, oto-sclerosis and Ménière's syndrome may all, at some time or other, benefit by physical treatment.

ACUTE OTITIS MEDIA

This follows an upper respiratory infection and sometimes it follows influenza, scarlet fever, measles and diphtheria. It usually originates from the nose or throat and reaches the tympanic cavity by way of the Eustachian tubes. The condition is characterized by inflammation of the mucous membrane lining the middle ear. A serous exudate is formed which often becomes purulent. One particular danger of this is that it may spread via the aditus into the mastoid antrum. The condition may subside with chemotherapy, but it is sometimes necessary to perform a myringotomy, that is to incise the ear drum in order to allow free drainage through the external auditory meatus. Even then pain and raised temperature may persist, suggesting retention of pus in the mastoid air cells. A cortical mastoid operation may then be necessary, to open and clear away these cells in order to prevent the spread of infection into the cranial cavity or elsewhere. The incision is made behind the auricle and the tympanic cavity is not approached.

For this acute condition physiotherapy is not indicated, though it may be of use if the ear continues to discharge (see later).

CHRONIC SUPPURATIVE OTITIS MEDIA

This condition may result from a variety of causes. A quiescent mastoiditis, necrosis of bone following one of the infectious diseases, failure of the acute condition to clear and constant re-infection from the nose or throat, may all be responsible. The condition is characterized by persistent discharge from the ear, varying degrees of deafness and often a visible opening in the ear drum. In almost every case, not only the tympanic cavity is infected, but also the mastoid antrum and air cells. Conservative measures aim at promoting free drainage and drying up the discharge, but, if these fail, then surgical treatment is necessary. This will be radical mastoidectomy, which may sometimes be modified in some degree. The air cells, antrum and tympanic cavity are converted into one large cavity. Neither cortical nor radical mastoid operations involve the inner ear and should not, therefore, result in vertigo, although occasionally the labyrinth is involved by the disease process. Other complications do occur.

Discharge from the ear may persist for some time after the operation, or the facial nerve may be damaged by disease or at the operation. In these complications, physiotherapy can prove of value. Persistent discharge sometimes yields to zinc ionization, combined with the dressings and chemotherapy carried out by the aural department. Zinc ionization may be applied in several ways, but the principle is that bactericidal effects are obtained by the formation of a layer of zinc albuminate over the mucous membrane of the walls of the tympanic cavity and attic. The zinc solution may reach this area through a special aural electrode, or by means of careful packing of the external auditory meatus with ribbon gauze soaked in a two per cent solution of zinc sulphate. About three milliampères may be given for ten minutes. This may be repeated weekly until the discharge ceases.

Facial palsy may readily occur because the facial nerve lies in very close connection to all three parts of the ear (see Fig. 13). It travels from the internal auditory meatus in a narrow bony canal outwards and backwards round the inner ear, down between the middle ear and mastoid, to leave the skull through the stylomastoid foramen.

In acute inflammation of the middle ear, oedema of the nerve, within the narrow confines of its bony canal, will cause paralysis by compression of the nerve fibres so that they cease to conduct. In chronic suppuration there may be direct erosion of the canal and the nerve. This is particularly liable to occur in a variety of chronic infections leading to a tumour-like formation of epithelial debris known as cholesteatoma. In the former condition the paralysis should clear following cortical mastoidectomy. Where the nerve is eroded by chronic disease, radical surgery will be required, and, if there is any break in continuity of the nerve, the missing part will be replaced by nerve graft, usually from the lateral cutaneous nerve of the thigh, and then recovery will not be expected for many months.

After operations on the ear, therefore, facial paralysis might occur at once if actual damage has taken place, or later if the nerve has become compressed by bleeding or exudate. In the first case the surgeon may decide to open the canal at once to relieve pressure, or repair the nerve; in the second case a waiting period may elapse, since spontaneous recovery is likely.

Physical treatment is of value whichever procedure is adopted, since in either case there will be a period before full recovery of facial muscles can occur, while regrowth of nerve takes place or recovery from compression occurs. During this period atrophy of muscles is rapid, owing to the gross diminution of their katabolic processes. In addition, owing to stagnation of blood and lymph, fibrosis will occur; and in these delicate muscles, muscle fibres will more rapidly be replaced by fibrous tissue, with its characteristic tendency to contract, than in coarse muscle. If a successful result is to be obtained, atrophy must be kept as slight as possible and fibrosis prevented. As soon as the paralysis is discovered, physiotherapy should be started. The circulation can be maintained and metabolic processes stimulated by the use of massage and radiant heat or inductothermy applied to the affected side of the face. This should be followed by electrical stimulation, using whatever current produces a comfortable contraction of the muscles. Care to prevent deformity, due to stretching of flaccid muscles and overactivity of healthy muscles, is important. To this end splintage is often used, the best being an acrylic mould attached to the upper teeth elevating the corner of the mouth. Appliances should be carefully checked and the skin watched by the physiotherapist. When the muscles begin to show signs of recovery, electrical stimulation may be omitted and active exercises substituted.

The surgeon will not consider decompression or nerve repair until he is certain that there is a complete paralysis. To be sure of this not only clinical tests, but also electrical examination of the condition of nerve and muscle are necessary, the latter usually being carried out by the physiotherapist.

OTOSCLEROSIS

This condition most commonly occurs in young women and is of unknown cause. Spongy bone gradually grows over the fibrous margin of the oval window and often encroaches on the foot plate of the stapes. Thus the movement of the stapes is progressively impaired, reducing movement of the fluid in the cochlear duct and the stimulation of the organ of Corti. As movement becomes less, deafness increases.

No means are known of checking the bony growth; consequently the patient has either to wear a hearing aid, or to undergo the operation of stapedectomy. The operation is performed under local or general anaesthesia through an incision in the external auditory meatus, part of the stapes is removed leaving the foot piece. A plastic piston is attached to the long process of the incus and fitted into a hole made in the foot piece. The piston will be moved up and down by the sound waves acting on the malleus and incus and this will cause movement of the inner ear fluid.

For the first twenty-four hours the patient lies flat in bed. Some surgeons prefer the patient to lie on his side with the affected ear uppermost. Sitting out of bed is usually possible by the fifth day, and about this time the small drain inserted at the time of operation is removed.

Two complications are liable to arise. One is a transient facial paralysis, its origin and treatment similar to that described in the discussion on chronic otitis media. The second is vertigo, which is almost invariably present to some degree after operation.

Vertigo appears immediately on recovery from the anaesthetic and may remain present for several weeks after operation. The giddiness is aggravated by any change of position and is particularly bad on sudden movements of the head or eyes. For this reason the patient tends to hold the head and eyes still and to move the trunk slowly and carefully. The neck and shoulder muscles therefore become tense and often remain so, long after the giddiness has permanently disappeared. Giddiness can usually be controlled by drugs, but occasionally it persists and physiotherapy is then ordered.

The object of physical treatment is to gain relaxation of tense muscles and to overcome the fear of giddiness, until it completely ceases and the patient is capable of carrying out normal activities with normal self-confidence. If these aims are not achieved, the tenseness continues and activities are limited through fear of the unpleasant sensation of vertigo.

The exact routine of exercise varies. Many surgeons like physical treatment to begin on the second post-operative day. Usually it is then carried out with the patient in bed. It is common to begin with eye movements, first slowly, then quickly, and then a combination of both. The use of long and short focus is also valuable. Provided that the head is supported, head bending forward and rotation may also be given. Head backward bending is often avoided as it seems to produce more vertigo. On the next day, the same movements may be practised in the long-sitting position and head rolling and head extension may be added, performed first with the eyes open and then with them closed. These movements should also be performed slowly at first and then quickly and then changing rapidly from one speed to another. Often the patient is allowed to sit out of bed on the fifth day. Shoulder movements to gain relaxation are now added and slow trunk movements. About the seventh day the patient can join a class of other patients, so that the spirit of competition may enter into the treatment. Exercises in sitting, stressing trunk and head flexion and extension, are given, and standing, trying to gain steady balance, is added. Progression is made daily by adding exercises in standing and by using changes of posture, first with the eyes open and then with them closed. Ball throwing makes a useful exercise to obtain balance and co-ordination. Ball work may be developed in standing and walking so that moving about freely is encouraged. Later balance walking, walking round objects and passing other people should all be used.

Patients vary in their progress and exercises must be chosen accordingly. The mental make-up of the patient has a great deal to do with the rate of recovery. The treatment should be pressed to the limit of tolerance of the individual, and encouragement given in order to restore confidence. The patient has to learn that a movement which makes him a little giddy has no untoward effects, and the next day that same movement may well fail to produce giddiness.

MÉNIÈRE'S DISEASE (or hydrops of the labyrinth)

This disease consists of recurrent attacks of severe giddiness often accompanied by severe prostration, vomiting and falling. Usually there is a history of tinnitus and gradually increasing deafness in one or both ears, followed by the onset of sudden attacks of severe vertigo, lasting from half an hour to several hours. In between these attacks, giddiness can sometimes be produced by sudden vigorous movements of the head. The symptoms are the result of dilatation of the endolymphatic system by increase of the amount of endolymph; but the syndrome, consisting of the symptoms of deafness, tinnitus and vertigo may occur in an acute labyrinthitis, or erosion of the capsule in chronic ear disease, and in tumours of the auditory nerve (acoustic neuroma). It is also present in certain toxic disorders of the labyrinth, such as that following therapy by streptomycin, and also in a form involving the vestibular mechanism alone, sometimes called 'vestibular neuronitis', possibly due to a virus inflammation of the vestibular ganglion.

In severe cases of Ménière's disease it is sometimes possible to cure the attacks of vertigo by destruction of the diseased labyrinth, usually accomplished by withdrawing the membranous lateral semicircular canal through a fenestra in the bony capsule; while occasionally alcohol is injected through the oval window by a fine hypodermic needle.

Labyrinthectomy produces a temporary severe vertigo, the degree depending on the amount of vestibular damage present before operation. It can be controlled by drugs. With drugs the patient soon becomes capable of maintaining normal balance with only one labyrinth functioning, and is free from vertigo.

Physiotherapy has therefore the same objects and is carried out if necessary in the same way as in the preceding condition.

THE NOSE AND ACCESSORY NASAL SINUSES

THE NASAL CAVITY

This lies between the cranium and the roof of the mouth. It is divided into two halves by a median septum, cartilaginous in front and bony behind. The two halves, known as the nasal fossae, communicate with the pharynx posteriorly. Opening into each are the orifices of the various sinuses. The lateral wall of each fossa is irregular and shows three scroll-like bones, known as the turbinates. The superior and middle of these are derived from the ethmoid; the inferior is a separate bone attached to the lateral wall of the cavity. Below the turbinate bones are grooves known as the superior, middle and inferior meatus respectively.

Each nasal fossa is lined by mucous membrane. This membrane consists of an upper olfactory part, containing the bipolar cells of origin of the fibres of the olfactory nerve, and a lower respiratory part. The olfactory portion is found lining the upper third of the nasal septum and the lateral wall of the fossa. The respiratory portion lines the lower two-thirds of the fossa and the air sinuses. The respiratory epithelium is a specialized structure, ciliated and containing mucous glands. The submucosa contains glands, connective tissue and blood spaces which are under control of the autonomic nervous system so that the thickness of the soft tissue can be altered from time to time, thus enlarging or narrowing the air pathways. The nose has three functions. It, together with the olfactory nerve and its central connections, is the organ of smell. It is responsible for the filtration of the air passing through it, and also for moistening and warming the air before it passes to the lungs. Should there be any nasal obstruction, these three functions may be upset.

THE ACCESSORY NASAL SINUSES

These are air spaces in the bones of the skull all communicating with the nasal cavity. It is usual to classify them into anterior and posterior groups. The anterior group open into the middle meatus and consist of frontal and maxillary sinuses, and anterior ethmoidal cells. The posterior and middle ethmoidal cells open into the superior meatus and the sphenoidal sinus into the spheno-ethmoidal recess above this (see Fig. 15). These sinuses are irregular in shape and vary in size at different ages and in different individuals. Their mucous membrane is in direct continuity with that of the nose, so that infection of the nasal mucous membrane is prone to lead to

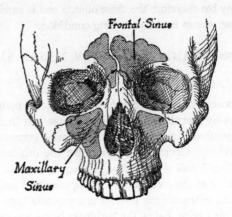

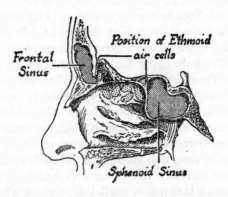

FIG. 15. THE ACCESSORY NASAL SINUSES

infection of that of the sinuses. The openings into the nasal cavity are small and are therefore easily blocked by swelling of the mucous membrane, and when this occurs, secretions will accumulate in the sinuses and not be able to drain into the nose.

The maxillary sinus is within the maxilla. It extends from the floor of the orbit to the roof of the mouth and from the lateral wall of the nasal cavity to the third molar tooth. The floor is the alveolar process of the maxilla and is in relation to the roots of the premolar and molar teeth. It may actually be perforated by the roots of the first two molars.

The frontal sinus lies behind the superciliary arch. It varies very much in size and shape in different individuals and is rarely symmetrical with its fellow. In many cases it extends upwards for a considerable distance into the frontal bone. The floor is formed by the roof of the orbital cavity, and the sinus itself may extend laterally to the level of the outer angle of the eye. Each sinus is separated from its fellow by a thin plate of bone.

The ethmoidal sinuses consist of a group of air cells in the lateral mass of the ethmoid. They thus lie at the upper part of the lateral wall of the nasal cavity and in the medial wall of the orbit.

The sphenoidal sinuses consist of a pair of cells lying in the body of the sphenoid behind the upper part of the nasal cavity. They are separated from each other by a thin septum of bone.

Diseases of the Nose and Sinuses in which Physiotherapy is of Value

Few diseases of the nose require treatment by physical means, though occasionally the condition of vasomotor rhinorrhoea is benefited by zinc ionization. Inflammation of the accessory nasal sinuses, sinusitis, is often considerably relieved by the use of short-wave diathermy or inductothermy.

VASOMOTOR RHINORRHOEA

This is a condition in which there appears to be undue sensitivity of the nerve fibres of the nasal mucous membrane. In some cases a definite irritant can be found; in others no known irritant provokes the onset of symptoms; but in some the individual is unduly sensitive to sudden changes in temperature.

The attack of rhinorrhoea is characterized by a pricking in the nose, a violent bout of sneezing and a profuse, watery discharge accompanied by intense lacrimation. The condition is usually treated by desensitizing injections or anti-histamine drugs. In some cases an attempt to reduce the sensitivity of the nasal mucous membrane, by the use of zinc ionization, is successful. The first treatment is usually given for five minutes and six milliampères should be tolerated. Three treatments are given and the time is progressed from five to seven and then to ten minutes. The course often proves successful in relieving the condition for a period of several months. It should be given in April or May and may be repeated after three or four months if necessary. In carrying out the treatment, care is necessary not to produce a haemorrhage, and very careful packing of the nasal cavities is required. This packing should be done in the ear, nose and throat department. Permanent loss of the sense of smell has been reported following zinc ionization.

NASAL SINUSITIS

This is an inflammation of the mucous membrane of the sinuses. It may be acute or chronic, and may involve one sinus only, all the sinuses of one side, or the sinuses of both sides, when it is known as a pansinusitis.

Acute sinusitis. This is often due to a virus causing the common cold. The swollen nasal mucous membrane blocks the opening from the sinus into the nose, mucus therefore stagnates in the blocked cavity and becomes a good breeding ground for bacteria. The stagnant mucus is converted into pus, the mucous lining of the sinus swells and the action of its cilia is depressed.

Partial blockage of an opening may also result from a deflected nasal septum or nasal polyps.

Owing to the retention of infected material, temperature, pulse and respiration rates rise; headache is usually present and is felt behind the eyes, if the ethmoidal sinuses are affected, and deep in the centre of the skull, if it is the sphenoidal sinuses which are involved. Pain is usually present, sometimes with tenderness on pressure. In the case of the maxillary sinus, this is in the region of the upper teeth; in frontal sinusitis it is just under the upper margin of the orbital cavity; and in ethmoidal sinusitis it is at the upper part of the sides of the nose. In most patients nasal discharge is mucoid at first, but after a few days purulent material appears in the nasal cavity. Once adequate drainage is established, relief of pain may be expected and within a few days the condition may be temporarily cleared and discharge ceases.

Treatment is usually directed towards providing adequate drainage by bringing about shrinkage of the swollen mucous membrane. For this, inhalations and ephedrine drops are most effective. Pain is relieved by sedatives and infection controlled by systemic antibiotics. Short-wave therapy may be ordered, but it must be given with great care if drainage is not yet established. Its purpose is to stimulate the circulation and vitality of the membrane without increasing the metabolism of the tissues or of the micro-organisms, and, for this reason, it must not produce heat. Mild doses are therefore given, and the electrodes are arranged in such a way that all the walls of the affected sinus are treated.

Sometimes the condition subsides with this combination of treatments. More often the pus becomes thinner, the mucous membrane shrinks and discharge commences. Short wave therapy is now more useful, since, with free drainage, there is less danger of increasing congestion and pain. Stronger thermal doses are now suitable. These should be repeated several times daily, though, as the discharge decreases, treatments need not be so frequent.

If the condition does not clear with conservative treatment the surgeon may decide to clear the pus by means of an antrum washout. In this a hollow cannula is inserted through the nose and the wall of the maxillary antrum the fluid is inserted under pressure into the antrum so that it returns through the normal opening. Several washouts may be needed and short-wave therapy may be continued until the sinuses are clear.

Chronic sinusitis. This develops if the treatment fails to clear the infected sinus. Sometimes the lining membrane is so badly damaged by the acute condition that the cilia never recover and secretions cannot be swept up towards the opening. Occasionally little pockets of pus form due to irregularity in the membrane. If systemic antibiotics, nasal drops and antrum washouts are not successful it may be necessary to make a new opening into the sinus. When this is done physiotherapy may be ordered. This will have three main objects: the improvement of general health; the stimulation of the circulation and nutrition of the lining membranes; and the promotion of good drainage. The fulfilment of these aims may be aided by the use of general light-baths, and the application of short-wave diathermy to the sinuses. Because the condition is a chronic one longer doses, thermal in nature, may now be used and should be given once daily.

THE PHARYNX

The pharynx extends from the base of the skull to the level of the cricoid cartilage and is divided into three parts. The naso-pharynx extends from the base of the skull to the soft palate and lies behind the nasal cavity. The oro-pharynx extends from the soft palate to the epiglottis and lies behind the cavity of the mouth. The laryngo-pharynx lies behind the larynx and extends from the epiglottis to the level of the cricoid cartilages. The naso-pharynx communicates with the nose by the posterior nares and with the mouth, and, in its lateral wall, is the opening of the Eustachian tube leading into the tympanic cavity of the ear. At the junction of the posterior wall with the roof of this part of the pharynx, in the midline, there is a large mass of lymphoid tissue known as the pharyngeal tonsil, or adenoid, present in childhood, but tending to disappear with age. A second mass of this tissue is found in the oro-pharynx, between the pillars of the fauces on each side. This is the oral tonsil. In both cases the function of the tissue is probably that of protection against infection and it is for this reason that it is much more developed in children.

Diseases in which Physiotherapy may be of Value

The only diseases in this region in which physiotherapy is likely to prove of real value are those affecting the lymphoid tissue. If the pharyngeal tonsil hypertrophies, the condition is known as adenoids and may require treatment. The oral tonsil may become acutely inflamed or chronically infected as in acute or chronic tonsillitis.

ADENOIDS

This condition is present when the lymphoid tissue of the naso-pharynx is hypertrophied. This may occur either as a result of chronic nasal congestion or of infection. The enlargement has several disadvantages. It is liable to obstruct the airway from the posterior part of the nasal fossae into the pharynx, causing mouth breathing. This means that the function of filtering, warming and moistening of the air, normally carried out by the nose, is lost, predisposing the patient to bronchial infections. Inefficient breathing also means shallow breathing; the chest becomes flat; oxygenation of the blood is reduced and mental and physical development are retarded. Mouth breathing causes difficulty in swallowing. Appetite becomes defective and nutrition impaired.

A second disadvantage of the enlargement of this tissue is the tendency to block the openings of the Eustachian tubes. This results in deafness and, in unfavourable cases, the spread of infection up the tubes to the ear, or forward into the nasal sinuses.

The obvious result of all this is a child of typical appearance, with narrow nostrils, underslung jaw, mouth perpetually open and a vacant expression; a child who is mentally and physically retarded and at a disadvantage with other children.

PRINCIPLES OF TREATMENT

Since obstruction is causing trouble it must obviously be relieved. This can be achieved conservatively in some cases. In others, removal of the tissue may be necessary. If the obstruction is not too great, resolution of inflammation and consequently shrinkage in size of the tissue will follow measures which improve the child's general health and resistance and improve the breathing habits. Both may be aided by the use of physiotherapy. Improvement in general health may be gained by a course of general ultra-violet light treatment and general exercises, including those which improve posture and stimulate mentality. Good breathing habits may be established by specific training of breathing. The obvious essential is to regain nasal breathing. All breathing exercises should start with clearing any nasal discharge. The child should be taught to blow the nose with the head bent forward and holding the bridge of the nose and not the nostrils. The child is then taught to breath in, with the mouth closed, and out, with it open. Once this is mastered, correct use of the chest is taught so that the child uses the bases and lateral regions of the lungs. Manual pressure and use of straps are of value. A good habit is acquired by carrying on the good breathing while performing simple exercises, games and everyday activities. The co-operation of the parents is obviously essential.

Should the obstruction be already extensive or complete, conservative treatment will be of little avail. The enlarged tissue is excised and immediate benefit seen. By this time, however, bad breathing will have become a habit, which will not be broken simply by removing the offending tissue. Physiotherapy follows excision, therefore, on the same lines as in the case treated conservatively. Work to mobilize the chest, improve posture, increase and stimulate metabolism is of great importance. Children are more successfully treated in groups, once individual training in good breathing has achieved a measure of success.

TONSILLITIS

This condition may be acute or chronic. Acute infection or irritation may cause an acute inflammation accompanied by fever and general illness. Occasionally the condition fails to clear completely and chronic inflammation results. In these cases the crypts of the tonsil become filled with pus and toxic absorption may be continuous, thus causing trouble elsewhere.

The most satisfactory treatment is the removal of the tonsil. In children chronic tonsillitis often accompanies the presence of adenoids and both masses of lymphoid tissue may be removed at the same time. Pre- and post-operative breathing and general exercises should be given but particular care must be taken because the main complication of tonsillectomy is haemorrhage, either at once, or later, between five and ten days, when slough on the tonsillar bed begins to separate. For this reason exercises are often postponed for ten days.

Very occasionally blood or septic material is inhaled into the lungs during the time the patient is unconscious. This is liable to produce broncho-pneumonia, lung abscess or pulmonary collapse. If signs of chest complications do arise, physiotherapy may be ordered and will be carried out on the lines discussed in Chapter IV.

MALIGNANT DISEASE OF THE
UPPER RESPIRATORY TRACT

Malignant growths may involve the nose, paranasal sinuses, the pharynx, larynx or ear. Treatment will be by radiotherapy or by surgery to remove the tumour and surrounding tissue. If the method of choice is surgery it may be the removal of the maxilla, laryngectomy, or pharyngo-laryngectomy according to the site and extent of the malignant growth. Radical neck dissection for removal of all lymphatic nodes in the neck may be carried out on its own or in combination with other operations.

In the operation known as pharyngo-laryngectomy the larynx and part of the pharynx are removed. Some part of the colon is used to replace the pharynx, one end being sutured to the upper end of the oesophagus and the other to the remaining part of the pharynx. This patient will therefore have both an abdominal and an anterior neck incision. A radical neck dissection is also carried out to remove all lymph nodes and other soft tissues in the posterior triangle of the neck, excluding the carotid arteries and brachial plexus. The accessory nerve may be either damaged or destroyed and both sterno-mastoid and trapezius will either be removed or considerably damaged. For this reason the shoulder region is usually painful for some days after the operation, and the shoulder tends to drop down and forward.

The patient is in the intensive care unit for the first twenty-four to forty-eight hours. When he returns to the ward he is nursed in the half-lying position and warned not to lean forward since this might occlude the airway. Usually tubes are removed about the seventh day and the patient is then allowed to get up. Walking is started the tenth day by which time the patient should be able to cough up secretions, and suction through the tracheostomy should no longer be necessary. The patient is discharged home the second or third week.

Physiotherapy

Breathing exercises and coughing are given every two hours while the patient is in the intensive care unit. Suction will be essential because at first the patient will be unable to cough up the secretions further than the lower end of the trachea. It must be carried out with great care (see Chap. VIII). Gradually the patient will learn to cough and get secretions up without suction. To do this he has to contract the abdominal muscles strongly. In the presence of an abdominal incision this is not easy. Help can be given by teaching the patient to use a broad strap round the abdomen to support the site of incision. The usual post-operative leg exercises will also be given. As soon as the patient is back in the ward gentle neck exercises are started. Full-range shoulder movements are also encouraged and the posture of the shoulder girdle is checked. When the tubes draining the sites of incision are removed, at about seven days, heat may be given if the shoulder is still painful and more shoulder exercises practised together with intensive training of shoulder girdle posture. Breathing exercises and coughing are continued, but suction should not be needed after about ten days. These patients cannot speak so a paper and pencil should be kept handy. Speech therapy is given and some patients eventually learn to speak though it is much more difficult than following a laryngectomy.

HYPOPHYSECTOMY

In some patients suffering from malignant growths of the breast or prostate the pituitary gland is removed. This gland produces hormones which influence the activity of other endocrine glands and it has been found that some breast and prostate cancers are affected by the hormones produced by the ovaries and adrenals. These cancers may regress after excision of the hypophysis.

A small incision is made in the side of the nose round the inner angle of the eye, the gland is excised through the sphenoidal sinus which is then packed with a piece of thigh muscle. The patient is nursed flat for the first twenty-four hours. Usually the sutures are removed at five days and the pack which holds the muscle in the sphenoid sinus at seven days. If there is no leakage of cerebro-spinal fluid the patient is allowed up at ten days. Cortisone therapy is started at once and thyroxine and Pitressin used as necessary.

One complication of this operation is leakage of cerebro-spinal fluid once the packs are out and during the first week there is a definite danger of meningitis.

Physiotherapy

Particular attention to the chest is often necessary since there may be secondary deposits in the lungs. Breathing exercises start at once but because of the danger of cerebro-spinal fluid leakage blowing the nose must be avoided and great care must be taken over coughing. Coughing should be used only if secretions are present and then must be done with as little strain as possible. The usual post-operative progressive routine of leg exercises, walking, etc., will be included. A careful watch should be kept as pathological fractures do occur due to secondary deposits in the bones and if these are present in the vertebral column a spinal support will be needed.

Chapter VIII

THORACIC SURGERY I

by A. SYMONS, M.C.S.P.
Introduction. Outline of Anatomy. Respiratory Function.
Incisions. Drainage Tubes. Tracheostomy. Respirators.
Physiotherapy Techniques

INTRODUCTION

Most surgeons consider that before and after chest operations physiotherapy is of great value in the prevention, minimization, or treatment of various complications.

The physiotherapist should therefore have a sound knowledge of the normal anatomy and physiology of the thorax and its contents and the changes which occur in abnormal conditions. She should also be familiar with the surgical and nursing procedures which are used, as team-work in treating these patients is essential.

The founder of physiotherapy in chest surgery in this country was Miss Winifred Linton. She started her work at the Brompton Hospital in 1934 having come from the Westminster Hospital where she had developed her interest in asthma and devised the breathing and relaxation exercises which are used throughout the world today.

Miss Linton's enthusiasm, patience and personality slowly overcame the surgeons' reluctance and resistance until the benefits of improved posture and control of breathing were understood and it was finally realized there could be no good chest surgery without physiotherapy.

OUTLINE OF ANATOMY

THE THORACIC CAGE

The walls of the thorax consist of bone, cartilage, muscle and other soft tissue, therefore they have elasticity and the muscles can move them. The posterior wall consists of the thoracic vertebrae and the posterior ends of the ribs. From the posterior angles, the ribs curve forwards and downwards to form the lateral walls while the anterior boundary consists of the sternum to which the ribs are connected by the costal cartilages. The thoracic inlet is the opening into the upper extremity of the thorax. It is comparatively small and slopes downwards and forwards and is formed by the first thoracic vertebra, first pair of ribs and the upper border of the manubrium sterni. The outlet is the lower opening and is considerably larger. It is formed posteriorly by the twelfth dorsal vertebra, laterally by the eleventh and twelfth ribs and anteriorly by the seventh to the tenth costal cartilages and the tip of the xiphoid process. The outlet is closed by a sheet of muscular and aponeurotic tissue, the diaphragm.

The shape of the chest differs considerably in different people as does the angle made by the diverging costal margins at the xiphisternum. Normally the lateral diameter of the chest is wider than the antero-posterior diameter. The latter is often increased in emphysematous subjects and, with a more horizontal run of the ribs this forms a 'barrel chest' deformity. Unusual depression or prominence of the sternum is caused by developmental anomalies.

The sternum consists of three parts: manubrium, body and xiphoid process. The bone segments are joined by cartilage which allows slight movement on respiration in young subjects but increasing ossification leads to increasing rigidity after puberty.

The ribs are placed obliquely one above the other, and the intercostal spaces between them are filled by fascia and intercostal muscles; the intercostal vessels and nerves run just below each rib. The width of the intercostal spaces increases with inspiration and is narrowed by expiration. Crowding of the ribs in kyphosis or where there is underlying pleural thickening severely limits rib movement and consequently respiration.

The upper ten ribs articulate by means of synovial joints with the bodies and transverse processes of the dorsal vertebrae and directly or indirectly with the sternum through their costal cartilages. The eleventh and twelfth ribs articulate only with the bodies of their corresponding vertebrae. Owing to these articulations, the ribs are able to move. The direction of movement is upwards and outwards, rather like lifting a bucket-handle, the greatest movement being by the long middle ribs (fifth to eighth inclusive). These movements also raise the sternum. Thus both the lateral and antero-posterior diameters of the chest are enlarged.

THE THORACIC MUSCLES

The floor of the thorax is formed by a single dome-shaped muscle, the diaphragm, which descends on contraction and increases the capacity of the thorax. It has been estimated that the action of the diaphragm is responsible for about 60 per cent of the volume of inspired air. Working with the diaphragm are the intercostal muscles, which also function in elevation of the ribs and sternum.

There are many other muscles which influence the thorax either by assisting respiratory movements or maintaining the best functional position and shape of the chest. These are the muscles which pass from the head, neck and shoulder girdle to the ribs. In relation to the posterior aspect of the thorax lie trapezius, latissimus dorsi, levator scapulae and the rhomboids. All these muscles acting together will hold the shoulders up and brace them back, thus lifting the anterior portion of the ribs. Deep to these muscles lies the sacrospinalis which, by steadying the thoracic spine, affords a better leverage for the movement of the ribs; also, by straightening the spine it helps to increase the size of the thorax.

The sterno-mastoid and pectoral muscles anteriorly and serratus anterior laterally play a part in fixing or elevating the ribs or shoulder girdle. The scalene muscles on each side of the neck are attached to the first two ribs and fix or elevate these.

Because so many of these muscles are passing from the head, neck and shoulder-girdle to the thorax, faulty carriage of the head and shoulders will affect their ability to lift the ribs. Also, weakness of these muscles following, for example, an incision, is liable to affect both posture and movement of the arm and shoulder girdle.

THE CONTENTS OF THE THORAX

The Pleurae. Within the thoracic cage are the two separate pleural cavities.

Each pleural cavity is a closed sac invaginated by the corresponding lung. Thus it consists of two layers, the visceral pleura covering the surface of the lung including the interlobar surfaces and the parietal pleura lining the walls and floor of the thorax. The visceral and parietal layers are in contact but move freely over one another, because the adjacent surfaces are kept moistened by a small amount of serous fluid.

Air may escape from the lungs between the two layers of pleura spontaneously or after injury or operation. The air-filled space so created is called a pneumothorax, and if much air collects under positive pressure (tension pneumothorax) the lung will collapse.

The pleural space is also a common site for the development of large amounts of liquid (effusion) in disease or infection. A localized collection of pus in the pleura is called an empyema.

The Lungs. The lungs are composed of a great number of lobules bound together by elastic connective tissue. Each lobule consists of a terminal bronchiole ending in a collection of air sacs called alveoli. Associated with

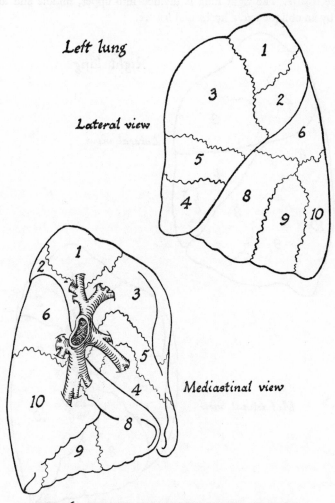

Left lung

Lateral view

Mediastinal view

FIG. 16A. THE LEFT BRONCHOPULMONARY SEGMENTS

Key to numbers referring to segments of the lobes

1. APICAL		6. APICAL	
2. POSTERIOR	UPPER	8. ANTERIOR BASAL	LOWER
3. ANTERIOR	LOBE	9. LATERAL BASAL	LOBE
4. INFERIOR LINGULA		10. POSTERIOR BASAL	
5. SUPERIOR LINGULA			

each lobule are nerves and blood and lymph vessels. The lobules are grouped together to form segments and collections of segments to form lobes.

The left lung is divided into upper and lower lobes by a long, deep oblique fissure. The right lung is divided into upper, middle and lower lobes by an oblique and a horizontal fissure.

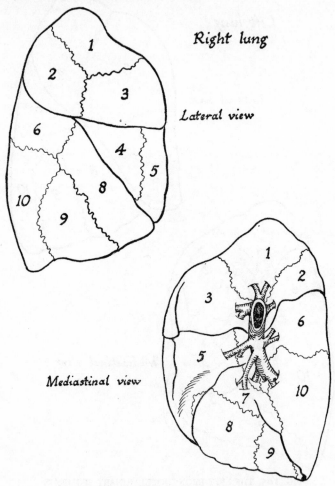

FIG. 16B. THE RIGHT BRONCHOPULMONARY SEGMENTS
Key to numbers referring to segments of the lobes

1. APICAL	UPPER	6. APICAL	
2. POSTERIOR	LOBE	7. CARDIAC (MEDIAL BASAL)	LOWER
3. ANTERIOR		8. ANTERIOR BASAL	LOBE
4. LATERAL	MIDDLE	9. LATERAL BASAL	
5. MEDIAL	LOBE	10. POSTERIOR BASAL	

On the left side the lower lobe occupies the lower and posterior part of the chest including the lower half of the lateral aspect, whilst the upper lobe lies in front and above it behind the anterior chest wall and at the apex of the chest and axilla. On the right side, the lower lobe occupies the same position as on the left but the remainder is divided so that the upper lobe is confined to the apex of the chest and lies behind the upper three or four ribs, the middle lobe occupying the lower part of the chest anteriorly.

The lobes consist of a number of broncho-pulmonary segments (see Fig. 16, A and B), each of which reaches the surface. Each segment is quite distinct and occasionally this may be apparent on the surface of the lungs by means of slight visible indentations. The right lung has ten segments and the left nine. (The correct positions to drain most of these segments are shown in Plates III, a–g.)

The Trachea and Bronchi (see Figs. 17, 18, 19). The trachea divides at its lower end into the right and left main bronchi. The sharp dividing line is known as the main carina and its deformity as seen on bronchoscopy is an important sign of inoperability in lung and oesophageal cancer.

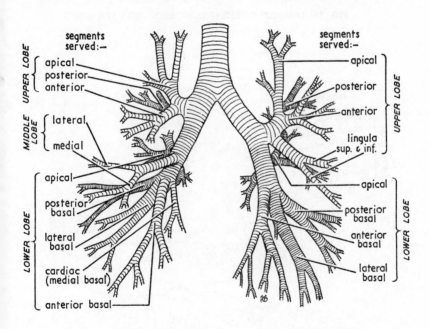

FIG. 17. ANTEROPOSTERIOR VIEW OF THE BRONCHIAL TREE

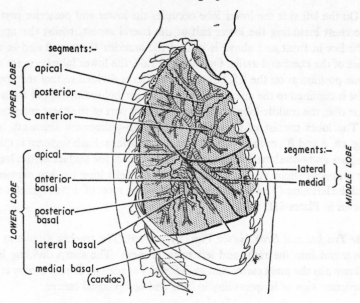

FIG. 18. DIAGRAM OF RIGHT LUNG SEEN FROM THE SIDE

Labels on right lung diagram:

UPPER LOBE — segments:-
- apical
- posterior
- anterior

MIDDLE LOBE — segments:-
- lateral
- medial

LOWER LOBE
- apical
- anterior basal
- posterior basal
- lateral basal
- medial basal (cardiac)

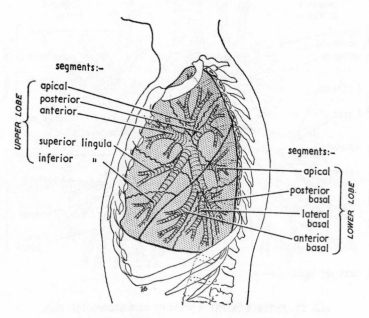

FIG. 19. DIAGRAM OF LEFT LUNG SEEN FROM THE SIDE

Labels on left lung diagram:

UPPER LOBE — segments:-
- apical
- posterior
- anterior
- superior lingula
- inferior "

LOWER LOBE — segments:-
- apical
- posterior basal
- lateral basal
- anterior basal

120

The right main bronchus branches off at an angle of about 45 degrees, being more nearly in line with the trachea than the left main bronchus, which curves more sharply to the left. Thus inhaled food and foreign bodies tend to fall into the right lung when the patient is upright.

The right main bronchus is relatively short (3 to 4 cm.) and broad (1½ to 2 cm.), giving off the upper lobe bronchus on its lateral wall at its distal end. It then continues in a straight line as the intermediate bronchus for two centimetres before giving off the middle lobe bronchus anteriorly and continuing thereafter as the lower lobe bronchus.

The lower lobe bronchus divides into four basal bronchi distally (medial, anterior, lateral and posterior), after having given off the apical or superior segmental bronchus posteriorly.

The middle lobe bronchus has two segments: medial and lateral. The right upper lobe bronchus divides into three segmental bronchi: apical, anterior and posterior.

On the left side the main bronchus is longer (5 to 6 cm.) and slightly narrower than on the right side and curves more sharply from the main carina as it runs beneath the arch of the aorta. At its distal end it gives off the upper lobe bronchus and continues as the lower lobe bronchus.

There is thus no intermediate bronchus and no middle lobe on the left side. There is also no medial basal bronchus on the left side since the heart occupies that volume. The left lower lobe consists of anterior, lateral and posterior basal segments, with the apical or superior segment above them.

The position of the separate right middle lobe is taken on the left side by the two lingula segments (superior and inferior) which are part of the upper lobe. The remaining upper lobe segments, as on the right side, are the anterior, posterior and apical segments.

There are nineteen segments in all. The bronchi of these segments repeatedly divide into smaller and smaller divisions until they end in a cluster of air sacs or alveoli.

All except the terminal bronchi are lined by ciliated epithelium and mucus-secreting cells. The cilia move rapidly and ceaselessly throughout life wafting a stream of mucus from the periphery of the lung to the trachea and pharynx where trapped dust and bacteria can be swallowed or expectorated.

Cilia may cease to work by reason of overwhelming secretion, secretion made too sticky by dehydration, cilia poisoned by drugs (morphine and anaesthetics) or damaged by operation or endotracheal tubes. Secretions are then retained, bronchial obstruction and pulmonary collapse follow and infection soon supervenes.

In these circumstances, the importance of maintaining ciliary activity by humidification of inspired oxygen and air (especially if the patient has a tracheostomy and loses nasal humidification) can be seen, also the necessity for effective painless coughing and postural drainage.

The Mediastinum. This is the area between the lungs outside the pleural cavity. It contains the heart and pericardium, the oesophagus, trachea, aorta, thoracic duct, the vagus and phrenic nerves and the thymus. There is also considerable connective tissue, lymphatic vessels and glands.

The mediastinum is supported by the even, elastic pull of the two lungs. Should one lung collapse the sound lung tends to shift to the affected side (mediastinal shift) and to undergo compensatory enlargement.

RESPIRATORY FUNCTION

Respiration is a complex function requiring:

(*a*) adequate ventilation of the lungs by diaphragmatic, intercostal and other muscle power and needing a clear airway (nose, pharynx, larynx, trachea and bronchi may all be sites of obstruction);

(*b*) the even mixing of fresh air within the lungs;

(*c*) the diffusion of oxygen into the blood and the equally important release of carbon dioxide across the alveolar-capillary membrane;

(*d*) a normal pulmonary circulation.

Inspiration is the active movement drawing fresh air into the lungs. Enlargement of the chest by muscular action reduces the pressure within the chest to less than that of atmospheric pressure. This can be measured by a fine recording needle placed between the two layers of the pleura, or down the oesophagus, and connected to a manometer. Normal inspiratory pressures are between 5 and 15 centimetres of water less than atmospheric (– 5 cm. to – 15 cm.), rising to pressure – 30 cm. or – 40 cm. on forced inspiration.

Expiration is usually a passive movement. After relaxation of the inspiratory muscles the elastic recoil of the lungs and chest wall expels the air with a positive (above atmospheric) pressure of 2–3 cm. of water. Expiration may be increased powerfully by contraction of the chest-wall, shoulder girdle and especially the abdominal muscles. This occurs particularly in coughing when the glottis is temporarily closed to build up pressure before the explosive forced expiration.

The diaphragm normally has an excursion of 2–3 cm. on quiet respiration rising to 6–8 cm. on very deep breathing. The liver lies beneath the right hemi-diaphragm which is at a slightly higher level than the left, below which lies the stomach.

If a careful watch is kept on the thorax during deep inspiration, the chest will be seen to enlarge in all diameters and in all its parts. The sternum moves slightly forwards and upwards, owing to the thrust on it of the anterior ends of the ribs which move forward as they rise. The thorax enlarges laterally by the outward movement of the ribs. The vertical diameter is increased by the descent of the diaphragm and elevation of the upper ribs.

Expansion and ventilation of the lungs may be hampered by:

(a) lung and pleural disease especially if fibrosis occurs;

(b) deformities or injuries of the thoracic cage;

(c) limitation of rib movement because of joint changes due to old age or diseases such as osteo-arthritis and ankylosing spondylitis;

(d) weakening or paralysis of the muscles as in neurological or neuro-muscular disease, or because of old age, poor posture, or general debility; or

(e) injury or metabolic or drug damage to the respiratory centre in the mid-brain.

The physiotherapist can help the patient improve his mechanics of ventilation. She can teach the patient to strengthen and control main and accessory muscles of respiration, to correct his posture and clear obstructions from his airways. Development of these skills can open up collapsed areas of lung, aid the interchange of gases, induce recession of infective processes and the absorption of pleural exudate. Pain caused by disease, injury or poor posture can be resolved and the improved chest contours and circulatory mechanics induce a feeling of well-being.

INCISIONS USED IN THORACIC SURGERY

Surgical entry into the thorax is known as thoracotomy. The type of incision will vary considerably depending upon the site of the lesion, the choice being based on the necessity to gain the best possible access to the lesion. After the incision is made, the gap may be widened by retracting the ribs. Whether the incision should be made through an intercostal space or through the bed of a rib will depend on the width of exposure required and the age of the patient. When a wide exposure is needed, much rib retraction will be necessary, so in patients over thirty years old when the ribs are more rigid and fracture easily rib resection (usually fifth, sixth or seventh rib) is the better method. In the case of children and people under thirty years old the ribs are soft and elastic and much retraction can be produced without fear of fracture.

Most incisions are made parallel to the ribs and therefore run obliquely round the lateral chest wall. A short vertical incision across the lines of the seventh, eighth and ninth ribs may be made for rib resection and drainage of an empyema.

STANDARD THORACOTOMY

The most common incision is a postero-lateral one and it is so often used that it is known as a standard thoracotomy. The level of this varies according to the operation. For a pneumonectomy it is through the beds of the fifth or sixth resected ribs, for an upper lobectomy the fourth or fifth and for a lower lobectomy the sixth rib is removed. The seventh and eighth ribs are removed for operations around the diaphragm such as for hiatus hernia and oesophageal growths.

THORACO-LAPAROTOMY

A thoraco-laparotomy incision is an extensive one and is employed on the left side for a total gastrectomy and oesophageal resection. It commences posteriorly in the bed of the seventh or eighth rib and continues forward to divide the costal margin and to cut the left external and internal oblique abdominal muscles, the transversalis and the rectus abdominis. The diaphragm may be divided in the line of the incision or at its periphery.

ANTERO-LATERAL INCISIONS

Sometimes an antero-lateral incision is used. This incision is carried from close to midline in front, below the breast to the post-axillary line (see Plate IV).

ANTERIOR INCISIONS

For some operations on the heart or other mediastinal structures an anterior approach may be used. This may be longitudinal, splitting the sternum, the two halves then being distracted; or it may be transversely across the chest just below the breasts and nipples through an intercostal space (usually the fourth), the sternum being divided across in the same line.

The significance of the type and site of incision to the physiotherapist lies in the fact that certain muscles have to be cut through in the process of operation. If post-operative care is not taken, an adverse effect on the posture of the head, spine, thorax and shoulders may occur, the exact nature depending on the muscles affected. In addition interference with muscles will have an effect upon the patient's willingness to perform full range movements. There will also be a natural tendency to lessen strain on the operation wound, as the patient unconsciously adopts the posture which will best fulfil this object.

In a standard thoracotomy the lower part of the trapezius and rhomboids are cut, also the latissimus dorsi and the serratus anterior muscles. Considerable interference with full elevation and retraction of the shoulder girdle follows. The patient also tends to elevate the hip and lower the shoulder on the affected side in order to relieve tension on the wound. This results in flexion of the trunk to the affected side.

THORACOPLASTY

The older type of thoracoplasty operation with more extensive incision of trapezius, rhomboids and scalene muscle attachments and extensive removal of ribs was used for tuberculosis and is still occasionally performed for this or for the obliteration of an infected pleural or pneumonectomy space. This can lead to severe scoliosis concave to the affected side. Compensatory cervical and lumbar curves will develop to the opposite side and there is often head tilting and apparent lateral shift to the operation side.

DRAINAGE TUBES

After most thoracic operations it is necessary for one, or sometimes two, drainage tubes to be retained for a few days to drain unwanted fluid or air from the chest. An apical tube drains mostly air and a basal one mostly liquid. Drainage is often necessary too after injury or for pleural disease when the fluid in the chest is too thick for aspiration by a needle.

Intercostal drainage (see Fig. 20). A rubber or plastic tube is inserted through an intercostal space, into the pleural cavity. The other end of the tube is attached to a glass tube inserted through the rubber cork of a Winchester bottle into water which half-fills the bottle. Another short length of glass tube passes through the cork but not into the water. This may be open or attached to a suction pump. The type of fluid draining from the chest may be seen in the bottle.

It is the duty of all staff to check that the drainage is satisfactory whenever they are attending to the patient. As the patient breathes, the level of water in the glass tube rises and falls because of the different pressures in the chest. If the tube is blocked or kinked this 'swing' will stop. Usually a change of position of the tube or 'milking' it will clear it of a blood-clot or other obstruction, but, if not, a surgeon may have to re-insert the tube.

After operations on the lung a stream of bubbles will normally appear from the tube into the water as the patient coughs or breathes. A very large loss of air may indicate that a larger bronchus has been divided or ruptured, a condition known as broncho-pulmonary fistula.

It is of the utmost importance that the end of the long glass tube remains under water so that air cannot enter the patient's chest and cause a pneumothorax.

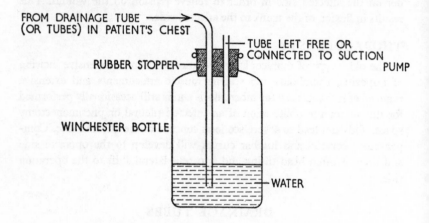

FROM DRAINAGE TUBE ⟶
(OR TUBES) IN PATIENT'S CHEST

TUBE LEFT FREE OR
CONNECTED TO SUCTION
PUMP

RUBBER STOPPER

WINCHESTER BOTTLE

WATER

FIG. 20. APPARATUS FOR INTERCOSTAL DRAINAGE

On no account must the bottle be raised from the floor unless the tube to the patient is clamped off, otherwise the contents of the bottle may drain back into the chest. Clamping off the drain may be necessary on moving or turning the patient, but there is no reason why he cannot walk around holding the bottle near the ground if his general condition permits this.

Closed drainage. When toilet of the pleural space is needed, usually to evacuate blood clot or infected fibrin, a larger calibre tube is used than for intercostal drainage. The chest wall is closed round the drainage tube to make an airtight seal and the tube is connected to the bottle as for intercostal drainage.

Open drainage. Open drainage is occasionally used for a very localized empyema where the rest of the pleural cavity is obliterated and there is no danger of pneumothorax. The pus drains through the chest-wall by a short tube into dressings preferably sealed off in a colostomy-type plastic bag. The danger of open drainage is infection from the wound to the ward or of organisms in the ward air re-infecting the wound.

126

TRACHEOSTOMY

Silver Tracheostomy Tube. Tracheostomy with insertion of a silver tracheostomy tube may be necessary if there is obstruction of any part of the upper airway or if the patient is not able to cough effectively and rid himself of secretions. The nurses and physiotherapists can then keep the airways clear by means of catheters attached to a suction apparatus. When passed down the trachea the catheter will also stimulate the cough reflex.

Cuffed Tracheostomy Tube. If the patient is also suffering from weakness of swallowing or there is danger that he may inhale infected matter after injury or operation to the upper chest, neck or face, a cuffed tracheostomy tube has to be inserted (see Fig. 21).

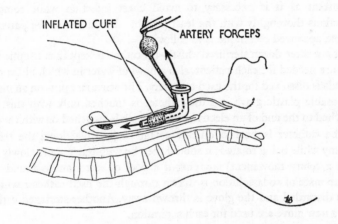

INFLATED CUFF ARTERY FORCEPS

FIG. 21. DIAGRAM SHOWING PATIENT WITH CUFFED TRACHEOSTOMY TUBE

With the cuff inflated and clamped off, although air can pass through the tube into the lungs, matter from the upper air passages, or regurgitated from the stomach, cannot be inhaled.

It is of the utmost importance to note that as long as swallowing is weak or the danger of inhalation exists, the cuff must be deflated *only* when the patient is lying on his side *and* is tipped head down at an angle of 45 degrees. The cuff is released for about one minute every four hours to relieve pressure on the lining of the trachea.

If a patient attached to a respirator is receiving negative as well as positive pressure (see section on Respirators, p. 128), the negative pressure must be turned off while the cuff is deflated to avoid inhalation of secretions. When the dangers of inhalation are over, the tube may need to be retained but the cuff can be deflated all the time.

Humidification. When a tracheostomy is performed air is drawn directly into the trachea, and the normal warming and humidifying in the upper air passages cannot take place. Secretions will become crusted and difficult to remove and so a humidifier must be used. This consists of a small tank of water which is electrically heated and thermostatically controlled. An electric fan blows the warm, moist air from the tank through a tube which ends in a cap lying loosely over the tracheostomy tube. Oxygen can, if necessary, also be led through the humidifier.

Suction of a tracheostomy. Secretions must be regularly and thoroughly removed through the tracheostomy tube. The technique used is extremely important as it is necessary to avoid chest infection while removing secretions thoroughly with the least possible discomfort to the patient.

One approved technique is as follows:

About three dozen sterilized whistle-tip catheters kept in antiseptic solution are needed for each patient, also a bowl of water in which bicarbonate of soda is dissolved for the used catheters. The attendant puts on an unused disposable plastic glove and the catheter is touched only with this. It is attached to the end of an electric sucker which is switched on with the foot.

The catheter is pushed quickly as far as possible down the tracheostomy while being rotated; it should then be withdrawn more slowly (still with a rotary movement) stopping if a pool of secretions is found. The bicarbonate of soda solution is drawn through the used catheter which is then discarded and the glove is thrown away. Another sterilized catheter and a new glove are used for each aspiration.

If the patient can cough at all, he should be encouraged to do this during suction procedure and the catheter will stimulate the cough reflex.

If the patient cannot breathe effectively and is attached to a respirator, suction must be performed quickly and a close watch kept as he may become distressed for lack of air if too long is taken. With a very ill patient it is preferable for a second person to detach and re-attach the connection from the patient to the machine while the first uses the sucker.

RESPIRATORS

Some form of artificial respiration is essential if a patient is unable to breathe adequately. This may be after any major chest surgery but especially thymectomy associated with myasthenia gravis or if paradoxical breathing occurs.

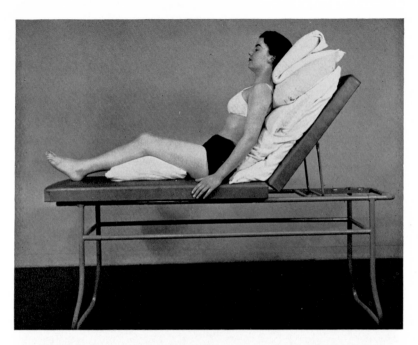

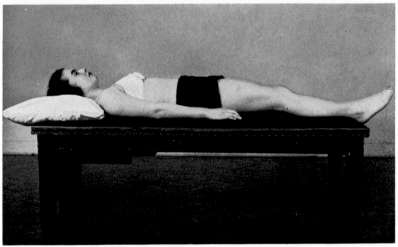

III. Positions for postural drainage (*see* p. 132)

(*a*) for drainage of apical segments of upper lobes

(*b*) to drain anterior segments of upper lobes

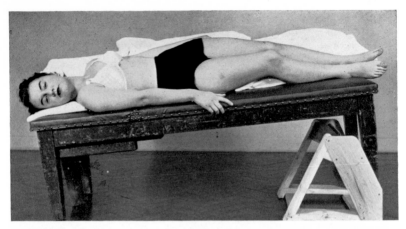

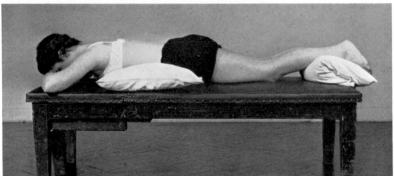

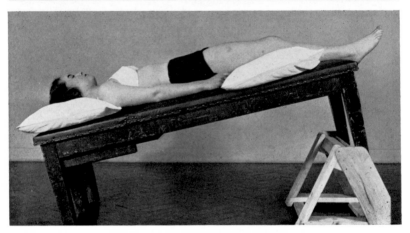

III.   (c) to drain lingular process
(d) to drain apical segments of lower lobes
(e) to drain anterior basal segments

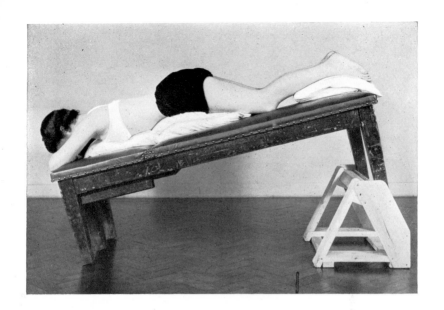

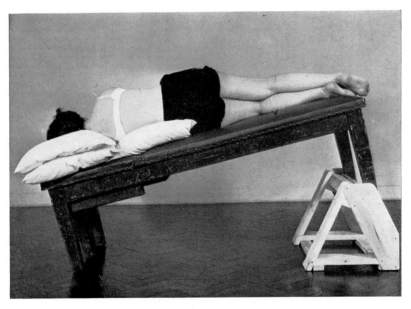

III. (f) to drain posterior basal segments
(g) to drain lateral basal segment of right lung

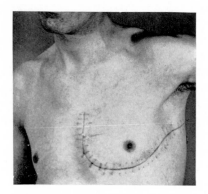

IV. Anterior thoracotomy incision
(*see* p. 124)

Respirators

Respiratory failure may also occur with severe chest injuries, polyneuritis, poliomyelitis, severe tetanus when curarization is needed, barbiturate poisoning, and a variety of rarer conditions.

Positive pressure, or positive-negative pressure, respirators incorporating humidifiers and attached to the patient through inflated cuffed tracheostomy tubes have largely superseded tank respirators. They are essential if swallowing as well as breathing is weak or absent, or if there is danger of inhalation of foreign matter into the lungs for other reasons. They are also more convenient for care of the patient in other cases of inadequate spontaneous respiration not associated with weakness of swallowing. Some of the respirators are mechanical, providing the patient with a fixed rate and depth of respiration. Others are 'patient-triggered', that is, the patient can use what little power of respiration he may have and the machine will supplement this to an adequate level.

Tank respirators can be used only if swallowing is normal, which occurs almost entirely in certain types of poliomyelitis. Cuirass and jacket types of respirators and rocking-beds may be required to assist inadequate breathing in the chronic stage of poliomyelitis only.

All staff attending patients attached to respirators must be familiar with the working of the machines and the steps to take in the event of electrical or mechanical failure. Modern respirators can be worked by hand or switched to a battery in an emergency. Extra hand pumps will also be available. A knowledge of artificial respiration by the expired air method and of external cardiac massage is also necessary for use if all mechanical aids fail or while waiting for the Emergency Resuscitation Team.

A patient with a respirator is unable to clear his chest of secretions unaided. It is the physiotherapist's responsibility to do this for him, but, as with all seriously ill patients, duties overlap and team-work with doctors, nurses and other hospital workers is essential.

The general nursing care and physiotherapy for the chest of a patient nursed with a respirator is the same regardless of the cause of his respiratory failure. He should be nursed on his side on a mattress with fracture-boards beneath it. The bed should be capable of being tipped up or down to an angle of 45 degrees (or adequate elevators to do this should be available). He should be turned to his other side every two hours, and allowed on his back for only very brief intervals, if at all, to avoid pooling of secretions in the posterior parts of the lungs from where it is difficult to remove them. Suction of the trachea is carried out whenever necessary which in the acute stage is probably every fifteen minutes.

Accurate postural drainage for the bases and apices and other parts of the lungs as necessary should be carried out four-hourly during the day and up to 10 p.m. The patient should not need physiotherapy during the night, but the two-hourly turning and regular suction continues throughout the twenty-four hours and a physiotherapist should be on call.

Physiotherapy for the chest is of first importance and the patient is never too ill for it. However occasionally the blood-pressure will be low or unstable and the head-up position may be omitted, but should be started again as soon as possible as collapse of the apices of the lungs is common. The one condition in which physiotherapy may be omitted is in barbiturate poisoning when the patient, if he survives, is likely to be attached to the respirator for a few days only and chest complications are unlikely to arise. On the other hand unnecessary disturbance may cause a fatal circulatory collapse.

The total time spent at one session of physiotherapy for these patients in the acute stage of any illness should not exceed one hour or the patient will be overtired. This calls for good judgement on the part of the physiotherapist as to how long to spend on any one area of the lungs, and the co-operation of a nurse to suck out the trachea and otherwise help the physiotherapist throughout the treatment.

As the patient recovers, he will need less physiotherapy to the chest and more active general exercises depending on the condition from which he is suffering. Except in poliomyelitis, recovery of the power of respiration and swallowing and 'weaning' from the respirator is usually a steady and not too difficult process.

It must be remembered that although the care of the chest is of first importance, leg and foot movements to try to prevent thrombosis, arm and shoulder movements after chest surgery and other exercises must still be undertaken even if a patient is attached to a respirator.

TECHNIQUES OF PHYSIOTHERAPY

Aims of Physiotherapy

Pre-operative aims will be:
- (a) to increase the efficiency of ventilation;
- (b) to clear excessive secretions;
- (c) to mobilize the joints of the chest, spine, neck, shoulders and shoulder-girdles;
- (d) to improve posture;
- (e) to explain and teach post-operative procedures.

Post-operative aims will be:
- (a) to try to prevent lung and circulatory complications;

(*b*) to maintain the efficiency of unaffected areas of the lungs;

(*c*) to re-expand affected areas of the lungs;

(*d*) to help the patient eliminate excessive secretions;

(*e*) to maintain or increase mobility of the shoulders and shoulder-girdle, chest, neck and spine;

(*f*) to maintain or improve good posture;

(*g*) to increase exercise tolerance.

BREATHING EXERCISES

Careful teaching of correct breathing is one of the most important of the physiotherapist's skills. It takes patience and practice. It is probably best for the patient to begin in the half-lying position where he can most easily relax his upper chest, shoulders, arms and neck. The 'contrast' method, aiding relaxation by first contracting the groups of muscles, can be used with advantage.

Quiet general breathing, first out through the mouth, then in through the nose should then be taught with relaxation. It should be pointed out that in the normal rhythm of breathing, there is a pause at the end of expiration before the next inspiration. Some people consider that a 'sniffing' type of movement should be discouraged as this leads to use of the upper chest and accessory respiratory muscles.

The next progression is diaphragmatic breathing. The patient is told to breathe out while letting himself narrow round the waist, then to expand in the same place, when he will feel air being drawn in. Relaxation of the upper chest must be emphasized throughout.

Although many surgeons now believe general deep breathing is sufficient, localized breathing is also usually taught.

Control of bilateral or unilateral breathing, using the lateral costal, upper costal and posterior basal areas as necessary should be mastered by the patient. The pressure of the physiotherapist's hands guides and controls the movements. Pressure must be firm enough so that the patient can move the chest against slight resistance but not so firm that movement is restricted.

It is easier for the patient if each exercise starts with expiration and if he thinks of moving his chest and not of expelling or drawing in air. Hurried changes from one breathing exercise to another are to be avoided.

The patient should be instructed in practising the exercises by himself several times a day. He can use his own hands or straps to provide pressure, but care must be taken that he relaxes his upper chest and shoulders, etc., as before.

Other positions than half-lying should be used as alternatives or progressions according to the condition of the patient. To increase exercise tolerance and breath control, breathing exercises in conjunction with general exercises, or walking on the level or up and down slopes and stairs can be used. The aim will be to perform controlled breathing during or after exercise of increasing length or strength.

Rhythmical breathing in time to walking is a useful exercise, for instance, taking two steps for inspiration and three for expiration and progressing the time and altering the speed of walking and breathing. The patient can also be taught to relax, if necessary leaning on a wall or banister, and to control his breathing if he becomes really 'short of breath'.

With very ill patients, inhalants or oxygen or both may be required before or during treatment. The physiotherapist will therefore have to learn how to use the particular apparatus and drugs ordered. Analgesics may be necessary in the early days after surgery or injury.

POSTURAL DRAINAGE

A patient with excessive secretions will need accurate posturing to assist the drainage of the lungs. The positions for draining the various segments are shown in Plate III, a–g. Pillows must be used carefully and purposefully, for instance, a pillow under the head should not also be under the shoulder.

With the patient in the correct position, efficient breathing and coughing must be performed. Emphasis on full expiration, but not very forced expiration with wheezing, helps move secretions and seems to stimulate coughing.

Periods over about twenty minutes in any one position at a time seem unnecessary. The physiotherapist will learn with practice by the 'feel' of the chest whether a part of the lungs is clear or not and therefore how long the patient needs. The number of treatments per day will vary according to the amount of the secretions. As a patient improves, little will be removed at too frequent treatments and some sessions may be omitted.

Percussion is not so much used nowadays except for bronchiectasis and lung abscess where surgery has not been undertaken. It is often too painful after surgery and traumatic conditions to be useful.

Shaking, vibrations and rib-springing are necessary for patients who are paralysed or unconscious or who, for other reasons, cannot perform breathing and coughing exercises actively. Rib-springing consists of increasing pressure of the physiotherapist's hands on the ribs over the area of lung treated while the patient is breathing out. At the end of expiration a firm extra pressure and release is given, then release of pressure during inspiration.

COUGHING

Effective but not violent coughing is an essential protective mechanism for keeping the air-passages clear. A patient suffering from any condition who will not or cannot cough is in grave danger of lung complications.

The patient should be taught to support his operation wound or other painful area and be assured that he will not harm himself though a cough will be painful. Support of the lower chest by the physiotherapist and firm pressure during the expiratory phase of a cough will also help him.

If a patient is not able to cough effectively, a catheter attached to a sucker passed down his nose will stimulate the cough reflex. Where a patient is unconscious or paralysed for any length of time, he will probably need a tracheostomy and, in some cases, a respirator so that secretions can be cleared by suction of the trachea. As the catheter passes down the trachea it will also stimulate the cough reflex if this is present.

OTHER EXERCISES

Leg exercises. When a patient is in bed after thoracic surgery, or indeed for any other reason, simple foot and leg movements are important to try to prevent thrombosis. It must be explained to the patient why these are necessary, and he must be encouraged to perform vigorous dorsi-flexion and plantar-flexion, and alternate knee flexion and extension many times a day. Passive movements, though not so effective, must be given if the patient cannot for any reason perform active movements.

Later, when the patient is up, leg exercises will be included in the general exercise scheme and in conjunction with postural exercises and re-education of walking.

Shoulder and head exercises. After thoracic surgery, restriction of shoulder and neck movement due to pain and division of the muscles will occur. From the first day after operation, full-range active movement must be encouraged several times a day. Resisted movements, especially with proprioceptive neuro-muscular facilitation techniques make it much easier for the patient to obtain less painful and full-range movement early.

Later more vigorous exercises including the use of apparatus in the gymnasium can be given and class games with balls, etc., played.

Trunk exercises. Trunk exercises are used in conjunction with postural training. Many kinds may be used. Klapp's crawling exercises are very useful for stiff joints in children and young people. Mobile joints of the thoracic spine, head and shoulder-girdle will increase mobility of the chest and facilitate breathing exercises.

Postural exercises. Postural training is undertaken in the pre-operative period and re-training begins on the first day after thoracic operation. When the patient is sitting up in bed, pillows must be arranged so that he is in a good position, that is, sitting with pelvis level and back against the pillows, with shoulders level and relaxed and head straight. Long mirrors should be available to place at the end of the bed so that the patient can check his position.

As the patient progresses to exercises sitting over the side of the bed or on a chair, posture must be corrected throughout the treatment, especially in conjunction with the shoulder, trunk and head exercises.

When the patient is standing or walking, firm shoes are a great help to good posture, and when all tubes are out, it is better for him to be fully dressed. It is usual for posture and walking to be very poor when a patient is in dressing gown and slippers.

Chapter IX

THORACIC SURGERY II

by A. SYMONS, M.C.S.P.

Introduction. Infection. The pre-operative period. Post-operative complications. Operations on the Chest Wall. Chest Injuries. Operations on the pleural cavity. Lobectomy and Segmentectomy. Pneumonectomy. Mediastinal Tumours

INTRODUCTION

Before and after thoracic surgery treatment and progression vary with the individual patient, the surgeon's wishes and the circumstances of the particular hospital. A usual routine is described.

Physiotherapy is not usually needed between 6 p.m. and 9 a.m. but arrangements should be made for evening treatment if necessary and a physiotherapist should be 'on call' to cover any emergency which may occur outside normal working hours. Treatment is necessary at weekends and holidays for recent post-operative and acutely ill patients.

The physiotherapist should attend the surgeon's ward rounds whenever possible so that she may be able to co-operate fully with him and the other staff.

INFECTION

Most patients needing thoracic surgery are not suffering from infectious diseases but staff should know how to protect themselves when an infectious disease is present, and should also beware of carrying infection to any patient.

Ideally no member of staff with a respiratory infection should attend patients, but if this is unavoidable an adequate mask should be worn. On the other hand, if a patient is known to be suffering from 'open' tuberculosis or other infection, masks must be worn by the staff who should also take other precautions (possibly barrier nursing) as necessary. They should have annual chest X-rays, and, if not re-acting positively to a tuberculin test, should be protected by B.C.G. vaccination.

The infectious patient must be taught to turn the head away from anyone else while coughing into a disposable tissue. Sputum and used tissues should be contained in closed cartons.

THE PRE-OPERATIVE PERIOD

Unless the operation is an emergency one, pre-operative treatment may take days, weeks or even months. Medical and nursing care will bring the patient's general condition to the highest possible level. Explanation of procedures should be given to the patient; the physiotherapist often being expected to explain the incisions and drainage he is likely to have.

Smoking should always be discouraged and is forbidden altogether in some units.

X-rays and blood tests will be taken. Records of respiratory function such as vital capacity, peak-flow readings and measurements of chest expansion will be started, usually by the physiotherapist. Satisfactory progress as shown in these tests is an important factor in deciding when an operation can be performed.

Bronchoscopy. A bronchoscope can be passed through the mouth to examine the pharynx, larynx, trachea and larger bronchi, as an aid to diagnosis. Through the bronchoscope retained secretions or inhaled foreign bodies may be removed. The procedure may be carried out under general or local anaesthesia.

Bronchograms. These are valuable aids to diagnosis and the planning of an operation. They determine the positions needed for postural drainage especially in bronchiectasis.

Before the procedure, the physiotherapist clears any excessive secretions from the patient's chest by means of postural drainage and after local or general anaesthesia has been administered, a radio-opaque iodine-containing dye is injected into the trachea; the patient is then postured so that the dye enters all the segments of the lung to be examined. It outlines all the smaller bronchi and bronchioles even as far as the periphery of the lung, and demonstrates on the X-ray film distortions, blocks, strictures and dilations.

After X-ray films have been taken and seen to be satisfactory, coughing and postural drainage are again performed to drain the dye from the lungs. Since the throat has been anaesthetized, the patient should not eat or drink for three hours after the examination in case he inhales material into his lungs.

Bronchograms can also be performed with a patient who has a tracheostomy by passing the radio-opaque substance through a catheter directly into the trachea.

Pre-operative Physiotherapy

Depending on the condition for which the patient will be undergoing surgery, various kinds of pre-operative physiotherapy will be necessary.

Breathing exercises appropriate to the condition must be taught and practised regularly by the patient under supervision and alone several times a day.

If excessive secretions are present, regular postural drainage will be given in addition. The sputum should be measured and recorded daily, as this is another factor in determining the timing of the operation. If fewer secretions are present, there is less risk of post-operative lung complications.

The physiotherapist must check the mobility of the patient's chest, back, neck and shoulders. Appropriate exercises to correct any defects in his posture will also be given. She must also teach him any other exercises which he will have to do after operation.

Explanation of the reasons for these exercises and for all pre- and post-operative procedures will do much to gain the confidence of the patient and ensure his full co-operation which is so necessary for a successful outcome.

POST-OPERATIVE COMPLICATIONS

These can usually be diminished by adequate treatment.

(a) Because of transfusion of blood during operation (usually 500–1500 ml.), *surgical shock* (that is excessively low blood-pressure) is rarely seen post-operatively unless there is sudden and serious bleeding into the pleural space. In these circumstances a collection of blood in the drainage bottle should be noticed.

(b) *Some oozing of blood and serous fluid into the pleura and wound* is normal, but excess is drained by a tube.

(c) *Leakage of air* is also normal when small bronchi have been divided. Again a drainage tube will remove any excess.

(d) *Collapse of segments or lobes of lung.* This complication is usually the result of retained secretions. Fear and pain combine to inhibit the cough and prevent adequate clearance of the bronchi.

(*e*) *Limitation of shoulder movements* should be avoided by early exercise. Occasionally a 'frozen shoulder' follows an operation and is due to idiopathic capsulitis.

Other stiff joints and poor posture can be prevented or corrected by adequate physiotherapy.

(*f*) *Anoxia and carbon dioxide retention.* Lack of oxygenation of the blood in the lungs, which, when severe is shown as cyanosis, may disturb the brain even before this stage is reached, the patient being restless and irritable; he may even suffer permanent brain cell damage. Oxygenation is maintained by a clear airway, the evacuation of bronchial secretion, adequate powers of ventilation and the prevention of areas of pulmonary collapse and infection. Added humidified oxygen may be needed temporarily or continually when the lungs have been severely damaged by disease, operation or post-operative complications.

A tracheostomy is another way of providing air or oxygen to the lungs more easily than breathing through the nose or mouth, as well as providing an easy means of sucking retained secretions from the bronchi.

It has been more recently recognized that inability to exhale carbon dioxide with its retention in the blood stream may lead to a similarly dangerous state, the patient often appearing warm and sweating, and with a misleadingly good peripheral circulation and blood pressure, before coma and cardiac arrest ensue. This state is most likely to be seen with severe ventilatory depression post-operatively, especially in patients with emphysematous lungs. For this reason patients undergoing thoracic surgery must be roused from anaesthesia before leaving the theatre and must not be allowed to sleep again until they have consciously demonstrated to the physiotherapist the adequacy of their ventilatory powers. Only then will sedation be allowed and this should never be so heavy as to prevent the patient from being awakened and instructed to breathe and cough.

The degree of suboxygenation can be estimated from blood samples if necessary, and the carbon dioxide retention can be assessed from the blood or more conveniently from expired air.

OPERATIONS ON THE CHEST WALL

THORACOPLASTY

This is the removal of sections of several ribs to collapse the underlying lung. It is now rarely performed as the primary treatment of pulmonary or pleural tuberculosis but is sometimes necessary in special circumstances. It may also be used occasionally to obliterate a non-tuberculous infected space such as may follow the development of bronchial fistula after pneumonectomy.

OPERATIONS FOR CONGENITAL DEFORMITIES

Operations to the chest wall to correct major congenital deformities may be undertaken. The usual deformities are caused by vertebral anomalies, or sternal or costo-chondral maldevelopment. These may lead to gross kypho-scoliosis or pectus excavatum (funnel chest—undue depression of the sternum) or pectus carinatum (undue prominence of the sternum). The capacity and mobility of the chest may be restricted. Anterior chest deformities can be dealt with by surgical reconstruction with gratifying improvement in appearance and with some benefit to cardiac displacement and pulmonary ventilation.

TUMOURS OF THE CHEST WALL

Portions of the chest wall may need to be resected when tumours grow from the ribs. Plastic repair with prostheses may be necessary.

THORACOTOMY

This is an incision through the chest wall and it may be undertaken to remove a foreign body, or repair a torn bronchus or bronchial stricture, with or without removal of some lung tissue.

Pre-operative Physiotherapy

Before operations on the chest wall, the most important skill to teach the patient is diaphragmatic breathing with relaxation. Localized breathing for the sound lung or both as necessary should then be attempted.

Exercises to mobilize the chest, neck, shoulders and back must be performed by patients about to undergo thoracoplasty, while for those with congenital deformities, attempts must also be made to improve posture by means of exercise.

Post-operative Physiotherapy

Breathing and coughing exercises will be started on the first day. The posture must also be corrected from the beginning. Pillows should be used to keep the patient in the correct position, and a mirror should be available for him to correct himself when sitting up.

When the patient is out of bed intensive postural training will be required to prevent deformity in the case of thoracoplasty and to maintain any improvement gained in the case of congenital deformity.

Thoracic Surgery II
CHEST INJURIES

Minor injuries of the chest involving one or two rib fractures are often associated with considerable pain and some pleural effusion. The quickest way to recovery is by adequate pain-killing drugs combined with controlled breathing exercises, and graduated arm and trunk exercises.

A largely discarded method of treatment leading to possible complications is to strap or bandage the area and confine the patient to bed. The older the patient, the more dangerous is this practice.

Major injuries of the chest are unfortunately common in traffic accidents. The injury may be so severe as to dislocate whole areas of the chest wall laterally or round the sternum. The fractured ribs tear the pleura and lung with extensive bleeding and escape of air into the pleura. Leakage of air into the overlying muscles and subcutaneous tissues produces a condition known as surgical emphysema. The lung itself may bleed into the bronchi which may be torn, as may the great arteries and veins and mediastinal contents. Injuries to other parts of the body may further complicate the picture.

When an adequate airway, ventilation and circulation have been established, a plan for further treatment can be made. The most severe chest injuries will call for tracheostomy, and an intermittent positive pressure respirator. This is particularly true when paradoxical breathing is present and adequate ventilation and normal breathing movements cannot be maintained. Paradoxical breathing means that when the patient breathes in and the relatively undamaged part of the chest expands, the negative intrathoracic pressure so created sucks in the disconnected segment of the chest wall. When the patient contracts his chest in expiration the internal expressive force blows out the damaged chest wall. The positive pressure respirator expands all parts of the chest equally so the normal movement and shape of the chest are restored.

If the patient has a tracheostomy, whether in conjunction with a respirator or not, he will need a routine of turning, posturing and suction of the trachea. Adequate fluid intake and humidification of inspired air are necessary to keep secretions moist. (See sections on tracheostomy and respirators.) Other injuries may prevent a full routine, but care of the chest is of vital importance.

Artificial respiration with a positive pressure respirator may be necessary for one to three weeks. It is used gradually less and less and the patient tries to breathe alone for longer and longer periods. Active breathing and coughing exercises can be added as soon as the patient can co-operate and these can be progressed rapidly once the respirator is unnecessary.

Operations on the Pleural Cavity

Pain is a marked feature of these injuries and inhibits breathing and coughing. Often the only effective way to relieve this is by epidural analgesia. A fine nylon catheter is passed between the mid-thoracic vertebral spines until it comes to rest just outside the dura mater round the spinal cord. Injections of local anaesthetic solution act on the issuing spinal nerves over many segments. This has the useful effect of killing pain before motor power is seriously affected.

When the patient is over the acute stage, it will often be found that rib movement and chest expansion are poor, that posture is affected and that wasting of chest and shoulder girdle muscles has occurred. A long and active period of rehabilitation will be necessary even if other injuries are not present.

OPERATIONS ON THE PLEURAL CAVITY

PLEURAL DISEASE

This is nearly always due to disease of the underlying lung. Tuberculosis and cancer both require exclusion as possible diagnoses. A collection of air and blood in the pleural cavity is a common complication in injuries to the chest wall.

Infection of the pleural space rapidly leads to fibrous thickening with subsequent contraction which draws in the rib spaces, crowds the ribs and reduces the volume of the hemithorax. Scoliosis, concave to the affected side also follows, as does contraction of the lung and restricted ventilation.

Investigations of pleural disease can be made by aspiration of fluid, biopsy and occasionally by thoracotomy. The pleural cavity can also be inspected through a thoracoscope inserted through an intercostal space after air has been injected to open the pleural space. This was a frequent operation when artificial pneumothorax was used in the treatment of tuberculosis and is still occasionally used to investigate spontaneous pneumothorax when air suddenly leaks from the lung to the pleural space.

Operations may therefore be needed to remove air, blood, pus or serous fluid or to divide adhesions. Closed intercostal drainage, rib resection with closed (or occasionally open) drainage and sometimes thoracotomy may be used to drain the pleural cavity. Suction to the drainage bottle is usually necessary.

EXCISION OF THICKENED PLEURA, PLEURECTOMY, DECORTICATION

These terms are all used to describe the peeling off of the thickened parietal pleura from inside the chest wall, and the thickened adherent visceral pleura over the lung, with or without the removal of any contained effusion, blood or pus. The diaphragm is freed peripherally if it has become adherent to the chest wall by organizing infection, which limits its descent and reduces ventilation. The chest is then drained by apical and basal intercostal drains until the lung is fully re-expanded.

Pre-operative Physiotherapy

If the operation is not an emergency, pre-operative physiotherapy will be needed. The usual explanations will be given and records started. Chest expansion measurement and peak-flow readings are of special significance. Emphasis should be placed on diaphragmatic breathing and lateral costal breathing for the affected side.

Posture must be corrected, and mobility of the joints of the thorax, neck and shoulders increased.

Post-operative Physiotherapy

First day. After the position of the patient and the drainage tubes have been checked, diaphragmatic breathing and localized breathing must be practised by the patient several times a day. Long periods lying on the sound side over pillows while moving the affected area of lung will be needed to expand this and open up the rib spaces.

The physiotherapist must make sure that the patient can cough efficiently whilst supporting the painful area. Retained secretions in the lobe of the affected lung is a possible complication, so postural drainage is probably necessary.

Foot and leg movements are needed to try to prevent thrombosis. Arm movements, especially of the affected side, should be started as the patient may be reluctant to stretch the site of operation. Posture needs checking whenever the patient is sitting up. The patient should be taught to move himself about the bed and into the different positions as this is much better for his physical condition and morale and is probably less painful. A rope tied to the foot of the bed will help him.

Second day. The patient will continue the same exercises but may sit over the side of the bed for some of them and may sit out in a chair for a short period. Postural drainage and breathing exercises lying on the sound side will be repeated also.

Gentle trunk movements can be added and postural training emphasized. Movement of the shoulder on the affected side is usually soon back to normal but graduated arm exercises will help expand the chest and increase exercise tolerance.

Third day. The patient can now walk a short distance carrying his drainage bottle if necessary. All other exercises and procedures can be continued and increased in duration and strength.

After the third day. Postural drainage will be continued as long as excessive secretions are present.

The length of time the drainage tubes are left in the chest will vary considerably, but quite vigorous exercises can and should be performed even while they are present as long as the physiotherapist continually checks that no jerking or strain on the tubes occurs and that drainage remains free.

When the tubes are removed, the patient can dress and increase the length of his walks. More strenuous exercises can be undertaken in the gymnasium.

Postural exercises and periods of lying on his sound side for localized breathing will continue throughout his stay in hospital. He must continue these exercises for some weeks as an out-patient with the physiotherapist and alone at home. The patient should also sleep at night on his sound side until full function and correct shape are restored.

LOBECTOMY AND SEGMENTECTOMY

Removal of a lobe or segment of a lung is commonly undertaken for localized bronchiectasis, tuberculosis, in less prosperous countries, and other persistent chronic infections. Less common conditions so treated are benign tumours, fungus infections, congenital and emphysematous cysts and hydatid cysts. Lobectomy may be performed for cancer but a more extensive operation is often needed.

Up to a total of half of both lungs may be resected but it must first be established that the patient has sufficient healthy lung to survive the immediate post-operative respiratory difficulties and to leave him without respiratory distress thereafter. Bronchitis, emphysema and pulmonary fibrosis may all contra-indicate resection in an otherwise operable case. Pulmonary function studies and experienced clinical judgement are needed to make a decision in difficult cases. A final decision may have to be deferred until bronchitis has been treated and the physiotherapist has taught the patient to use to the maximum his ventilatory power, a process which may take up to several weeks.

The place of resected lung tissue is taken by expansion of the remaining parts of the lung, mediastinal shift to the operated side and by the raising of the diaphragm thus reducing the size of the hemi-thorax.

Thoracic Surgery II

Pre-operative Physiotherapy

This will follow the usual lines for all patients undergoing thoracic surgery. For patients with bronchiectasis who are young and otherwise reasonably fit, the regime must include regular postural drainage of the affected lobes and the rest of the lungs several times a day. Carefully taught localized breathing and vigorous general exercises should be given to improve pulmonary efficiency, mobility of joints, posture and general condition. Older patients and those suffering from other conditions may need a slightly less vigorous routine; intensive teaching of localized breathing will be the most important factor. Some postural drainage will probably be necessary.

Post-operative Physiotherapy

First day. Breathing exercises and coughing while supporting the affected side should be started as soon as the patient is sufficiently conscious after the operation. Movement of the ribs over the area of the resected area of lung must be started straight away so as to encourage the remaining parts of the lung to expand and fill this space. After a few hours, postural drainage two or three times a day will be added and foot, leg and arm movements started. The posture of the patient when sitting up must be corrected and the patient encouraged to move around the bed by himself with care not to pull on the drainage tubes.

Second day. Exercises are continued, but increased and the patient may sit over the side of the bed. Trunk movements are added.

Third day. The patient should be out of bed and walking around the ward. If the tubes have been removed, he can dress himself, if not, he can carry bottle and drainage tubes with him.

Fourth day onwards. Unless drainage tubes are still necessary, the patient will now be fully dressed and may attend the gymnasium for more vigorous exercises.

The further progression of exercises will depend on the age and condition of the patient but young people after operations for bronchiectasis should be able to do a full scheme of class exercises by the fifth day. Postural drainage will continue as long as excessive secretions are present.

Continued care to maintain good posture and to increase the ventilation of the lungs will continue for at least six weeks after operation though the patient may be at home after ten days and should attend as an out-patient.

PNEUMONECTOMY AND PLEURO-PNEUMONECTOMY

Removal of a whole lung with or without removal of the pleura is most often undertaken for carcinoma of the bronchus but may be performed for benign tumours or for any condition which destroys the function of one lung whilst the other remains healthy enough to support life.

The operation may be very extensive and include dissection of the mediastinal glands, the phrenic nerve and left recurrent laryngeal nerve. If these nerves are cut, half the diaphragm will be paralysed and there will be inability to approximate the vocal cords, so the ability to cough is seriously impaired. Areas of the chest wall, the pericardium and atrial wall of the heart may also have to be excised.

When a lung has been removed, the chest wall falls in and the space is further greatly reduced by the mediastinal shift and raising of the hemi-diaphragm which occurs. The remaining space becomes filled with blood-clot which slowly organizes and contracts leading to further mediastinal displacement and tracheal shift to the operated side.

Pre-operative Physiotherapy

This will follow the usual lines before any chest operation. Breathing exercises with the sound lung are of great importance. Bronchitis is often present and postural drainage may be necessary to remove secretions from the diseased or the sound lung. These patients are often not very fit but exercise tolerance and general condition can be greatly improved with more efficient ventilation and a decrease in sputum.

Post-operative Management

There are different opinions about the early post-operative care of these patients. Some surgeons prefer their patients to remain in the half-lying position for forty-eight hours, so that fluid in the chest is less likely to wash over the stump of the bronchus. Others do not consider this an important factor and allow the patients to change position frequently from half-lying into side-lying on the operated side, and lying on the back; and possibly on the sound side as well.

Drainage tubes are not usually used after this type of operation, as the space must be allowed to fill with blood-clot. If, however, a tube is not inserted, pleural pressure in the pneumonectomy space will need to be regulated by means of aspiration in order to balance the mediastinum.

COMPLICATIONS

Bronchopulmonary Fistula

Serious leakage following breakdown of the stump is a major complication which may occur 7-14 days after the operation. The patient will become distressed and dyspnoeic and will cough up dark fluid. He must immediately be turned on to the operated side. Further surgery will be needed.

Cardiac Complications

Cardiac arrhythmia (atrial fibrillation) and heart failure may occur.

Lung Complications

Bronchitis is common and the patient may have great difficulty in clearing secretions. Atelectasis may follow and lead to anoxia and carbon dioxide retention. The patient may need intermittent oxygen for the first forty-eight hours or more after operation.

To overcome these complications when it is beyond the patient's strength and the physiotherapist's skill to do so, bronchoscopy may be used. Occasionally tracheostomy and even the use of a positive pressure respirator may be necessary, so that the lung can be cleared and be kept clear of secretions.

Physiotherapy will continue in spite of complications but progress will be slower than usual. If the patient is nursed with a respirator, the usual routine for respirators will be followed.

First and second day (for the patient with no serious complications). Breathing exercises must be started as soon as the patient is conscious and continued for several short periods throughout the day, whatever the position of the patient. He may need intermittent oxygen. Coughing may or may not be allowed. Postural drainage for the base of the lung is not usually given but is occasionally necessary.

Foot and leg movements must be given to try to prevent thrombosis, and shoulder movements for the affected side started. Posture must be corrected frequently while the patient is in the half-lying position.

Third day. As the condition of the patient improves oxygen will be needed less or not at all. The patient may sit over the side of the bed for some of the exercises. Gentle trunk movements can be added. Breathing and coughing exercises must be continued several times a day.

Fourth day. The patient will be allowed to sit out of bed and exercises can be increased.

Fifth day. In addition he can now walk a short distance and can dress himself.

Sixth day onwards. Exercise will gradually be increased, including walking longer distances and eventually, up and down slopes and stairs. Breathing exercises and postural training must be continued as long as the patient is in hospital. Some surgeons like the patient to practise movements of the ribs on the operated side of the chest after a week, so as to maintain to some extent the contour of the chest which assists in good posture.

SURGERY FOR MEDIASTINAL MASSES

Mediastinal masses may partially or completely block the bronchi, the oesophagus or the superior vena cava and its tributaries. Obstruction of or pressures on these structures may endanger life or cause pain.

The following conditions may be responsible:

(*a*) tumours and other obstructions of the oesophagus;

(*b*) mediastinal lymph node involvement from carcinoma of the bronchi, or (less commonly) stomach or breast;

(*c*) primary lymph node tumours of which Hodgkin's disease and lympho-sarcoma are the commonest;

(*d*) swelling of lymph nodes due to tuberculosis (especially primary) or sarcoidosis;

(*e*) tumours of the thymus with or without myasthenia gravis;

(*f*) intrathoracic goitres;

(*g*) neurogenic tumours, especially neuro-fibroma;

(*h*) bronchogenic and enterogenous cysts arising from maldevelopment of bronchi or oesophagus; and

(*i*) dermoid or teratoid cysts due to embryonic maldevelopment.

Surgery is nearly always needed for these conditions. To diagnose them various procedures will be necessary—X-rays, tomograms, barium swallow, bronchoscopy and oesophagoscopy.

SCALENE NODE BIOPSY

Exact pathology of common lymph node enlargements may be revealed by excising a gland above the clavicle. These glands drain the mediastinal lymph and therefore their pathology may reveal the disease within this area in cases of carcinoma, tuberculosis, sarcoidosis, lymphomas and reticuloses.

GENERAL TREATMENT

The conditions involving the oesophagus, great vessels and diaphragm are dealt with in another chapter.

Mediastinal lymph-gland involvement by carcinoma of the bronchus renders the condition inoperable and treatment is by radiotherapy which is also used for primary lymph node tumours in combination with chemotherapy. Tuberculosis and sarcoidosis of the glands are also usually treated medically.

Intrathoracic goitres are usually continuations of the lower poles of the thyroid gland and can be excised from the neck, but occasionally the tumour extends too far down for this and thoracotomy is necessary.

Neurogenic tumours (usually benign) arise along the sympathetic chain lying outside the pleura, and can be removed by resecting a rib over the affected area.

Other forms of cysts and tumours may call for removal because of pressure symptoms or to ascertain their exact nature.

Pre- and Post-operative Physiotherapy

This will be along the general lines for any lateral thoracotomy, though sometimes a midline vertical incision with sternal splitting is used.

MYASTHENIA GRAVIS AND THE THYMUS GLAND

Myasthenia gravis is a disorder in which there is a defect of the transmission of the nerve impulses across the myoneural junction by the chemical transmitter acetyl-choline. There is rapid fatigue of striated muscle without wasting. In the early stages, spontaneous recovery after rest, and spontaneous remissions occur.

Life may be endangered later by weakness of respiration and swallowing followed by inhalation of pharyngeal secretions or foreign matter. Weakness of coughing and inadequate ventilation cause further trouble. Most myasthenics respond to neostigmine or related preparations given by mouth or injection, as these drugs maintain the effective action of acetyl-choline.

Unfortunately, a few patients do not respond adequately and may need a tracheostomy with a cuffed tube and a positive pressure respirator with the usual routine for patients so treated.

For reasons not fully understood myasthenia gravis may occur in the presence of tumours (benign or malignant) of the thymus gland. If these are removed, improvement of symptoms may occur. Sometimes removal of a normal thymus may also help. Radiotherapy may be used before or after removal of a malignant tumour of the thymus. Thymectomy is performed through a vertical incision splitting the sternum.

Pre-operative Physiotherapy

If the operation is not performed as an emergency, pre-operative physiotherapy will take the form of explanations and the teaching of localized breathing. Since the patient will almost certainly suffer from increased myasthenic weakness and respiratory failure after operation, the probability of tracheostomy and a period during which he will be nursed with a respirator should also be discussed.

Post-operative Treatment

The usual routine for patients attached to respirators will be followed. Active movements of legs and arms can be done by the patient from the beginning and he should be encouraged to move as much as he is able. Exercises will not, of course, strengthen the muscles but mobility and circulation are maintained.

General and breathing exercises will be increased as the patient improves. When he is free of the respirator for some of the time, he will be encouraged to walk about the ward and care for himself as far as possible.

A myasthenic crisis with gross weakness of all muscles including those of breathing and swallowing may continue for weeks or months before the patient is entirely free of the respirator, stabilized with doses of neostigmine and able to lead a normal life. Retrogressions are common and very depressing for the patient and disappointing for the staff. However, eventually stabilization occurs though an occasional patient may have crises periodically for his whole life. Patients who have had malignant growths may suffer from metastases causing further complications.

Chapter X

OPERATIONS ON THE PERICARDIUM AND HEART

by S. A. Hyde, M.C.S.P.

Ten years ago cardiac surgery was a subject to be approached with some awe and certainly open heart surgery still evoked considerable respect and a sense of the dramatic. In the past decade there have been many advances in this field and in consequence the physiotherapy for this group of patients has changed to meet the demand. It is important to remember that the physiotherapist is part of a team which comprises physicians, surgeons, anaesthetists, nurses, technicians and radiographers, all of whom are interdependent and all share a common goal.

The object of this text is to provide a guide for the treatment of these patients but it must be stressed that each individual patient will be treated as his or her condition demands.

The heart is operated on by either a closed or open procedure. Closed operations do not interfere with the circulation to the heart and the defect is corrected through an incision in the heart which is only large enough to allow the passage of a finger or instrument so that the surgeon does not have a direct view of the lesion. An 'open heart' operation is, as the name implies, one in which the surgeon has a clear view of the interior of the heart and this is made possible by an incision in the wall of the heart. It is immediately apparent that in order to perform such surgery the heart must be excluded from the circulation and yet the myocardium and all body tissues must be maintained in a viable condition. Induced hypothermia and/or extra-corporeal circulation with a heart-lung machine accomplish this, the method of choice being predetermined by the anticipated length of time needed for surgery.

Prior to surgery many investigations are undertaken and, whilst it is

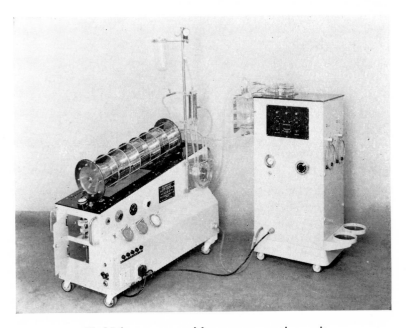

V. Melrose pump with coronary suction unit
(*see* chapter X)

obviously unnecessary for the physiotherapist to concern herself with the details of these, it is advisable to be familiar with the most common ones. These will be:

1. X-rays.
2. Cardiac Catheterization: a tube is passed into the heart chambers so that pressure gradients across the valves can be recorded and blood samples taken to determine oxygen saturation in different parts of the heart.
3. Angiocardiography: injection of a contrast medium to show the path taken by blood through various chambers of the heart.
4. Electrocardiography.
5. Blood tests: for haemoglobin and electrolytes.

Some of the investigations occur whilst the patient is an out-patient but it is usual for him to be admitted several days before surgery and during this time he will receive pre-operative physiotherapy.

EXTRA-CORPOREAL CIRCULATION

This is a method of excluding the heart from the circulation by a cardio-pulmonary bypass. The functions of the heart and lungs must now be undertaken by artificial means; this is done by a heart-lung machine. The blood is withdrawn from the patient via cannulae from the superior and inferior vena cavae, oxygenated by the machine and then pumped back into the femoral artery, although sometimes it may be pumped into the aorta itself. If the aorta is opened to expose the aortic valve, the aorta is clamped distal to the incision and the coronary arteries are then perfused separately. The blood is treated with heparin to prevent clotting.

There are three methods of effecting gaseous interchange in the machine.

1. Filming of blood by spreading it in thin films over a large area and exposing it to gases by means of:
   (a) Rotating discs
   (b) Vertical stationary screens
2. Bubbling of oxygen through blood.
3. Semi-permeable membrane: A membrane which is permeable to gases but not fluids is interposed between a thin layer of blood and gas. This method is still under development.

The temperature of the blood is carefully controlled by a heat exchanger; this is of great importance since the oxygen requirement of the tissues varies with their temperature. When the heart is cold it is possible to temporarily interrupt the coronary circulation without causing irreversible damage.

Operations on the Pericardium and Heart

PROFOUND HYPOTHERMIA

Blood is circulated through a heat exchanger whilst two pumps replace the two ventricles of the heart and so maintain the systemic and pulmonary circulations. When the body has cooled to 12°C to 15°C, the pumps are turned off and surgery performed on the arrested heart. At this temperature the tissues remain viable for up to one hour. The pumps are then re-started and the body is rewarmed to 37°C; the heart is restarted and the pumping circuit removed.

PHYSIOTHERAPY FOR CARDIAC SURGERY PATIENTS

It has been established for many years now that physiotherapeutic measures are of benefit to these patients both in the pre- and post-operative phases. The rationale of such treatment is based upon an understanding of the condition, the methods used to correct the deficiency or abnormality but most of all on the appreciation of the physiological changes that occur.

The main purposes of respiration are oxygenation and elimination of carbon dioxide from the body. The body needs energy to sustain life and the energy is obtained from the combustion of carbohydrate for which oxygen is absolutely essential. All the functions in the body can be performed only when the internal environment of the body is kept stable at a given level. Body temperature and acidity are two of the most important criteria. Acidity is controlled by the kidneys and respiration: the normal is pH 7.4. Carbon dioxide is one of the decisive factors in determining the value of pH of the body and for these reasons adequate respiration is important for the maintenance of life.

The respiratory mechanism is very complex but an understanding of its anatomy and physiology is essential for the intelligent use of physiotherapy in the pre- and post-operative care of a patient who has undergone cardiac surgery. It is not within the scope of this text to detail these mechanisms but it is perhaps worthwhile to consider some aspects.

Pulmonary Ventilation

There are three essential factors to maintain the physiological process of gaseous exchange in the lungs:

1. The total pulmonary ventilation and the proportion of this reaching the alveoli.
2. The matching of ventilation and blood-flow in the alveoli.
3. The presence of right to left intrapulmonary shunts.

It is important to remember that since gaseous interchange only takes place at the alveoli, it is the alveolar ventilation that is most important in respiration. This is always less than the total volume of air entering the upper respiratory tract, because part of the inspired air ventilates the trachea and bronchi and therefore takes no part in gas exchange. Furthermore part of the air going to the alveoli ventilates alveoli which have little or no blood supply. In lung disease this 'dead space' increases so that a smaller proportion of each breath reaches the alveoli which are supplied with blood and so takes part in gas exchange. Hence ventilation in lung disease is very inefficient.

When lung disease is present, some alveoli receive very little ventilation and the blood passing through them is not properly oxygenated. Furthermore some blood may pass through collapsed alveoli which receive no air. This blood remains desaturated and so constitutes a right to left shunt. Both these sources of desaturated blood cause arterial hypoxaemia, but the former can be eliminated by breathing an oxygen-enriched atmosphere. This therefore improves the oxygen saturation of the arterial blood.

Chemical Control of Respiration

The chemical composition of the blood influences the rate and/or depth of respiration in two principal ways:

(a) Direct action on the respiratory centre.
(b) Influence on the chemoreceptors in the carotid and aortic bodies.

Therefore any change in carbon dioxide tension (pCO_2), oxygen tension (pO_2) or pH in the blood is critical.

The respiratory centre is stimulated by pCO_2 above 40mm. Hg at which level the patient starts to become comatose. The respiratory centre can be damaged by a reduction in the blood supply which may result from hypotension, cardiac arrest, or poor perfusion during bypass and this will impair or arrest respiration. Severe lack of oxygen will have the same effect.

Respiratory depressant drugs temporarily reduce the sensitivity of the respiratory centre to pCO_2 so that higher levels are required to drive it. Gross overdosage will cause apnoea.

Respiratory failure or malfunction in the post-operative period occurs as a result of some of the above. Depression of respiration and cough reflex may cause small areas of atelectasis and allow retention of secretions, this will in turn cause an increased arterial desaturation. Atelectasis decreases lung compliance and the presence of secretions in the airways increases resistance and therefore the work of respiration. The failure to cough may also be as a result of inhibition because of pain, or fatigue. The anaesthetic may also have depressed the ciliary activity, or the secretions may have become so viscid as to prevent the wave-like motion of the cilia, which normally assists removal of secretions.

In patients who undergo cardiac surgery there are additional factors predisposing to post-operative respiratory problems. Patients may suffer right or left heart failure or both. Right heart failure will cause oedema of the limbs, a high venous pressure, large liver and pleural effusions. Left heart failure will cause pulmonary oedema. The latter is often less obvious and may only be diagnosed from X-ray and the lowering of the arterial pO_2 which it causes. The patient undergoing surgery often has a much enlarged heart which tends to compress the lung and left main bronchus.

The final and most specific cause of respiratory failure is the post-perfusion lung syndrome in which there is a haemorrhagic exudate on the alveoli. It appears to result from damage to the blood as it passes through the oxygenator.

In summary the causes of respiratory failure post-operatively are:

1. Depression of the respiratory centre—anoxia, drugs, carbon dioxide retention.
2. Neuromuscular block caused by prolonged action of muscle relaxants.
3. Muscle weakness and pain.
4. Increased resistance to inflation caused by:
   (i) Pneumothorax, Haemothorax.
   (ii) Lungs—atelectasis, pulmonary oedema, post-perfusion lung syndrome pneumonitis and pneumonia.
   (iii) Airways—bronchospasm, pulmonary oedema.

In consideration of the physiological process involved therefore, the aims of physiotherapy will be:

1. To maintain or gain full expansion of all parts of the lungs.
2. To prevent retention of secretions.
3. To maintain good systemic circulation to prevent venous complications.
4. To correct postural faults.
5. To maintain full range of motion of joints.

PRE-OPERATIVE PHYSIOTHERAPY

Once the patient has been admitted for surgery the physiotherapist begins the pre-operative regime. This will include evaluation of the patient's normal breathing with particular reference to lower costal and diaphragmatic breathing. It is also important to gain the patient's confidence and co-operation. Over the next few days the patient is instructed in unilateral and bilateral breathing of all parts of the chest. The patient will be taught to practise these exercises in half-lying and alternate side lying because these will be the positions in which he may be treated post-operatively. When positioning the patient it is important to watch for signs of distress in breathing and an adequate number of pillows provided to support the patient. In fact many patients are unable to lie down because of heart failure and indeed in patients with mitral valve disease lying flat may precipitate left heart failure.

In order to expectorate secretions that may have collected in the lungs the patient is taught to cough. The necessity for a deep basal cough is stressed as it is obvious that following surgery the act of coughing may be inhibited by pain. Short, sharp expiratory breathing 'huffing out' is often used to re-educate a cough, and the patient should be instructed to hold or support the incision site.

In some cases it will be necessary to institute relatively vigorous physiotherapy at this stage to clear the lungs of secretions that may already have collected.

Since it is known that in the post-operative phase it is important to prevent venous complications, the patient is shown the leg and arm movements that it will be necessary for him to perform to maintain circulation.

During the pre-operative phase the physiotherapist will examine the patient's posture and emphasize certain aspects of correct posture according to the anticipated incision site in order to prevent post-operative deformity. Children and young adults often find it more difficult to regain their postural sense than older people.

An accurate record of all these findings, i.e. chest expansion, vital capacity, range of motion of shoulder joints and cervical spine, posture together with the patient's exercise tolerance to walking on flat ground, negotiating stairs should be noted in order that it may be used for post-operative comparison.

It is essential that the physiotherapist establishes a good rapport with the patient during this pre-operative period and with the surgeon's knowledge and approval, it is helpful to explain some post-operative details. The patient should know that he will awake in the Intensive Care Unit, that there will be drains and drips in situ and that he will have a Ryle's tube.

Many of the open heart surgery cases, particularly the valve replacements, tetralogy of Fallot, and ventricular septal defect will be nursed initially on a ventilator and if the patient's pre-operative condition makes this a probability then the patient is told that he may have an endotracheal tube and possibly a machine attached to this to assist his breathing.

Warning is given that speaking will not be possible temporarily but that his requirements will be understood by the staff.

The pre-operative approach will obviously have to be adapted according to the mental age of the patient. Various activities are used to teach young children and whilst expiratory breathing by blowing cotton-wool balls is of use, it is also important to teach the child to take a deep inspiration.

There will be a daily ward class which the patient will take part in during both the pre- and post-operative phase. It normally takes between twenty and thirty minutes and the patient is allowed to rest between exercises if necessary. It is rare for a cardiac patient to be unable to join in at least part of the class.

Guide to Typical Ward Class of Cardiac Patients

A typical scheme of exercises would be:

(*a*) Bilateral lower costal breathing.

(*b*) Shoulder shrugging.

(*c*) Head and neck rotation, flexion and extension.

(*d*) Foot and ankle exercises.

(*e*) Diaphragmatic breathing.

(*f*) Arms bend, elbow circling.

(*g*) Alternate hip and knee flexion and extension for bed patients, and an adaptation of this for patients sitting on stools.

(*h*) Unilateral right lower costal breathing.

(*i*) Neck rest, elbow pressing back with shoulder girdle retraction.

(*j*) Quadriceps contractions for bed patients, or alternate knee extension and flexion for up patients.

(*k*) Unilateral left lower costal breathing.

(*l*) Relaxed forward sitting and correction of posture on active extension.

(*m*) Alternate trunk rotation with relaxed arms swinging.

(*n*) Alternate trunk side flexion localized to the thoracic spine using hands as fulcrum with breathing.

(*o*) With straight arms, hands clapping, alternately on stool (or bed) and overhead, starting with one clap on stool and one overhead, progressing to two and upwards to five, then down to one again.

(*p*) Bilateral lower costal breathing.

POST-OPERATIVE OBSERVATIONS

The physiotherapist should make a note of the following because they will influence the treatment that is given.

Operations on the Pericardium and Heart

Incisions

1. *Anterior Thoracotomy*
   (a) Median sternotomy. This is a mid-line vertical incision extending from the suprasternal notch to mid-way between xiphoid and umbilicus.
   (b) Transverse sternotomy.
2. *Anterolateral Thoracotomy*
   Through fifth rib interspace.
3. *Posterolateral Thoracotomy*

Drains

When the chest has been opened it is necessary to put in drainage tubes from the pleura, mediastinum and pericardium. These tubes leave the chest via small stab wounds and are connected to underwater seal drainage with Roberts suction pumps; the number of drainage tubes will vary. The tubes will be removed as soon as leakage has stopped but meanwhile the volume of liquid passed will be carefully measured so that the fluid output can be counterbalanced with input.

Fluid Balance

This refers to the patient's total input and output of fluid and will be frequently recorded by the nursing staff. It is an attempt to equate output from kidneys and chest drainage with input from drips, Ryle's tube and oral fluids.

Electrocardiograph

The patient will always be connected to an oscilloscope by E.C.G. wires and, although it is not necessary for the physiotherapist to concern herself with the details, it is wise to be familiar with the more important wave patterns and in particular the resting pattern for the individual patient in order that any major change may be observed.

Blood Gases

Normal value for pO_2 100 mm. Hg
pCO_2 40 mm. Hg

The arterial pCO_2 is the most important of all acting directly on the respiratory centre and the slightest change in pCO_2 brings an almost immediate response. pCO_2 indicates the balance between carbon dioxide and alveolar ventilation, so that hypo-ventilation results in an increased pCO_2 whilst hyper-ventilation causes a decreased pCO_2.

157

Hypoxaemia, that is a low pO_2, excites the chemo-receptors and whilst a pO_2 of 60 mm. Hg is tolerable for normal patients a pO_2 60 mm. Hg may harm cardiac patients causing arrhythmias and impaired cardiac function, and a pO_2 of 25 mm. Hg would be lethal.

The normal pH of blood is 7.4 and indicates a balance between the respiratory component of acid-base balance, the pCO_2 and the non-respiratory component, the bicarbonate or base excess. Thus for example an increased pCO_2 will cause a low pH. If one component changes the other component will change to bring the pH back to normal.

POST-OPERATIVE PHYSIOTHERAPY

Consideration of the post-operative physiotherapy must fall into two main categories:

A. Those patients not on a Ventilator

These patients will be returned to the Intensive Care Unit and in all cases will be receiving continuous oxygen by mask. Within the first two or three hours the physiotherapist should see the patient and institute the following routine:

(i) *Breathing exercises*

The patient will be nursed flat and should not be turned at this time. Deep generalized breathing is encouraged and by careful but firm positioning of her hands the physiotherapist encourages the patient to expand the lungs fully. The patient is able to localize touch, responding to the proprioceptive stimulus, particular emphasis is given to the bases and if there is a pleural drain it is essential to attempt expansion of that side. If possible the patient should be encouraged to cough although expectoration is unlikely at this stage.

(ii) *Leg exercises*

Active or active-assisted foot movements and alternate knee flexion, extension exercises are performed approximately ten times. Patients receiving oxygen by mask, or rarely in the case of children by oxygen tent should only have this interrupted to allow coughing and expectoration.

The nursing routine at this early stage will involve quarter- or half-hourly observations of blood pressure, pulse, drainage and drips (fluid balance). Evacuation of drainage tubes will be carried out at regular intervals. It is important for the patient's comfort that the physiotherapist co-ordinates her visits with these other activities, especially if pain-relieving drugs are being regularly administered.

Operations on the Pericardium and Heart

First to third post-operative day

It is during this time that any post-operative lung complications will manifest themselves. Before starting treatment the physiotherapist should look at the patient's charts with reference to temperature, pulse, respiration rate and blood pressure. It is also worth noting the resting wave pattern on the oscilloscope.

Breathing. General and localized breathing is performed, the physiotherapist encouraging maximum expansion of the lungs with the patient in half lying, forward sitting or alternate side lying positions. Coughing is often easier in the forward sitting position. Vibrations and chest shaking are used on expiration to help loosen secretions and aid expectoration.

Positioning of the patient for chest treatment. Positions for postural drainage of the lungs are well documented elsewhere, the patient being placed in such a position as to facilitate drainage of secretions for the various segments of the lung. However, patients who have undergone cardiac surgery are rarely able to tolerate the head down or tipped position, in fact some will not cope with the supine or side lying positions without three pillows (45°). Therefore it is necessary to compromise and where secretions have collected in the bases the patient is placed in the side lying position. The position in which the patient is treated will depend upon the condition and from the doctor's comments of the day's X-ray. Any changes in the patient's position will obviously be mediated by blood pressure observations.

Adult patients should always have two people to move them in the early post-operative stage. If patients are sitting up it is easier to lower them on to two or three pillows first, one person supporting while the other arranges the pillows, prior to turning. There should be minimum discomfort for the patient if both assistants lift him slightly to one side of the bed, moving first the head and shoulders. At the same time the under arm is eased forward for comfort.

There may be several drainage tubes to take care of and these must not be allowed to pull on the chest. Rotation of the trunk should be avoided as the patient is turned, because this places strain on the operation wound and drains causing pain. Pillows are so placed as to relieve the strain.

The patient is encouraged to breathe deeply while gentle chest vibrations are given on expiration. The physiotherapist places one hand on the anterior and one on the posterior aspects of the side of the chest being treated, working on all parts of the lung, starting with the bases. Care must be taken to avoid the incision site and drains, but she should move her hands to support the incision during coughing. It is often necessary to lay patients on their pleural drains, so the pillows are adjusted to prevent them from pressing into the chest wall. The patient may remain in the side lying position for at least ten to fifteen minutes. Depending upon the actual operation and upon the patient's condition, he may then be turned so that both sides are treated at one session. If secretions are particularly tenacious it may be necessary to use gentle percussion. When percussion is used on these patients we prefer to use a method in which the patient is percussed with one hand through the other.

The patient is normally treated three or four times during the day. When the morning's X-rays and blood gas results have been evaluated, it may be decided that the patient needs more frequent treatment directed to the specific areas of the lung that have shown diminished air entry or consolidation.

Leg exercises. As explained pre-operatively.

Arm exercises. Gentle shoulder movements are given and should receive particular attention in patients who have undergone lateral thoracotomy.

Third to fifth day

Many of the patients will return to their own wards during this time and treatment will continue as previously described two or three times a day. Most of the patients will start joining in the daily ward class at this stage.

Fifth day onwards

The patient will continue to be treated in half lying, forward sitting and alternate side lying positions, depending upon how good the expansion of the lung is and how much sputum he is expectorating.

Depending upon the operation and the individual surgeon's wishes patients will sit out of bed in a chair any time after the third day (for details see under individual conditions). When patients have sat out of bed for an hour in the day, they may progress to sitting on stools to join the ward class. Stair climbing is commenced a few days before he is discharged, beginning the first day with three to six steps and progressing over the next three or four days to a flight. Patients seldom have any discomfort from this but some tend to be apprehensive before attempting it.

Possible complications

1. Respiratory complications.
2. Pleural effusion.
3. Pericardial bleeding or effusion leading to tamponade.
4. Post-operative haemorrhage.
5. Pulmonary, cardiac or cerebral emboli.
6. Arterial or venous thrombosis.

7. Kidney complications.
8. Cerebral damage.
9. Heart block.
10. Cardiac arrest.

B. Patients on a Ventilator

It is increasingly common for patients to be returned to the Intensive Care Unit on a ventilator attached by means of an endotracheal tube and they may remain on this for the first 12 hours whilst they stabilize. However, a patient who has not needed a ventilator at this early stage may later require mechanical assistance to ventilation as a result of complications.

Indications for Mechanical Ventilation are:

1. If ventilation is inadequate due to abnormal reaction to drugs or cerebral damage.
2. Because they have developed signs of incipient pulmonary oedema (low pO_2) during operation.
3. Because they have had serious pre-operative impairment of cardio-respiratory function (pulmonary oedema, or pulmonary hypertension) or previous chronic lung disease.
4. Because of cardiovascular instability when it is especially important to ensure ventilation is adequate.
5. Because they may need re-opening for bleeding.

If renal function becomes impaired and peritoneal dialysis is required it may be necessary to ventilate the patient because the fluid injected in to the peritoneum pushes up the diaphragm and throws an extra load on an already impaired respiratory system.

In general, patients requiring mechanical assistance to ventilation for twelve hours to three days are attached to the ventilator by means of an endotracheal tube. If ventilation is required for longer periods it is necessary to perform a tracheostomy.

It is important for the physiotherapist to know the reason for the use of the ventilator as it should not be assumed that such patients are necessarily 'chesty' and therefore presenting a problem that necessitates increased frequency of treatment. Indeed in patients with a low cardiac output and low blood pressure vigorous chest physiotherapy may prove extremely detrimental to their condition.

Physiotherapy for patients on Ventilators

Patients on ventilators should only be treated upon the specific instruction of the surgeon or anaesthetist. The method of treatment will depend upon:

(*a*) the patient's general condition, i.e. blood pressure, pulse, cardiac output.

(*b*) the day's clinical examination and chest X-ray which will denote the presence of atelectasis, diminished air entry or collapse.

(*c*) blood gas results.

(*d*) the individual unit.

(i) If the general condition is poor but the chest is showing signs of presenting problems, increased secretions and poor air entry into some segments, chest shaking is given in time with the ventilator during the expiratory phase of respiration. The patient will preferably be turned to alternate side lying because the change in position will help drainage of secretions which will then be removed with tracheal suction.

(ii) If the general condition is satisfactory but the chest is full of secretions and X-ray examination demonstrates areas of collapse a technique of 'bag squeezing' may be employed. The technique is used to ensure full expansion of the lungs and produce an artificial cough. The technique is as follows:

The patient is disconnected from the ventilator by the anaesthetist who then proceeds to inflate the lungs with oxygen by means of a Water's bag and canister (the latter is not always used). The bag is released quickly to allow elastic recoil of the lungs and at this precise moment the physiotherapist applies chest shaking or vibrations, the combination of these two forces simulating a cough and moving secretions. This procedure is repeated several times until the sputum can be heard rattling in the trachea or main bronchi. The secretions are then cleared by tracheal suction via the tracheostomy or endotracheal tube. All areas of the chest are treated but if one segment is known to be collapsed it will obviously receive more attention and the patient will be turned into the appropriate position.

The physiotherapist should support the patient's chest whilst suction is carried out because if a cough reflex is present it will be stimulated by the presence of the catheter in the trachea.

Tracheal suction is performed as a strict aseptic technique, sterile catheters are passed with forceps or gloves and the same catheter is never used more than once.

The sterile catheter is attached to the sucker and then occluded at its proximal end whilst being passed into the tracheostomy. It should be inserted as far as possible. The catheter is then withdrawn with a rotatory action intermittently occluding it to prevent damaging the delicate mucous membrane of the trachea. It should be remembered that whilst the suction is being applied air is also being withdrawn from the lungs so that the whole procedure should take less than 20 seconds since the patient is not being ventilated during this period. The suction is more normally performed by a nurse. If the secretions are very thick and tenacious a sterile solution of sodium bicarbonate or sterile normal saline may be injected down the tracheostomy to help loosen them and make removal with suction possible.

Treatment may be given three or four times a day if there are copious secretions or air entry into a particular segment is diminished but the individual need of each patient must be evaluated and the physiotherapist aware of the risk of hyperventilation. The latter combined with expiratory vibration produces large falls in cardiac output and blood pressure in some patients and therefore the technique of 'bag squeezing' should only be used, in patients with known poor cardio-vascular function, when there is a definite indication and the effect on the cardio-vascular system monitored.

(iii) In patients where it is not contra-indicated 'bag squeezing' may be employed as a prophylactic measure, to ensure full expansion, in which case the procedure will be used less frequently.

When the patient's condition improves the anaesthetist will start to wean the patient from the ventilator, the rate at which this can be accomplished will vary; possibly the patient may only breathe for five minutes in the hour on his own in the early stages. However, during this phase the physiotherapist will probably increase the number of visits since it is extremely important to achieve maximum and efficient ventilation so secretions must not be allowed to accumulate in the chest; frequent blood gas evaluations will determine the success of the patient's efforts. It is important to remember that during periods off the ventilator the patient will receive continuous oxygen and humidification of the inspired gas.

As the patient regains strength he will need less assistance from the physiotherapist to clear secretions, and his response to suction will be an indication of the success in weaning him from the ventilator.

Physiotherapy for patients with Tracheostomy

These patients do not require special treatment but will be encouraged to do generalized and localized breathing exercises with chest shaking or vibrations and will be positioned as the condition of the chest denotes. Secretions will be cleared by suction as described previously.

Since the patient's own method of humidifying and warming inspired air has been by-passed, it is necessary to provide a substitute. Humidity is therefore maintained either by use of a heated water bath when gases are saturated with water vapour; or by gas-driven or ultrasonic nebulizers which provide cold air full of water droplets, which are deposited on the tracheal mucosa and also evaporate to maintain full saturation of the air as it is warmed by the trachea. This is also important to prevent crusting of secretions over and in the tube so blocking the airway. Therefore patients must not be left without humidification for any longer than necessary.

As the chest condition improves the tube is removed and an airtight dressing applied over the wound which heals in about 5 to 8 days. Coughing and expectoration are often difficult for patients during this period and the original technique must be relearnt in order to clear the secretions past the wound. The patient must be instructed to hold the wound firmly in the initial stages when he coughs and may need help from the physiotherapist to do this. During the first 48 hours following removal of the tracheostomy tube it will be necessary to increase the frequency of treatment in order to ensure that there is no accumulation of secretions.

The use of the Bird Ventilator

The Bird Ventilator (intermittent positive pressure breathing) is a type of artificial respirator whereby the patients own inspiratory effort is assisted by the ventilator. Administration of oxygen without assisting ventilation may achieve oxygenation to a certain extent in severe respiratory distress or in advanced chronic pulmonary disease but elimination of carbon dioxide and improvement in ventilation is just as important.

The Bird Ventilator is indicated before the patient goes into ventilatory failure and, it is hoped, may prevent him from requiring full assistance from a ventilator. It is also of assistance in the first days after the patient has dispensed with other types of ventilators.

The main use of the Bird is to increase tidal volume. It provides improved alveolar ventilation, and may, with the use of a nebulizer, provide the most efficient means of forcing chemical agents deep into the alveoli. The Bird, because it assists the patient's inspiratory effort, reduces the work of respiration.

The Bird is indicated where there is

(a) alveolar hypoventilation produced by central respiratory depression, atelectasis, tiredness, inhibition of respiration due to pain.

(b) severe disturbance in the ventilation perfusion ratio with hypoxia caused by: atelectasis (retention of secretions, collapse), occlusion of major bronchi.

The main disadvantages of the Bird are that there is:

(a) No airtight fit with the trachea.

(b) Difficulty in obtaining optimal adjustment of the flow rate, sensitivity and pressure.

164

SPECIFIC HEART CONDITIONS
PATENT DUCTUS ARTERIOSUS

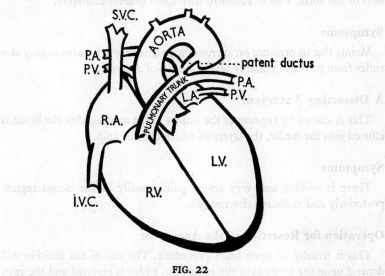

FIG. 22

This is the persistence of the embryological connection between the pulmonary artery and aorta and is usually diagnosed in childhood.

Symptoms

If this condition is present there will be breathlessness on exertion, fatigue, and retarded growth.

Operation—Ligation of Patent Ductus

Closed procedure.

Incision—Left posterolateral thoracotomy

At operation the patent ductus is either permanently tied off or divided, the results are good especially when performed early in childhood, at about 5 years of age. Complications are rare and the prognosis is good.

Pre- and Post-operative Physiotherapy

As previously described, the whole course usually requiring ten to fourteen days before discharge.

Operations on the Pericardium and Heart

AORTIC ANEURYSM

Aneurysms of the aorta are caused by trauma, or inflammation from syphilis, or atherosclerosis. They may be saccular, due to localized weakness of the aortic wall or fusiform with more general dilatation.

Symptoms

Mainly due to pressure on surrounding structures but patients may also suffer from pain and possibly severe attacks of dyspnoea.

A Dissecting Aneurysm

This is caused by rupture of the intima of the aorta so that the blood is effused into the media, the layers of which become split.

Symptoms

There is sudden and very severe pain, usually in the dorsal region, posteriorly and radiating downwards.

Operation for Resection of the Aneurysm

This is usually an open heart procedure. The site of the incision will depend upon the location of the aneurysm, which is resected and the ends are either anastomosed or joined by a Dacron graft.

Pre-operative Physiotherapy

This consists of very gentle breathing exercises only, the patient should not be allowed to join the ward class because of the danger of rupturing the aneurysm.

Post-operative Physiotherapy

These patients will often be ventilated for the first 12 to 18 hours after surgery. It is unlikely that they will need 'bag squeezing' but should receive routine prophylactic physiotherapy, as described earlier. They will normally start getting up on the fourth or fifth day and be ready for discharge to convalescence during the third week.

COARCTATION OF THE AORTA

Coarctation of the aorta is a congenital anomaly in which there is stricture or narrowing of the aorta. It is most commonly found just below or in the vicinity of the left subclavian artery, the decrease in the lumen preventing an adequate supply of blood from reaching the lower half of the body.

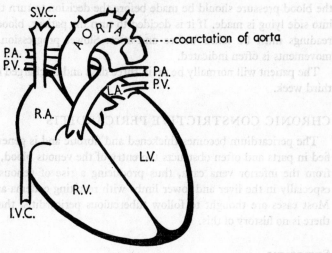

FIG. 23

Symptoms

There may be no symptoms, the condition being diagnosed in a routine examination, or the patient may complain of headache, dizziness, tinnitus, epistaxis, palpitation and insomnia. These are due to hypertension in the upper limbs and increased circulation to the upper limbs and head. The blood pressure in the legs is lower than that in the arms but this does not necessarily imply a normal or hypotensive level, and hypertensive levels may often be reached. Patients may have symptoms due to diminished circulation in the legs including cold feet and intermittent claudication. The femoral pulse is weak and may even be impalpable, however, when it is possible to palpate it will be delayed compared with the radial pulse.

Operation—Resection of the Co-arctation of the Aorta

This is a closed procedure.

Incision

The chest is opened via a left lateral thoracotomy, the co-arctation is excised and the two ends are either anastomosed or joined with a graft.

Pre- and Post-operative Physiotherapy

This will be as for a standard left thoracotomy but because there is often persistent hypertension the patient will be treated in the half lying position. Should the patient develop atelectasis of a lung a careful evaluation of the blood pressure should be made before the decision to turn the patient into side lying is made. If it is decided to turn the patient, blood pressure readings must be taken before and after. Slower progression with arm movements is often indicated.

The patient will normally be up in three days and discharged during the third week.

CHRONIC CONSTRICTIVE PERICARDITIS

The pericardium becomes thickened and fibrotic and is generally calcified in parts and often obstructs the entry of the venous blood, especially from the inferior vena cava, thus producing a rise of venous pressure, especially in the liver and lower limbs with resulting oedema and ascites. Most cases are thought to follow tuberculous pericarditis, though often there is no history of this.

Symptoms

Increasing dyspnoea followed by oedema of the legs, ascites and hepatic enlargement, and sometimes pleural effusion.

Operation—Pericardectomy

Closed procedure.

Incision—Left thoracotomy or anterior thoracotomy

As much of the thickened and calcified pericardium as is possible is resected.

Pre-operative Physiotherapy

This is particularly important because the ascites and pleural effusions will have impaired thoracic function. It may be necessary to treat the patient two or three times a day and it must be remembered that in severe cases the patient will not tolerate less than four pillows.

Post-operative Physiotherapy

This must be instituted as soon as the patient regains consciousness but it should be remembered that because the myocardium is in a state of disuse atrophy, as a result of prolonged restriction of activity, the patient must be prevented from over-exerting himself.

The patient may get up from the fifth to the eighth day and will be discharged during the third week.

PULMONARY STENOSIS

Pulmonary stenosis is a congenital abnormality in which there is an obstruction to the flow of blood from the right ventricle to the lungs. The obstruction may be in the valve (valvar stenosis) where the cusps are joined together forming a membranous cone with a circular perforation; or infundibular stenosis, where the outflow tract of the right ventricle may be narrowed by muscular and fibrous overgrowth.

Symptoms

Physical development is usually normal and there may be no symptoms but if present they will be fatigue and breathlessness on exertion. The right ventricle will hypertrophy first, and this will lead to hypertrophy of the right atrium.

Operation—Pulmonary Valvotomy

This is now almost always performed under total cardio-pulmonary bypass.

Incision

Median sternotomy.

Post-operative Physiotherapy

The patient will probably be allowed up on the third to fifth day and will be discharged during the third week.

ATRIAL SEPTAL DEFECTS

There are two types of defect of the atrial septum occurring at different stages in the embryological development:

1. *Persistent Ostium Primum* type occurs because of failure of the septum primum, which grows from the dorsal wall of the atrium, to fuse with the endocardial bar. This type is often associated with other abnormalities such as mitral incompetence or ventricular septal defect and presents greater problems than the ostium secundum type.

2. *Ostium Secundum* type is usually a solitary defect occurring as a result of arrested growth of the septum secundum. This type is easier to deal with surgically.

Symptoms

There may be no symptoms or the patient may complain of fatigue and breathlessness on exertion. Patients have poor physical development and the condition is often associated with skeletal deformities such as arachnodactyly or Marfan's syndrome. Blood is shunted from the left to the right atrium through the defect, resulting in enlargement of the right atrium and right ventricle, and an increased blood flow to the lungs causing dilatation of the pulmonary arteries.

Operation

The repair of the atrial septal defect. This is an open procedure.

(a) *Ostium primum type of atrial septal defect*

Incision—Median sternotomy

The operation is performed under a bypass. The heart is entered via the right atrium and the defect repaired by direct suture or with a Teflon patch, associated defects may be repaired at the same time.

(b) *Ostium secundum type*

Incision

Right anterolateral thoracotomy or median sternotomy.

Operation

The repair is as described above but may not necessitate bypass in which case hypothermia will be used.

Pre-operative Physiotherapy

As routine.

Post-operative Physiotherapy

More frequently the post-operative course is uncomplicated and the physiotherapy will be routine. However, where closure of the atrial septal defect causes such significant changes in the pressure gradients as to cause embarrassment to the pulmonary circulation, pulmonary oedema may result and ventilation may be required.

If the course is uncomplicated the patient will be up on the third or fourth post-operative day and discharged at approximately the fourteenth day.

VENTRICULAR SEPTAL DEFECT

The interventricular septum consists of a muscular and membranous part. The commoner form of ventricular septal defect is due to non- or maldevelopment of the membranous septum. Less commonly defects are situated in the lower muscular septum. Ventricular septal defects are often associated with other defects, most commonly pulmonary stenosis.

Symptoms

Occasionally there are no symptoms, but usually the infant will not thrive and frequently suffers recurrent respiratory infections. In adulthood there is a risk of developing severe pulmonary vascular disease.

Operation

The repair of ventricular septal defect. This is an open procedure.

Incision—Median sternotomy

The operation is performed under cardiopulmonary bypass, the defect is approached via the right ventricle and repaired either by direct suturing or Teflon patch.

Pre-operative Physiotherapy

As routine.

Post-operative Physiotherapy

Often ventilated initially and will be treated accordingly. The patient may get up on the third to fifth day and probably be discharged during the third week.

TETRALOGY OF FALLOT

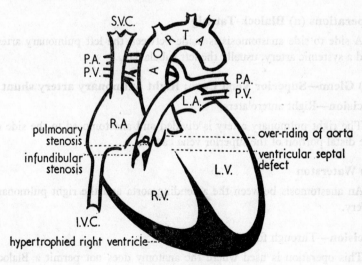

FIG. 24

171

This is the commonest form of congenital heart disease associated with cyanosis. The anomaly consists of

1. Pulmonary stenosis.
2. Ventricular septal defect.
3. Dextro-position and consequent over-riding of the aorta.
4. Right ventricular hypertrophy.

Symptoms

The child is usually undersized and cyanotic. The cyanosis becomes more apparent with effort and is accompanied by dyspnoea and a spontaneous desire to squat. The cyanosis is caused by the admixture of unsaturated and saturated blood in the systemic circulation which occurs as a result of part of the right ventricular output being shunted into the left ventricle and aorta through the ventricular septal defect. The cyanosis is further aggravated because as a result of the shunt part of the unsaturated blood from the right ventricle by-passes the lungs and remains unoxygenated. There is associated clubbing of fingers and toes.

Surgical intervention in the problem of Fallot's Tetralogy should be considered as either an initially palliative procedure to alleviate the condition or as a one stage total correction of the abnormality.

The following four procedures are palliative and would more normally be undertaken in infancy.

Operations (a) Blalock-Taussig

A side to side anastomosis is made between the left pulmonary artery and a systemic artery, usually the left subclavian.

(b) Glenn—Superior Vena Cava: Right pulmonary artery shunt

Incision—Right anterolateral

The right pulmonary artery is divided and anastomosed to the side of the distal portion of the superior vena cava.

(c) Waterston

An anastomosis between the ascending aorta and the right pulmonary artery.

Incision—Through fourth rib interspace

This operation is used where the anatomy does not permit a Blalock to be performed and because the shunt is more readily corrected at the time of total correction.

(d) Pott's

A side to side anastomosis between the aorta and the left pulmonary artery. This operation is not often performed now because of the difficulty of closing the shunt if total correction is undertaken later.

Closed Pulmonary Valvotomy and Infundibular Resection—Brock's Procedure

Incision—Posterolateral thoracotomy

The pulmonary valve is incised and dilated and the infundibular muscle resected. The operation may be regarded as final or it may be the first stage towards complete correction.

Post-operative Physiotherapy for Babies and Infants

The prophylactic treatment of babies and infants in the post-operative phase is of great importance because, due to the small lumen of the trachea and bronchi, whole lobes of the lungs can very rapidly become collapsed as the bronchi become blocked by secretions. It is advisable to treat the infant at least four-hourly in the immediate post-operative phase.

If the infant is being ventilated a Jackson-Rees tube will most likely be used and suction should be carried out quarter- or half-hourly. When using suction it is advisable to pass the catheter before attaching it to the sucker and then withdraw the catheter quickly with a rotary action. This method is a precaution against collapsing the lung by sucking out all the air.

If 'bag squeezing' is indicated, it is obvious that a much smaller bag must be used to inflate the lung; chest shaking or vibrations should not be too vigorous. It is also important to ensure that the lungs are completely inflated before re-attaching the patient to the ventilator.

Complete Anatomical Correction

This is the operation of choice and is usually performed when the child is about five years of age.

Incision—Median sternotomy

If a previous anastomosis has been performed it must be closed before the intracardiac repair is performed. The right ventricle is then opened and an infundibular resection or pulmonary valvotomy is carried out. The ventricular septal defect is repaired either by direct suture or by use of a Dacron patch.

Operations on the Pericardium and Heart

In a few cases the outflow via the pulmonary valve is still not wide enough so that it may be necessary to insert a gusset, made of pericardial material, to relieve obstruction.

The intracardiac part of the operation will be performed with the aid of a cardio-pulmonary bypass.

Post-operatively the patient may often be receiving ventilatory assistance initially.

Pre-operative Physiotherapy

As previously described, but since the majority of these patients will be children the physiotherapist's approach must be adapted to suit their age. It must be remembered that the child will often adopt the squatting position to conserve his oxygen supply for the brain so that he should not be discouraged from doing this. In some cases where cyanosis is severe the child will not tolerate a ward class.

Post-operative Physiotherapy

This will depend upon the need for assistance with ventilation and the age of the patient. Young children are normally allowed to get up earlier than adults but in all cases should be discharged in three weeks.

COMPLETE TRANSPOSITION OF THE GREAT VESSELS

This is a congenital abnormality in which the aorta arises from the right ventricle and the pulmonary artery from the left ventricle, so that venous blood is pumped through the systemic circuit and oxygenated blood through the pulmonary. It is usually associated with one or more other defects, for example atrial septal defect, patent ductus arteriosus. It is obvious that in order to survive there must be a communication between the systemic and pulmonary circulations, it is the presence of the associated defects that provides the communication and acts as a corrective factor.

Symptoms

The child will be cyanosed and will soon demonstrate clubbing of fingers and toes. The heart is enlarged and in particular the left ventricle. He will be poorly developed and will be breathless on exertion.

Operations

Various procedures are used to attempt to correct the abnormality but basically there are two ways of approaching the problem.

1. The anomaly of the aorta and pulmonary artery is accepted and an attempt is made to compensate for it by transposing the venous flow.
2. An attempt is made to correct the anomaly of the outflow tract.

The surgery will necessitate cardiopulmonary bypass and the incision more commonly used is a median sternotomy, although a right lateral thoracotomy is sometimes used.

Pre- and Post-operative Physiotherapy

This is routine. The patient will almost certainly be ventilated immediately following surgery.

MITRAL STENOSIS

Mitral stenosis, that is narrowing or blocking of the mitral valve orifice, occurs as a result of rheumatic disease, the cusps of the valve becoming contracted during the resolution of the inflammatory stage of the disease. As the outlet between the left atrium and ventricle has been decreased, congestion will occur in the pulmonary capillary bed, pulmonary artery and right ventricle. Hypertrophy of the left atrium will occur and atrial fibrillation may be present.

Symptoms

Shortness of breath and dyspnoea on exertion are the most outstanding features and result from the pulmonary congestion and decreased cardiac output. The more severe cases of dyspnoea may occur at rest, this paroxysmal dyspnoea is due to acute pulmonary congestion and will result in pulmonary oedema. Haemoptysis may also occur as narrowing of the valve progresses and there is more impedence of blood flow from the left atrium to the left ventricle.

Operation—Mitral Valvotomy

Incision

Left posterolateral thoracotomy usually through the fifth rib interspace. It will involve the trapezius, rhomboids and latissimus muscles.

The procedure is more often a 'closed heart' one and the heart is entered through the auricular appendage of the left atrium; the commisures are then split, either manually or with a mechanical dilator.

The operation is rarely curative but affords marked relief from symptoms which may last for many years.

The drainage tubes are normally removed 12 to 24 hours after surgery. Atrial fibrillation may persist after surgery and, in this event, the surgeon will defibrillate the patient.

The advances made in anaesthetics and the technology of producing mechanical valves have so reduced the risk of open heart surgery that the surgeon may well decide to perform the operation under perfusion preferring a sternotomy split in order that he may proceed to mitral valve replacement if it seems indicated at the time.

MITRAL INCOMPETENCE

In mitral incompetence the bicuspid valve of the left side of the heart fails to close properly during systole of the left ventricle, the left atrium is then forced to dilate to accommodate the blood which has regurgitated. The condition is usually acquired as a result of rheumatic disease but may be congenital.

Symptoms

These are fatigue, due to inadequate general circulation, and dyspnoea from the increased pulmonary capillary pressures. Pulmonary oedema will also be present. The symptoms may be only minimal initially but will increase rapidly as the condition progresses.

It is frequently found that mitral stenosis and incompetence co-exist in the same patient.

In all such cases or where the cusps are much thickened and heavily calcified mitral replacement is indicated.

Operation—Mitral Valve Repair or Annuloplasty

This is indicated where the valve is nearly normal but perhaps the valve ring is dilated, or there is isolated moderate involvement of the cusps. The annulus is narrowed by sutures and Teflon used to secure them.

Mitral Replacement

The operation is performed under cardiopulmonary bypass.

Incision

Either (a) Median sternotomy, or (b) Right thoracotomy.

The mitral valve is approached via an incision in the left atrium; it is excised and the mechanical valve secured. The most common mechanical valves used are the ball in cage, or flat disc varieties. The Starr Edward is an example of the former; it consists of a silicone rubber ball enclosed in a vitallium alloy cage.

The mounted homograft valve is now also being used by some surgeons. A human aortic valve may be mounted in a ring and sutured in the mitral position.

Pre-operative Physiotherapy

As routine.

Post-operative Physiotherapy

These patients are particularly prone to pulmonary and biochemical problems and so will more frequently be returned from the theatre receiving ventilatory assistance for the first few hours in order to stabilize. This may, however, take a few days.

The 'low output syndrome' is particularly prone to develop in patients with high pulmonary vascular resistance; the signs will be cyanosis and low venous oxygen saturation.

Progress is usually a little slower than with those conditions previously described, but the patient may start to get up as early as the third post-operative day depending entirely upon the view of the surgeon. It is usual for these patients to be discharged to convalescence at the end of the third post-operative week.

AORTIC STENOSIS

Aortic stenosis may be congenital or aquired as a result of arterio-stenosis or rheumatic heart disease. The thickening or calcification of the cusps of the valve prevents them from opening properly during the left ventricular systole, thereby causing an obstruction to the outflow of blood from the left ventricle. Obstruction may also be caused by the formation of fibrous, muscular or fibromuscular bands above or below the valve (supra-aortic or subaortic stenosis). The condition is intractable to medical treatment because the problem is one of functional interference with the mechanics of the heart and because there is progressive hypertrophy of the left ventricle.

Symptoms

These are syncope, fatigue, angina and effort dyspnoea.

Operation—Aortic Valvotomy

This procedure is rarely used now because of the high risk of emboli from the calcium. However, where it is used it would always be done as an 'open' procedure under perfusion in order that the surgeon might proceed to replacement if necessary. Aortic valve replacement is more frequently the elective procedure.

AORTIC INCOMPETENCE

Aortic incompetence or regurgitation occurs where there is failure of the cusps of the valve to close properly during diastole; this may be due to shrinkage, perforation or rigidity of the cusps. Alternatively there may be dilatation of the aorta with consequent separation of the cusps from each other.

The condition may result from syphilis, bacterial endocarditis, trauma or is sometimes associated with Marfan's syndrome.

The mechanical manifestations of the valve's failure are that the left ventricle receives blood from the left atrium and aorta at the same time causing left ventricular hypertrophy.

Symptoms

The patient complains of dyspnoea on effort and angina, the latter caused by the inadequate amount of oxygenated blood in the coronary arteries.

Operation—Aortic Valve Replacement

The procedure is an 'open' one and performed under cardiopulmonary bypass.

The homograft valve is now the most commonly used replacement for the aortic valve; it has the added advantage of reducing the risk of thrombo-embolism.

It is still possible that a mechanical valve replacement may be used depending largely upon the availability of homografts.

Pre-operative Physiotherapy

As previously described.

Post-operative Physiotherapy

The patient will often be returned to the Intensive Care Unit on a ventilator and will remain on this for a few hours but is less likely to have pulmonary complications than the mitral valve replacements.

He will probably get up on the third day and be discharged to convalescence during the third week.

Multiple Valve Replacement

The advances in the realms of anaesthesia, the consequent reduction of the risk of cardiopulmonary bypass, combined with technological advances in the production of valve prostheses now enable surgeons to perform replacement of more than one valve at one time.

The operation will be performed under total cardiopulmonary bypass.

Incision—Median sternotomy

Pre- and Post-operative Physiotherapy

The same principles of physiotherapy apply as for mitral valve replacements but, of course, progress may be considerably slower.

CARDIAC MYXOMA

This is a fairly rare condition. A tumour, more commonly of the left atrium, grows from the interatrial septum and may grow through into the left ventricle.

Symptoms

These are the same as for obstruction of the mitral valve. Symptoms are intermittent.

Operation—Excision of the Tumour

This is an open procedure.

Surgery is performed under perfusion, the heart being opened via the right atrium and the root of the tumour is cut out with the septum to which it is attached and the myxoma is then drawn through into the right atrium and removed. The hole in the septum is then repaired.

Pre- and Post-operative Physiotherapy

As for ostium primum atrial septal defect.

HEART BLOCK

Heart block is the name given to the condition in which the bundle of His has been destroyed by disease or a complication of surgery. There is a dissociation between the atrial and the ventricular rhythm, the ventricles beating slowly and the atria normally. In the early stages of the disease the block may be incomplete.

Symptoms

Dizziness, feeling of faintness and dyspnoea on exertion. These may lead to Stokes Adams attacks, i.e. the pulse suddenly stops, there is blanching of the face and loss of consciousness. If this is prolonged, it is followed by convulsions, then suddenly the pulse returns.

These patients will be given artificial pacemakers. Initially, they are attached to an external pacemaker, one wire of which is attached to the heart via a suitable vein such as the cephalic or jugular. The second lead will be placed on the patient's skin at any convenient place. If continued assistance is necessary an internal pacemaker will be inserted.

Operation—Insertion of Internal Pacemaker

The chest is opened by a left thoracotomy and one wire sutured to the heart, preferably to the left ventricle. A second incision is made to insert the pacemaker either behind or in front of the rectus abdominis muscle or below either axilla.

AORTO-CORONARY GRAFT

This procedure is now being used for some patients who have suffered a coronary or who have intractable angina. The operation is only successful in those patients who have a block in the proximal end of the coronary artery, that is where it is widest near its origin. There must also be a good anastomosis between the two coronary arteries.

Operation—under cardio-pulmonary bypass

Incision—Median sternotomy

The long saphenous vein is used for the graft to bypass the block, it must of course be reversed so that the valves are in the correct position.

The procedure is still being developed.

Pre-operative and Post-operative Treatment

This is as routine but in the post-operative phase the patient is disturbed as little as possible.

SUMMARY

It cannot be sufficiently stressed that although it is possible to generalize and establish a guide to treatment, in the event each patient must be individually evaluated and treated as his condition permits.

The exact technique used and the expected rate of normal progress will vary from unit to unit depending largely upon the surgeon's preference for early ambulation.

However, it should also be remembered that at each stage the physiotherapist treats the condition that presents ensuring that there is sound physiological reason for what she does. It is of great importance that an accurate record of treatment and the patient's progress is made at frequent intervals.

In many parts of the world and in all spheres of surgery changes are continually being made in techniques; this is certainly true in the field of cardiac surgery. It is therefore apparent that the operations described in this text may soon be modified or outdated but nevertheless the general principles will still apply as far as the physiotherapy is concerned.

OPERATIONS ON THE OESOPHAGUS

by B. SHOTTON, M.C.S.P.

As these operations involve the opening of the thorax, they are being discussed in this section, but in some instances the operation is extended to the abdomen. Operations for children and adults will be considered.

CONGENITAL OESOPHAGEAL ATRESIA

Within a few hours of birth, persistent regurgitation of 'frothy' saliva may indicate malformation of the oesophagus, which can be confirmed by X-ray following Lipiodol swallow.

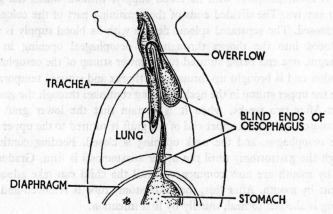

FIG. 25. CONGENITAL OESOPHAGEAL ATRESIA

The lower part of the oesophagus, as shown in Fig. 25, is not of course apparent in the X-ray, since the Lipiodol will not penetrate as far as this. The lower defect can only be ascertained during exploratory operation.

Approximately 85 per cent of cases show an upper oesophageal stump, and a fistula between the trachea and the lower part of the oesophagus. Another 10 to 12 per cent show no fistula.

DIRECT CLOSURE

This should be performed within a few hours of birth if at the exploratory operation it is discovered that the gap can be closed.

GASTROSTOMY followed by COLON TRANSPLANT

If it is found that the gap cannot be closed by approximation of the two ends of the oesophagus, an opening is made through the abdominal wall into the stomach, and the child is fed by a tube through this opening. The upper end of the oesophagus is brought to the surface at the left side of the baby's neck. Saliva will be seen to trickle out of this opening in the neck, which will be protected by a dressing. But it is essential that he is given opportunity to suck and later to swallow in order to train his swallowing reflex, for if he was fed only through the gastrostomy, this reflex would later prove defective.

This state continues for approximately eighteen months, during which time his parents may be able to care for the child at home. He will then be re-admitted to hospital for colon transplant. The splenic flexure of the colon is used, complete with its blood supply, without which the graft cannot survive. The divided ends of the remaining part of the colon are anastomosed. The separated splenic flexure with its blood supply is now introduced into the thorax through the oesophageal opening in the diaphragm, one end being sutured to the lower stump of the oesophagus. The other end is brought up through the thorax and sutured temporarily beside the upper stump in the neck. Feeding continues through the gastrostomy. After two weeks, when it is certain that the lower graft has anastomosed firmly, the upper end of the graft is sutured to the upper end of the oesophagus, and the neck opening is closed. Feeding continues through the gastrostomy until the upper anastomosis is firm. Graduated feeds by mouth are now commenced until the child can take adequate amounts by mouth. After this, the gastrostomy tube is removed and the opening is allowed to heal, usually by first intention.

Physiotherapy

Pre- and post-operative breathing exercises or percussion could be given at the time of the graft operation, but usually the child is too young to be able to co-operate.

Operations on the Oesophagus

ADULTS

Similar operations may be performed on adults when part of the oesophagus has to be removed as a result of stricture, either due to recurrent oesophagitis or to carcinoma.

DIRECT CLOSURE

This will be performed if the remaining ends of the oesophagus can be approximated. In regurgitant oesophagitis, the lower end is most commonly involved, an oesophago-gastrectomy being performed. A transthoracic incision is used, being on the left side if the lower third of the oesophagus is involved, but possibly on the right if the lesion is higher.

COLON TRANSPLANT

If direct closure is impossible, a colon graft is undertaken immediately.

No gastrostomy is needed, as the patient can probably start taking fluids by mouth twenty-four hours after operation. The incision will be on the left side of the thorax. It is not always continued into the abdominal cavity, since the operation on the gut may be performed through the thoracic incision by opening the diaphragm.

Physiotherapy

Routine pre- and post-operative treatment should be given, with special attention to the lung bases and to the circulation in the legs. The physiotherapist should not give the patient any fluids by mouth unless permission has been given.

Chapter XI

SURGICAL NEUROLOGY I

by M. C. BALFOUR, M.C.S.P.
Cranial Surgery

INTRODUCTION

By means of extensive research more has become known of the central nervous system, although much remains to be discovered. Increasing knowledge of brain areas, pathways, spinal cord tracts and function has opened up new fields in surgical neurology. Improved equipment, techniques, anaesthetics, drugs and antibiotics contribute to reduce the operating time and minimize post-operative complications.

Early diagnosis and submission to a neuro-surgical unit is essential to ensure maximum benefit as delay may cause irreparable damage with resultant risk of permanent disability.

It must be remembered that arising from brain lesions, motor and sensory defects may be accompanied by other defects which have a direct bearing on the capabilities of the patient, such as defects in sight, hearing, intellect and speech. Spinal lesions may also be accompanied by some degree of psychological disturbance which requires full understanding and suitable management.

Team work is essential in the over-all aim to rehabilitate the patient for normal living. The team includes surgeons, nursing staff, physiotherapists, occupational therapists, speech therapists, psychologists and medical social workers. Interchange of knowledge between members of the team allows a full understanding of the particular problems of each patient. Encouragement, patience and perseverance are of paramount importance during the rehabilitation period, which can be said to begin immediately the patient enters hospital.

Introduction

SPEECH THERAPIST

A wide range of speech disorders arise from lesions in the brain and can have a psychological as well as a neurological basis. The following are some of the disorders found:

1. Complete loss of speech.
2. Difficulty in finding the correct word.
3. Understanding what is said but unable to reply.
4. Inco-ordination of speech exists with cerebellar lesions.
5. Voice volume loss and accelerated speech is found with Parkinsonism.

A patient with a speech disorder can become very distressed and frustrated, thus guidance from the speech therapist on how to deal with the problem is very important. Information regarding speech recovery is essential to the occupational therapist and physiotherapist. The speech therapist is helped by reports from other departments on how much the patient attempts to speak and how well he makes himself understood. It is important to the patient that he can communicate with people, thus some time should be devoted to speaking to him and to giving him the opportunity and time to reply.

Certain types of speech disorders affect the patient's ability to co-operate with the various therapists. A patient may be unable to understand the spoken word but may understand and respond to written commands. A demonstration by the therapist may be necessary if the patient cannot comprehend the spoken or written word. Great patience is thus required by all members of the rehabilitation team in order to gain full co-operation from the patient.

PSYCHOLOGIST

Information and advice from the psychologist can be invaluable as he plays an important part in assessing the patient's mental state, which is not always easy to do in general conversation. A large range of psychological disturbances is associated with brain lesions and requires to be understood in order to be dealt with successfully and to make allowances for the patient.

In lesions of the dominant cerebral hemisphere (left side in a right-handed person) various types and degrees of loss of motor skills can exist with retention of adequate voluntary power and comprehension, they present as clumsiness or odd errors, which may improve with retraining. In right cerebral hemisphere lesions 'body scheme' and visual perceptual disorders can exist leading to odd behaviour such as difficulty with dressing and finding the way about. Patience and persistence in re-training usually meets with improvement unless the lesion is a progressive one.

A general disturbance of cerebral function has a general effect on behaviour, appearing as poor intellect, memory, concentration and grasp of the situation. Associated with these disorders may be a loss of normal control of emotional reactions. This includes undue tendencies to distress and irritability, often alternating with periods of excessive cheerfulness. To gain the patient's co-operation for physiotherapy treatment, firm, tactful management is essential.

OCCUPATIONAL THERAPIST

The work of the occupational therapist is closely linked with that of the physiotherapist. The patient's programme of treatment is such that the retraining of motor and sensory defects along functional lines is shared by both departments. The occupational therapist may require information as to the return and degree of voluntary power to enable her to select an appropriate activity. In turn the physiotherapist is informed of any par-ticular difficulty the patient experiences when attempting these activities, she can then concentrate on the re-education of the specific defects.

When a neglect phenomenon is the main feature, bimanual tasks are given to encourage the use of the neglected limb. These tasks are also given when a homonymous hemianopia is present so encouraging the patient to compensate for loss of visual field by head movements. Loss of sensation in the hand is re-educated by teaching the patient to appreciate objects of different sizes, weights and textures. Writing difficulties are associated with certain brain lesions, notably Parkinsonism, the tendency being for the writing to decrease in size. Some speech disorders are accompanied by loss of the ability to write. The physical re-education of writing deficiencies is undertaken by the occupational therapist.

Remedial sports such as skittles, darts, table tennis and archery are use-ful for the re-education of balance and co-ordination. The patient with a spinal lesion derives particular benefit from archery which strengthens the shoulder girdle muscles and improves balance, and table tennis, which aids balance and co-ordination.

To regain the patient's independence, feeding and dressing are en-couraged and gadgets provided when necessary. Kitchen facilities are provided to enable the housewife to practise her culinary skills and adjust to her disability, need for modifications or the use of certain gadgets in her own kitchen may become apparent. A home visit by the occupa-tional therapist and the physiotherapist to advise as to modifications in all parts of the home is important. Heavy workshop activities which include woodwork are provided for male patients.

Work assessments are carried out as a guide to the type of employment the patient is suited for when his rehabilitation programme is complete.

MEDICAL SOCIAL WORKER

Resettlement problems are dealt with by the medical social worker working, as do other members of the medical and rehabilitation staff in close collaboration with the consultant, who directs investigations and treatment.

The patient who has residual physical and mental defects may be unable to return to his former employment. It may be possible for the medical social worker in co-operation with the Local Authority to arrange for the provision of certain modifications in the home, such as ramps, rails at strategic places in bathrooms, banister rails, etc., which have been recommended by the physiotherapist. In certain cases it may even be possible to have the patient and his family rehoused.

A patient less severely handicapped may require help to find a suitable re-training scheme for employment within his capabilities. The medical social worker may help to gain the co-operation of his current employer to re-employ the patient in a job suitable to his capabilities. Financial difficulties can also arise and the medical social worker may be able to help and advise. Whenever it is possible the patient resumes some form of employment thus helping him to regain confidence in himself and in his ability to live independently, or relatively so.

During the course of physiotherapy treatment the patient may confide his worries and difficulties or give the impression of being worried and depressed. The physiotherapist should then advise him to see the medical social worker. There are various occasions when a report on the patient's progress and capabilities in occupational therapy and physiotherapy are useful to the medical social worker when making appropriate arrangements for employment and housing. It is often in co-operation with the medical social worker that an optimum discharge date can be decided upon.

When a patient has derived maximum benefit from his physiotherapy treatment and finds it difficult to break this contact, usually due to feelings of insecurity or even loneliness, the medical social worker may be able to suggest alternative interests such as clubs for the disabled and other organizations interested in the welfare of the disabled.

Surgical Neurology I

ANATOMY AND PHYSIOLOGY

For the purpose of description, the brain may be divided into cerebrum, mid-brain, pons, medulla oblongata and the cerebellum, which lies behind the two last-named. It must be remembered that the entire mechanism is highly complex, no one part works as a separate entity, and the response of the brain is a result of the integrated action of its various systems.

The following is a brief guide to the effect of a lesion at various levels throughout the brain:

THE CEREBRUM (see Figs. 26 and 27)

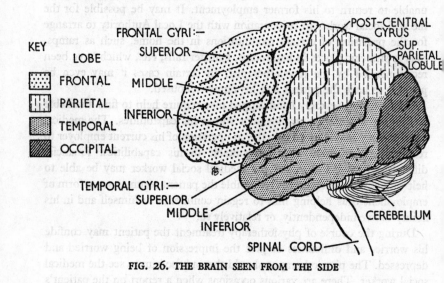

KEY
LOBE

FRONTAL
PARIETAL
TEMPORAL
OCCIPITAL

FRONTAL GYRI:—
SUPERIOR
MIDDLE
INFERIOR

POST-CENTRAL GYRUS
SUP. PARIETAL LOBULE

TEMPORAL GYRI:—
SUPERIOR
MIDDLE
INFERIOR

CEREBELLUM

SPINAL CORD

FIG. 26. THE BRAIN SEEN FROM THE SIDE

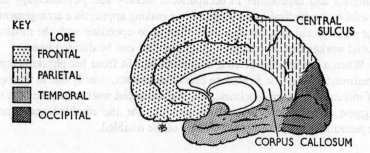

KEY
LOBE

FRONTAL
PARIETAL
TEMPORAL
OCCIPITAL

CENTRAL SULCUS

CORPUS CALLOSUM

FIG. 27. SAGITTAL SECTION OF THE BRAIN

Anatomy and Physiology

The cerebrum is the largest part of the brain, it consists of two hemispheres connected by bundles of nerve fibres, the corpus callosum. The surface of each hemisphere, covered by layers of cells, constitutes the cerebral cortex. This represents the highest centre of function and can be roughly mapped into areas, each concerned with a specific function. To facilitate reference each hemisphere is divided into four lobes namely, frontal, temporal, parietal and occipital. The right hemisphere controls the left side of the body, the left hemisphere usually controls speech function, and the right side of the body.

FRONTAL LOBE

Area	Function	Effect of a Lesion
(A) Motor area (which gives rise to the cerebro-spinal tracts)	Controls voluntary movement of the opposite half of the body which is represented on the cortex in an upside down position	Flaccid paralysis. A lesion between the hemispheres produces paraplegia
(B) Pre-motor area	Localization of motor function	*Spastic paralysis. Psychological changes
(C)	Controls movements of the eyes	The eyes turn to the side of the lesion and cannot be moved to the opposite side
(D)	Motor control of larynx, tongue, and lips to enable movements of articulation	Inability to articulate
(E) 'Silent Area'	Believed to control abstract thinking, foresight, mature judgement, tactfulness	Lack of a sense of responsibility in personal affairs

* The effects of a lesion in the pre-motor area vary with the rate of onset; a lesion which occurs suddenly, such as a head injury or a haemorrhage will result in a flaccid paralysis initially, spasm gradually developing over a variable period of time. A lesion which has a slow mode of onset, such as a slowly growing neoplasm will produce spasm in the early stages.

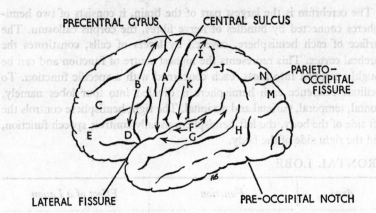

FIG. 28. DIAGRAM SHOWING SOME CORTICAL AREAS OF THE BRAIN

TEMPORAL LOBE

Area	Function	Effect of a Lesion
(F and G)	Hearing and association of sound	Inability to localize the direction of sound
(H) Auditory Speech Area	Understanding of the spoken word	Inability to understand what is said

Other areas on the medial aspect of the temporal lobe are associated with the sense of smell and taste. The optic radiations sweep through the temporal lobe to reach the occipital lobe and these may also be damaged by a lesion of the temporal lobe giving rise to a homonymous hemianopia.

(See diagram on Visual Pathways, Fig. 31.)

PARIETAL LOBE

Area	Function	Effect of a Lesion
(I, J and K)	Sensory receptive areas for light touch, two point discrimination, joint position sense and pressure	Corresponding sensory loss giving rise to a 'neglect phenomena'. 'Body image' loss is associated with lesions of the non-dominant hemisphere

190

Anatomy and Physiology

Visual defects arising from lesions in the parietal area may be highly complex and the patient unaware of them. Sensory loss gives a severe disability, which is out of proportion to any associated voluntary power loss

OCCIPITAL LOBE

Area	Function	Effect of a Lesion
(L)	Receptive area for visual impressions	Loss of vision in some areas of the visual fields. (See diagram on Visual Pathways.)
(M and N)	Recognition and interpretation of visual stimuli	Inability to recognize things visually

All nerve fibres to and from the cerebral cortex converge towards the brain stem forming the corona radiata, on entering the diencephalon they become the internal capsule. When the cerebral cortex is removed the remainder, or central core, is termed the brain stem. Its components from above downwards are:

1. The diencephalon.
2. The basal ganglia.
3. The mesencephalon or mid-brain.
4. The pons.
5. The medulla oblongata.

The nuclei of the cranial nerves are scattered throughout this area.

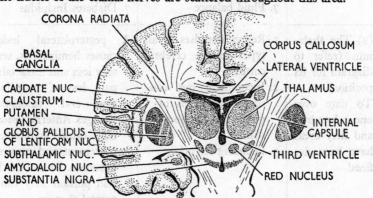

CORONA RADIATA

BASAL GANGLIA

CAUDATE NUC.
CLAUSTRUM
PUTAMEN AND GLOBUS PALLIDUS OF LENTIFORM NUC.
SUBTHALAMIC NUC.
AMYGDALOID NUC.
SUBSTANTIA NIGRA

CORPUS CALLOSUM
LATERAL VENTRICLE
THALAMUS
INTERNAL CAPSULE
THIRD VENTRICLE
RED NUCLEUS

FIG. 29. A DIAGRAMMATIC VIEW OF THE BRAIN IN CROSS SECTION

THE DIENCEPHALON (See Fig. 29.)

Components	Function	Effects of a Lesion
(A) Hypothalamus lies in the grey matter near the floor and lower walls of the third ventricle	1. Influences respiration, heart rate and blood pressure	1. Alterations in respiratory and heart rate and blood pressure
	2. Due to its connection with the reticular formation, it influences the conscious level	2. Pathological sleep
	3. Influences the pituitary gland	3. Refer to pituitary gland dysfunction
	4. Influences appetite	4. Appetite may be increased or decreased
	5. Has some influence over emotional behaviour	5. Effects on emotional behaviour are very variable
	6. Regulation of body temperature	6. Increase in body temperature
	7. Fluid balance	7. Diabetes Insipidus
(B) The thalamus (refer to diagram for its position) To date over one hundred and fifty areas have been defined	1. Relays impulses of all types to the cerebral cortex 2. Incomplete but conscious awareness of peripheral sensory stimuli 3. Focusing attention	A posterolateral lesion causes hemiparesis, sensory loss and intractable pain, loss of co-ordination and vasomotor changes. Anterior lesions may cause involuntary movements and impaired sensation. Lesion of the mid portion may cause mental changes

Basal Ganglia

Broadly speaking the basal ganglia include the (1) caudate nucleus, (2) putamen, (3) globus pallidus, (4) amygdala, (5) claustrum, (6) substantia nigra, (7) sub-thalamic nucleus. The corpus striatum and extrapyramidal motor system refers to the caudate nucleus, putamen and globus pallidus. The subthalamus and substantia nigra are closely related in function to the extrapyramidal motor system.

Lesions of the extrapyramidal system can be divided into two types, hyperkinetic and hypokinetic.

Hyperkinetic

  (a) Chorea characterized by quick jerky purposeless movements.
  (b) Athetosis which gives slow, writhing movements of the limbs.
  (c) Hemiballismus causing continual wild, flail-like movements usually confined to one arm.

Hypokinetic

  (a) Parkinsonian syndrome which will be described later.

Mid-brain, pons and medulla oblongata

The mid-brain, pons and medulla oblongata also act as a funnel for tracts passing from higher levels downwards to the spinal cord and for sensory tracts from the spinal cord passing upwards to higher centres. In view of it being a relatively small area, any lesion can give rise to widespread effects. Involvement of any of the following are likely:

  (a) Cerebellar function due to interference of the efferent and afferent pathways.
  (b) Sensation of all types as the fasiculi gracilis and cuneatus terminate in nuclei in the medulla oblongata. Nerve fibres then arise from these nuclei, cross the midline and continue upwards to the thalamus in the medial lemniscus. The spino-thalamic tracts which cross in the spinal cord pass directly upwards through the brain stem.
  (c) Loss of motor function occurs if the cerebro-spinal tracts are damaged. These pass downwards from the internal capsule to decussate at the lower end of the medulla oblongata.
  (d) The conscious level can be depressed if there is damage to the reticular formation which is scattered throughout the brain system.
  (e) Vomiting and disturbed respiratory rate can occur with pressure on the vomiting and respiratory centres in the medulla oblongata.
  (f) Cranial nerve nuclear lesions with characteristic palsies. (See table on cranial nerves.)

THE CRANIAL NERVES (See Fig. 30.)

Cranial Nerve	Function	Effect of a Lesion
1. Olfactory	Sense of smell	Loss of sense of smell
2. Optic	Vision	Various visual field defects (refer to diagram). Visual acuity
3. Oculomotor	Innervates medial, superior, inferior recti and inferior oblique muscle and voluntary fibres of levator palpebrae superiorus. Carries autonomic fibres to pupil	Outward deviation of the eye, ptosis, dilation of the pupil
4. Trochlear	Motor supply to the superior oblique eye muscle	Inability to turn the eye downwards and outwards
5. Trigeminal	(a) Motor division to temporalis, masseter, internal and external pterygoid muscles	(a) Deviation of the chin towards the paralysed side when the mouth is open
	(b) Sensory division: touch, pain and temperature sensation of the face including the cornea on the same side of the body	(b) Loss of touch, pain and temperature sensation and of the corneal reflex
6. Abducent	Innervates the external rectus muscle	Internal squint and therefore diplopia
7. Facial	Motor supply to facial muscles on the same side of the body	Paralysis of facial muscles

Cranial Nerve	Function	Effect of a Lesion
8. Acoustic	Sensory supply to semi-circular canals. Hearing	Vertigo. Nystagmus. Deafness
9. Glosso-pharyngeal	Motor to the pharynx Taste: posterior one-third of the tongue	Loss of gag reflex. Loss of taste in the appropriate area
10. Vagus	Motor to pharynx Sympathetic and para-sympathetic to heart and viscera	Difficulty with swallowing. Regurgitation of food and fluids
11. Accessory	The cranial part of the nerve joins the vagus nerve	
12. Hypoglossal	Motor nerve of the tongue	Paralysis of the side of the tongue corresponding to the lesion, thus it deviates to the paralysed side when protruded

THE CEREBELLUM

The cerebellum lies in the posterior cranial fossa of the skull connected to the pons and medulla oblongata by the cerebellar peduncles. The surface is corrugated and consists of cells forming the cerebellar cortex. It is divided into two cerebellar hemispheres which join near the midline with a narrow middle portion called the vermis.

The cerebellum controls co-ordinate action of muscle groups throughout the body to allow movement to be performed smoothly and accurately. Cerebellar lesions give the following characteristic signs:

1. Ataxia

(a) The disturbance of posture and gait. A unilateral cerebellar lesion causes the patient to overbalance to the side of the lesion.

(b) When performing a movement which involves several joints, the joints tend to move separately instead of together in a synchronized movement.

(c) When reaching out to pick up an object the hand stops before the object is reached or over-shoots it.

(d) There is an inability to stop one movement and follow it immediately by a movement in the opposite direction.

(e) When speaking, the spacing of sounds is irregular with pauses in the wrong places, termed dysarthria.

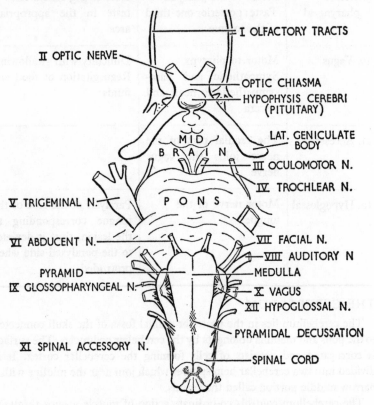

I OLFACTORY TRACTS

II OPTIC NERVE

OPTIC CHIASMA

HYPOPHYSIS CEREBRI (PITUITARY)

MID BRAIN

LAT. GENICULATE BODY

III OCULOMOTOR N.

IV TROCHLEAR N.

V TRIGEMINAL N.

PONS

VI ABDUCENT N.

VII FACIAL N.

VIII AUDITORY N

PYRAMID

MEDULLA

IX GLOSSOPHARYNGEAL N.

X VAGUS

XII HYPOGLOSSAL N.

PYRAMIDAL DECUSSATION

XI SPINAL ACCESSORY N.

SPINAL CORD

FIG. 30. THE BRAIN STEM AND CRANIAL NERVES SEEN FROM THE FRONT

2. Hypotonia

Tendon reflexes are decreased on the affected side.

3. Asthenia

The muscles affected by cerebellar lesions are weaker and tire more easily than normal muscles.

4. Tremor

Intention tremor is present.

5. Nystagmus

This may be due to:

(*a*) irritation of vestibular fibres in the cerebellum, or

(*b*) pressure on the vestibular nuclei of the brain stem.

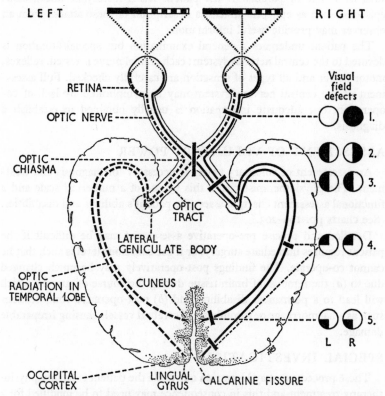

FIG. 31. DIAGRAM TO SHOW THE EFFECTS OF INJURY ON THE VISUAL PATHWAY

1. Shows blindness in one eye.   2. Bitemporal hemianopia.
3. Left homonymous hemianopia.   4 and 5. Quadrantic defects.

EXAMINATIONS AND INVESTIGATIONS

Before surgery can be considered extensive examinations and investigations may require to be carried out to localize the lesion and decide upon its nature and likely prognosis.

EXAMINATIONS

A history of the patient's present illness, previous illnesses and any relevant family illness is noted, social circumstances, occupation, drinking and smoking habits are taken into account. This information is obtained directly from the patient whenever possible, but if the patient's conscious level or language function is disturbed the family history and relevant details will probably have to be obtained from other convenient sources, such as a wife or parents. If the patient has a history of unconscious episodes, such as epileptic attacks, a description of these attacks from an observer may provide useful information.

The patient undergoes a general examination but special attention is devoted to the central nervous system; each cranial nerve is tested, reflexes, motor power and all types of sensation are carefully checked. Full assessment of the central nervous system may be complicated by lack of co-operation, but adequate information is usually obtained to establish a diagnosis.

ASSESSMENT OF VOLUNTARY POWER

An assessment of voluntary power is necessary for diagnosis and treatment. The physiotherapist charts this by use of a numerical scale and a functional assessment chart, to assess the patient's abilities and disabilities. (See charts pp. 199–203.)

Detailed and precise pre-operative assessment may be difficult if the patient requires immediate surgery, or if the conscious level is such that he cannot co-operate. The findings post-operatively may be much changed due to (a) the removal of brain tissue during the course of surgery which will lead to a permanent disability, and (b) post-operative complications such as a haemorrhage or thrombosis of cerebral vessels causing irreparable damage.

SPECIAL INVESTIGATIONS

These procedures may be carried out while the patient is having physiotherapy treatment and this in consequence may need to be modified for a few days.

1. Lumbar puncture

A needle is inserted in the subarachnoid space between the third and fourth lumbar spinous processes; pressure of the cerebrospinal fluid is determined and a sample of fluid taken for diagnostic purposes. Following lumbar puncture the patient is nursed lying flat in bed for twenty-four hours and active physiotherapy can be given in any of the lying positions.

Examinations and Investigations

PHYSIOTHERAPY DEPARTMENT
PHYSICAL DEMANDS OF DAILY LIVING

NAME... AGE...... DIAGNOSIS.....................

ADDRESS...................................... DISABILITY ....

BED ACTIVITIES	Date			Comments
1. Moving place to place in bed				
2. Rolling to L. and then to R.				
3. Sitting erect in bed				
4. Turn and lie on abdomen				
5. Remove objects from side table				
6. Sitting on edge of bed				
TOILET ACTIVITIES				
1. Manipulating bedpan				
2. Manipulating urinal				
3. Get on and off toilet				
4. Get in and out of bath				

PHYSIOTHERAPY DEPARTMENT
PHYSICAL DEMANDS OF DAILY LIVING

NAME..   AGE...... DIAGNOSIS.....................

ADDRESS...................................   DISABILITY ....

ELEVATION ACTIVITIES	Date			Comments
1. Bed to erect				
2. Erect to bed				
3. Wheelchair to standing				
4. Standing to wheelchair				
5. Standing up				
6. Sitting down				
7. Easy chair to erect				
8. Erect to easy chair				
9. Erect to toilet				
10. Toilet to erect				
11. Down to floor				
12. Up from floor				
13. Pick things up from floor				

Examinations and Investigations

NAME.. AGE...... DIAGNOSIS....................

ADDRESS.. DISABILITY..............................

WALKING ACTIVITIES	Date			Comments
1. Standing				
2. Walking forward				
3. Walking backward				
4. Running				
5. Opening and closing door erect position				
GAIT				
1. Four point alternate				
2. Swing to				
3. Swing through				
4. Two point alternate				
CLIMBING ACTIVITIES				
1. Up ramp				
2. Steps: Handrail No handrail				
3. Kerbs				
4. Bus step				

OCCUPATIONAL THERAPY DEPARTMENT—ASSESSMENT FORM 1

NAME...   R/L HANDED............

DAILY LIVING ACTIVITIES	Pre-operative date	Post-operative date
Eating		
Eat with spoon		
Eat with knife and fork		
Able to cut meat		
Able to butter bread		
Able to drink from feeder/cup/glass		
Washing		
Turn water taps		
Wash and dry hands		
Wash and dry face and neck		
Bath self		
Dry self		
Clean teeth, dentures		
Shave/use cosmetics		
Brush/comb hair		
Dressing		
Underclothes		
Shirt/blouse		
Trousers/skirt		
Jacket/overcoat		
Socks/stockings		
Suspenders		
Shoes/shoe laces		
Tie		
Fastening: buttons/hooks/zips		

Examinations and Investigations

OCCUPATIONAL THERAPY DEPARTMENT—ASSESSMENT FORM 2

NAME... R/L HANDED...............

MANUAL DEXTERITY	Pre-operative date		Post-operative date	
	Right handed	Left handed	Right handed	Left handed
Dexterity board, replace 12/24 pegs				
Match from box and strike it				
Thread 12 washers on rod				
Screw lid off and on jar				
Open and close safety pin				
Pick 12 pins up and stick in cushion				
Fold and envelope letter				
Open letter				
Manage book and turn pages				
Turn newspaper inside out				
Take 3 coins from purse/pocket				
Turn door handle, knob, lever				
Insert door key and turn lock				
Ability to use scissors				

A severe headache may develop after a lumbar puncture, which can be relieved by elevating the foot of the bed for several hours when no physiotherapy treatment is given.

2. X-ray

Plain films of the skull are usually necessary and can be supplemented by special views of various areas. A note is made of any intracranial calcification and possible displacement of a calcified pineal body. General X-ray examination may be indicated and chest X-rays are always taken.

3. Echo-encephalography

By means of ultrasonic waves echoes from midline structures can be obtained and mass lesions causing displacements can be detected easily and safely and may serve to indicate the need for further appropriate investigations.

4. Lumbar Air Encephalography

Small quantities of air are injected after lumbar puncture with the patient seated erect. Films are taken with the patient successively erect, supine and prone. The whole ventricular system, the basal cisterns and the sub-arachnoid spaces are displayed showing any displacements or deformities, thus accurately indicating the site of any lesions. Nursing care and physiotherapy treatment are the same as following lumbar puncture.

5. Ventriculography

A burr hole is drilled in the skull allowing insertion of a needle into a lateral ventricle. Myodil, a radio-opaque solution, or air, is then introduced and manoeuvred into the third and fourth ventricles. This procedure is often used to demonstrate lesions in the posterior fossa, and is a routine measure during stereotaxic surgery, when it is used to outline appropriate cerebral landmarks. This allows accurate measurements necessary for the introduction of electrodes into chosen positions. Nursing care and physiotherapy treatment are as previously described.

6. Cerebral Angiography

This is an extremely important procedure, which is usually carried out under a general anaesthetic. Injections of radio-opaque solutions into the carotid or vertebral arteries are followed by taking films of the arterial, capillary and venous phases of the circulation. Displacement of the blood vessels shows the site of intracranial masses such as clot, tumours, abscesses or cysts. In a proportion of tumour cases, the circulation of the tumour itself may also be seen and may give an accurate assessment of its pathological type.

Angiography is of great value in cerebral vascular disease. The site of arterial stenosis or occlusion is easily seen. In spontaneous intracranial haemorrhage the site of an aneurysm or arteriovenous anomaly can only be determined by angiography. Post-operative angiography is a useful means of checking the efficiency of surgical treatment of aneurysms and anomalies.

Indirect methods of angiography are now more frequently used. A catheter is inserted into the femoral or axillary artery and its tip passed into the aortic arch. Large quantities of contrast medium injected under pressure allows the display of all major cerebral arteries.

Following angiography the patient is nursed flat for twenty-four hours, then allowed to sit up and get out of bed if no headache is present. Physio-therapy treatment consists of breathing exercises and maintenance exercises. If the femoral or axillary artery have been used, care must be taken to ensure that the patient maintains full range hip or shoulder joint movement.

(*See* new note on **Radio-isotope Encephalography**, p. 236.)

ELECTRO-ENCEPHALOGRAPHY

The electro-encephalograph amplifies and records the electrical activity of the brain, but it can only give a measure of the extent of the disorder of brain function. No abnormal E.E.G. pattern is specific to the disease which produces it, thus interpretation of records requires an appreciation of the clinical problems involved and close liaison between the interpreter and the clinician. An E.E.G. can be recorded within forty-five minutes, with no danger or discomfort to the patient.

Many problems exist which E.E.G. cannot at present solve, however there are groups of cases in which it can be of real value. It must be appreciated that E.E.G. does not give a definitive diagnosis, but merely provides information which is of help in the final clinical evaluation of any particular case. Some of the useful applications to surgical neurology are:

1. The screening of out-patients, particularly those suffering from head-aches and bizarre psychiatric symptoms. An unsuspected organic lesion in a silent area of the brain may be divulged which can then be dealt with surgically.

2. To help to distinguish between cerebral tumours and cerebro-vascular accidents. In the former the E.E.G. abnormality is usually out of proportion to the clinical signs, the reverse being the case in cerebro-vascular accidents.

3. To provide positive evidence of a sub-dural haematoma.

4. In order to select those patients with intractable epilepsy who may be helped by surgical excision of a part of the brain. Such patients are those with essentially normal E.E.G.s, who show a defined focus of abnormality in an area of the brain which it is possible to remove surgically.

5. Electro-corticography, the recording from the exposed brain at operation, may help particularly in cases of epilepsy, to decide which areas are abnormal and responsible for the patient's fits.

Surgical Neurology I

GENERAL SIGNS AND SYMPTOMS OF CEREBRAL LESIONS

RAISED INTRACRANIAL PRESSURE

Intracranial pressure depends upon the volume of the skull contents. In a child under the age of eighteen months, any slow increase in volume will result in an increase in the size of the head. In individuals over the age of eighteen months there is no increase in the size of the head, thus the effects of raised intracranial pressure will produce a disturbance of cerebral function more rapidly. Increased volume may be caused by a space occupying lesion, such as a tumour or abscess, a blockage in the cerebrospinal fluid pathways or by haemorrhage from an aneurysm.

SYMPTOMS OF RAISED INTRACRANIAL PRESSURE

With raised intracranial pressure the soft walled veins become compressed, giving rise to oedema and subsequent lack of oxygen to the brain tissue, the symptoms vary with the degree of raised pressure. The most common factors arising are as follows:

1. Headache

This is probably due to abnormal tensions in the cerebral blood vessels. In the early stages this may be paroxysmal, occurring during the night and early morning, with continued increase in pressure it becomes continuous and is intensified by exertion, coughing and stooping. The headache usually becomes worse when the patient is lying down and is relieved when sitting up.

2. Papilloedema

This is oedema of the optic discs which can cause enlargement of the blind spot and subsequent deterioration of visual acuity and complete blindness.

3. Vomiting

This occurs when the headache is most severe and tends to be projectile in nature.

4. Pulse and blood pressure

Acute and sub-acute rises in pressure cause a slowing of the pulse rate, but if pressure continues to rise the pulse rate becomes very rapid. A rapid increase in intracranial pressure causes a rise in the blood pressure but a chronic rise does not affect it, and in some lesions below the tentorium cerebelli the blood pressure is below normal.

5. Respiratory rate

This is not affected by a slow rise in pressure but a sufficiently rapid increase in pressure which produces a loss of consciousness, usually results in slow deep respirations. This may change after a period and become irregular of the Cheyne Stoke type.

6. Mental symptoms

These can vary from confusion and disorientation to complete loss of consciousness.

7. Epileptic convulsions

Generalized fits may occur but it is not clear whether these are caused by the raised intracranial pressure or by the actual lesion itself.

EYE SYMPTOMS

It is essential to realize that eye symptoms are often present with a brain lesion and they can directly affect a patient's capabilities during his rehabilitation. Among those most commonly found are:

1. *Damage to the optic nerve, optic chiasma or optic tracts* which cause field defects. (See Fig. 31, p. 197.)

2. *Damage to the third cranial nerve* can cause a ptosis, an inability to open the eye.

3. *Nystagmus.* This is frequently present in cerebellar or brain stem lesions and is an involuntary jerky movement of the eyes.

4. *Diplopia or double vision.* This is present if there is any imbalance of the eye muscles and can be overcome by covering alternate eyes on alternate days until the imbalance adjusts itself.

EAR SYMPTOMS

Deafness may be caused by tumours of the eighth cranial nerve such as acoustic neurinomas; these tumours may give rise to vertigo.

SPEECH DISORDERS

These have already been briefly mentioned in relation to the role of the speech therapist. They are mainly associated with lesions of the temporal lobe on the dominant side.

THE LEVEL OF CONSCIOUSNESS

Numerous factors can be responsible for alteration in the level of consciousness. Several of the factors are as follows:

1. Certain types of trauma producing a craniocerebral injury.
2. Space occupying masses causing increased intracranial pressure.
3. Operational trauma.
4. Post-operative complications such as oedema or haemorrhage.

The following are a guide to assessing the patient's conscious level:

1. The patient is fully conscious.
2. The patient is disorientated to time and space but can answer questions.
3. The patient can obey commands but cannot answer.
4. The patient responds to painful stimuli but not to the spoken word.
5. The patient is completely unresponsive.

To accurately assess the patient's conscious level any disturbance of hearing, vision and speech function must always be taken into account, and suitable measures taken to ensure the patient is given every opportunity to understand what is expected of him.

CRANIAL SURGERY

Conditions which may be improved with surgery are as follows:

1. Cerebral trauma—craniocerebral (head) injuries.
2. Cerebrovascular disease.
    (A) Haemorrhagic lesions
        (a) intracranial aneurysms.
        (b) intracranial angiomatous malformations (arteriovenous anomalies).
    (B) Ischaemic lesions
        (a) Carotid artery stenosis.
3. Cerebral infections—intracranial abscesses.
4. Neoplastic lesions.
        (a) cerebral tumours.
        (b) cerebellar tumours.
        (c) acoustic neurinomas.

5. Dyskinesias—Parkinsonism.

6. Hydrocephalus.

7. Epilepsy.

The preparation of a patient for a cranial operation is extremely important. In the majority of operations involving the brain, the hair must be totally removed and the scalp carefully prepared. The female patient may require reassurance if she becomes distressed at the prospect. Most operations are performed under general anaesthetic and take a considerable period of time to complete. During the course of surgery a bone flap may be turned back, but this is usually replaced at the end of the operation.

Post-operative Treatment

On return from theatre the patient will have a pressure bandage on the head to control swelling; this may be extended to include the eye on the side corresponding to the operational site, for the same purpose. Eyes are very vulnerable to swelling and do so as a result of operational trauma, the position of the patient on the operating table may also be a contributory factor, hence for the first two or three post-operative days the patient may be unable to open either eye. Any intravenous infusion set up in theatre may be continued for the first post-operative day.

Care must be taken to restrain a restless, confused patient, as he may attempt to remove head dressings, which will allow easy access of infection and meningitis may result. Padding and bandages on the hands, which may need to be tied down, reduces this danger. Cot sides should be attached to the bed in the early post-operative phase. It is important to replace hand bandages and cot sides after any treatment.

A Bone Flap. This may be removed if the brain is very swollen during operation, or if the skull is splintered as a result of a head injury. Replacement of this flap is advisable once oedema has subsided, as the patient tends to suffer from headache, dizziness when stooping and is afraid of damage from a bump to the area. Following head injury the bone may be so badly damaged it has to be discarded, the defect is then filled with plastic material.

When bone has been removed the patient is not nursed on the affected side until he shows signs of recovery of his conscious level. The young active male patient who is once more ambulant may be provided with a protective metal plate inside a cap to prevent further trauma, until the defect is repaired.

Ventricular drainage. The patient may return from theatre with ventricular drainage if there are signs of blocked cerebrospinal fluid pathways at operation. A catheter is introduced into a lateral ventricle by means of a burr hole in the skull and the cerebrospinal fluid drained into a flask; the height of the flask is dependent upon the pressure of the cerebrospinal fluid. Care should be taken when treating the patient to ensure that the level of the head is not altered in relation to the flask as this alters the drainage pressure.

If the doctor's permission has been given for postural drainage the height of the flask must be adjusted as the bed is tipped and re-adjusted on its return to the horizontal, this being done under medical supervision.

Lumbar drainage. This may be set up several days post-operatively if there are signs of a continued raised intracranial pressure. The needle is placed as for a lumbar puncture and rubber tubing connects it to a drainage flask the height of which is dependent upon the cerebrospinal fluid pressure. If the drainage is to be continuous the patient is nursed in side lying, well supported by pillows. Turning is done by lifting the patient from side to front, to his other side.

During the first few post-operative days intensive nursing care is required, the patient's condition being carefully observed and charted. Deterioration can occur very rapidly due to post-operative complications, any change must be reported immediately as it can be a matter of life and death.

COMPLICATIONS

Apart from the complications arising from brain damage the following may also arise:

1. A cerebrospinal fluid leak following the original operation, which may require further surgical repair.
2. Post-operative oedema, thrombosis or haemorrhage from cerebral blood vessels, occur in a small number of patients.
3. Thrombosis elsewhere and pulmonary embolus.
4. Epilepsy may develop after a variable period of time.
5. Respiratory complications are fairly common.

RESPIRATORY COMPLICATIONS

Post-operative oedema can cause pressure on the respiratory centre and the vagus nerves in the medulla oblongata, causing alteration in the respiratory rate and loss of the cough reflex, the ability to swallow may also be lost, thus there is a constant danger of aspiration of mucus and vomit. Until the ability to swallow returns the patient is artificially fed by means of a Ryle's tube passed down the nose into the stomach to prevent aspiration of food or fluids.

Dealing with chest complications following cranial surgery is made more difficult by postural drainage being contra-indicated immediately after operation, as it will cause an increase in intracranial pressure. Changes in blood pressure may also govern the position in which the patient must remain and it is imperative to check the patient's chart. If the patient has a raised blood pressure, his head may be elevated about 30 degrees in an attempt to control this, and he must remain in this position. Permission to begin postural drainage should therefore be obtained from the surgeon.

When the conscious level is disturbed one must constantly try to gain the patient's co-operation. Deep breathing must be encouraged and use of pressure on the sides of the chest when the patient breathes out is helpful. Clear orders to cough should be given accompanied by pressure of the hands on the sides of the chest as the patient breathes out. A demonstration of a cough by the physiotherapist can be helpful.

Suction

When a patient's conscious level is depressed, or he is conscious but incapable of coughing, suction may be necessary to remove secretions. Shaking, clapping and rib-springing help to loosen secretions. A patient who requires suction is most successfully treated by two people, a physiotherapist and a nurse or two physiotherapists, one using the suction apparatus while the other assists the patient with breathing and attempts to cough.

TRACHEOSTOMY

This may be necessary if the patient has carbon dioxide retention due to respiratory insufficiency, or a clear airway cannot be maintained by use of a mouth airway and suction. Tracheostomy is also required to deal with the hyper-secretions associated with mid-brain damage following a head injury.

The removal of secretions from a patient with a tracheostomy should be regarded as an aseptic technique, the physiotherapist masked and gowned and the hands well scrubbed before touching the suction catheters.

Chest work with a patient who has respiratory complications can be very time-consuming and it may take almost constant attention throughout the day, but it is well worth the time and effort. An 'on call' system for physiotherapists is necessary when a patient has respiratory complications, this allows the patient to have chest care at any time throughout a twenty-four hour period.

GENERAL PHYSIOTHERAPY TREATMENT

Aims

1. To prevent chest complications.
2. To maintain circulation.
3. To make any pertinent assessment of the patient.

Methods

1. The patient must be told that the anaesthetic may act as an irritant, causing the production of excess chest secretions. Breathing exercises are taught and he is told to practise them hourly before operation and as soon as he recovers from the anaesthetic. A check must be made on the patient's ability to cough. It should be tactfully suggested that smoking is cut down or stopped for a few days.

2. The patient must be told to keep his legs moving after operation to maintain his circulation. Maintenance exercises are then taught which he may practise before operation and at hourly intervals post-operatively. This minimizes the danger of deep venous thrombosis. Passive movements are substituted when the patient has a loss of voluntary power.

3. Assessment of voluntary power loss, degree of ataxia, and type of gait is carried out where the patient's condition allows.

These general principles apply to all conditions in this chapter and the following one; they are modified and adapted to the patient's specific needs. The physiotherapy treatment following each of the conditions listed will therefore be confined to specific points.

CRANIOCEREBRAL INJURIES

Two distinct mechanisms are recognized by which injury to brain tissue occurs. The first is when a large traumatizing object strikes the static head, accelerating it in space; the second, when the moving head strikes a fixed or relatively immobile object and becomes rapidly decelerated. Both mechanisms may produce damage to the scalp and fracture of the skull.

Mechanism 1

A traumatizing object of variable size, shape and weight delivered with a variable force strikes the static head. This group includes crush injuries, which are rare, bullet wounds and stab wounds.

Craniocerebral Injuries

The skull may remain intact following this type of injury, but structural damage to the underlying brain tissues may be severe.

When a fracture is produced it can cause stretching and tearing of cranial nerves with characteristic palsies, and of blood vessels, giving rise to complications such as extradural haemorrhage. Bony fragments may be depressed, with laceration of the dura and underlying brain. Small traumatizing objects impelled with great force may penetrate the cranial cavity carrying infection with them and causing extensive brain damage.

Mechanism 2 (See Fig. 32)

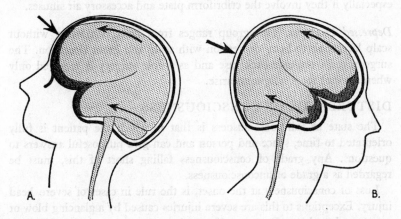

A.

B.

FIG. 32. DIAGRAM SHOWING THE MECHANISM OF A COUP CONTRECOUP INJURY

When the moving head strikes to a sufficient degree a fixed solid object a coup contrecoup injury results. The sudden impact causes:

(a) Compression distortion of the skull maximal at the site of the blow.

(b) Immediately at the opposite side the soft brain is thrust against the irregular promontories on the interior of the skull, producing contusion of the local cortex or haemorrhage within the region.

A fracture may be subadjacent to the site of the injury, or because of distortion, some distance from it.

The common source of brain injury is from rotational and linear acceleration forces, which occur when the head is suddenly accelerated or decelerated in space; these forces determine direct injury to the brain and its superficial blood vessels. Of greater significance, is the indirect injury to important basal brain structures, the hypothalamus, basal ganglia and

213

stretching of the perforating branches from the circulus arteriosus which affects the conscious level.

Complications likely to arise are subdural and intracerebral haematoma and contusional brain swelling.

SKULL FRACTURES

Linear Fractures. These are of little consequence in themselves apart from the concomitant brain injury.

Compound Linear Fractures. These allow a means of entry for infection, especially if they involve the cribriform plate and accessory air sinuses.

Depressed Fractures. This group ranges from bony depression without scalp laceration to bony depression with scalp and brain laceration. The surgeon must evaluate each case and as a rule surgery is required only when obvious focal symptoms arise.

DISTURBANCE OF CONSCIOUSNESS

The state of full consciousness is that in which the patient is fully orientated to time, space and person and can give purposeful answers to questions. Any grade of consciousness falling short of this, must be regarded as a grade of unconsciousness.

Loss of consciousness at the onset, is the rule in cases of severe head injury. Exceptions to this are severe injuries caused by a glancing blow or a penetrating object. Recovery of conscious state occurs in the following sequences:

1. Complete paralysis of cerebral function, which may extend momentarily to the vital centres.
2. Pulse and respiration having returned, there is a flaccid paralysis and absence of reflex action.
3. Reflex function returns. The patient may respond to command.
4. Voluntary movement and speech return without control or direction. The patient is confused, restless and often violent. Gradually he quietens but confusion persists.
5. Automatism. The patient will respond naturally to simple questions and perform accustomed actions in an orderly effective manner. He is still dazed and imperfectly aware of his surroundings.

Return of cerebral function thus begins at the lowest level, highest functions being last to recover. The process of recovery whether rapid or slow is always gradual.

DEGREES OF INJURY

1. Slight

(*a*) The patient is slightly concussed for a period then fully recovers. A period of complete amnesia exists both of the injury and subsequent events to the moment of recovery.

(*b*) There is a complete loss of consciousness for a few minutes followed by a rapid return of consciousness often with amnesia of events immediately preceding injury and for a period afterwards.

2. Moderate

This group includes those who do not recover consciousness within five minutes of injury but begin to do so within two or three hours. No focal signs are usually present.

3. Severe

In this group no recovery of consciousness takes place within two or three hours of injury. Focal signs may be present.

MANAGEMENT OF CRANIOCEREBRAL INJURIES

Any patient admitted to hospital as a result of head injury falls into one of three categories:

1. The patient who was not unconscious.
2. The patient who was unconscious for varying intervals of time.
3. The patient who is unconscious.

1. The patient who was not unconscious

A scalp laceration may be present which requires appropriate care and a thorough neurological examination is necessary. Few in this group require hospitalization; they are regarded as individuals with potential brain injury. If sent home their general practitioner should be informed in case of any deterioration in their condition.

2. The patient who was unconscious

A careful assessment must be made of the patient's mental state, details obtained of the nature of the injury, and the extent of the loss of consciousness. Thorough physical and neurological examinations are carried out and the results recorded; this group may later develop signs and symptoms of extradural or subdural haemorrhage. Hospitalization for observation is advisable as these complications may require emergency surgery.

3. The patient who is unconscious

(*a*) A clear airway must be ensured and the head turned to the side to prevent the tongue from obstructing respiration and mucus and vomit removed by suction. A mouth airway or tracheostomy may be life-saving measures.

(*b*) Shock caused by severe blood loss is combated by transfusion of blood or plasma.

(*c*) Examination follows to assess any serious damage apart from the head injury followed by a detailed neurological examination.

SURGICAL TREATMENT

Indications for surgery are:

1. Extradural haemorrhage.
2. Subdural haematoma.
3. Intracerebral haematoma.
4. Penetrating wounds.

It must be remembered that a patient with a severe head injury whether treated surgically or conservatively still presents essentially the same problem for the physiotherapist.

TREATMENT OF THE UNCONSCIOUS PATIENT

Careful nursing care is of paramount importance. The patient's charts must be marked up at fifteen-minute intervals for the first two to three days in case of any deterioration. Two-hourly turning and at least daily bathing is essential to prevent pressure sores developing.

The patient is artificially fed if unable to swallow; this minimizes the danger of aspiration. The position of the patient is important, nursing on the back is contra-indicated as the tongue tends to fall back and block the airway. Side lying is thus chosen, the patient is placed on his side with the underneath leg straight, the top leg flexed at hip and knee and supported by two pillows and a pillow behind the back. The top arm is supported on the pillow behind the back.

The three-quarter prone position is helpful for draining chest secretions and may be used as a nursing position if the patient remains unconscious for any length of time. Care should be taken to see that the underneath shoulder is in a comfortable position when the patient is lying on his side as painful shoulder joints can occur from bad positioning.

Pillow packs are used if the skin shows any sign of breaking down as they serve to remove pressure entirely from pressure points at the shoulder and hip.

PHYSIOTHERAPY TREATMENT

1. Breathing exercises, clapping, shaking and rib-springing and suction when necessary as described in the section on respiratory complications. Once the acute danger is passed it is still important to continue to check the patient's breathing at each treatment.

2. Passive movements are carried out twice daily to maintain the circulation and the nurses are taught to do full-range movements when turning the patient. These are continued until the patient's conscious level improves and he can take over active movement.

3. Passive movements and careful positioning prevent contractures developing. A patient may remain unconscious from a matter of days to months depending upon the severity of brain damage. The prognosis is bad if a patient shows no significant improvement in his conscious state after a six-month period.

SPASM

This can be a very troublesome entity during the period of depressed consciousness especially if the brain stem has been damaged which gives rise to decerebrate rigidity unilaterally or bilaterally depending upon the extent of the injury. Gentle passive movements can be done in a range which does not distress the patient. It has been found that as the conscious level improves the rigidity abates, usually with minimal loss of joint mobility, which can rapidly be regained by intensive physiotherapy directed to this means.

Spasm can develop at any time in hemiparetic limbs, certain spasm inhibiting positions are useful for providing a temporary relief, application of 'cold' gives longer periods of relief. Wet ice can be used safely in the majority of cases and is applied over the whole of the spastic muscle, giving immediate relief of spasm. The wet ice can be left in contact with the muscle for two to three minutes. Several applications may be necessary to gain maximum relief. Re-education can take place while the ice is being used.

As the patient's conscious level improves the physiotherapist must use her initiative to gain some measure of co-operation, even for a brief period. The patient is allowed to get up as soon as his general condition will allow. The ideal of treatment is as follows:

PROGRESSION OF TREATMENT

1. From passive movements the patient is graduated to active exercises as his conscious level improves. Facilitation techniques are used to initiate

contraction where muscle weakness exists and to aid swallowing. Short treatments several times a day prevent the patient becoming over-fatigued and allows maximum co-operation as he can only concentrate for a short period. Each treatment can be directed towards a different aim:

(a) Re-education of muscle weakness.

(b) Re-education of functional activities in bed such as rolling from side to side to help the patient to turn in bed. Hip-raising, so that he can use a bed-pan. Sitting up in bed and being able to maintain this position thus beginning balance re-education. Moving up or down the bed in a sitting position to enable him to alter his position.

Once he has regained his ability to swallow, the patient may need to be taught how to feed himself. When he is allowed to get up balance re-education can continue in sitting over the edge of the bed with the feet supported progressing to balance when sitting in a chair, then standing. He should be taught to dress himself at this stage.

Mat work

2. Functional re-education can continue on the mat. Rolling can be progressed to rolling from side to front to the other side. Sitting up from lying down and moving up and down and from side to side on the mat, using the arms to lift the buttocks off the mat. From prone lying practice in getting to the hands and knees position, sitting over from side to side and practice in crawling in all directions. From the hands and knees attaining the kneeling positions then half kneeling and from this position to sitting on a chair, then from a chair to half kneeling. From half kneeling the patient can also be taught to stand up and to kneel down again and lie down. From sitting on a chair he can be taught to stand up and sit down again.

Practice in standing up and sitting down is first started with the patient sitting on a chair facing the wall bars and using these for support to pull himself upright and to steady himself when sitting down. When he can do this successfully he can progress to standing up and sitting down between the parallel bars and also walking between the bars.

3. Walking re-education. In the early stages two physiotherapists may be required to support the patient at either side, the patient thrusting down with his arms against the resistance of the physiotherapists. Progress can be made by the patient using the parallel bars for support. If a hemiparesis exists a walking aid may be necessary in the form of a tripod or walking stick. All walking re-education is aimed towards the patient being able to walk independently with or without a walking aid depending upon his disabilities.

Stairs. Once standing balance has improved and the re-education of walking is progressing satisfactorily the patient must be re-educated in going up and down stairs.

4. Class work is useful when the patient is allowed to remain out of bed for longer periods. The presence of other patients in the class acts as a stimulus and with help from the physiotherapist he can join in the activities. Progressively less help is required and the patient will gradually be able to co-operate more fully. Occupational therapy treatment begins about this stage with simple activities and is gradually progressed.

From a practical point of view this outline of treatment has to be modified to the patient's capabilities. A patient who is slow to regain his conscious state may be allowed to sit up in a chair while still drowsy and confused. His treatment will have been directed towards the re-education of muscle weakness and functional activities as previously described but balance re-education taught as a specific entity does not meet with much success. Therefore, once he is allowed to get out of bed, and sit in a chair attempts should be made to stand him up, progressing rapidly to walking.

Walking re-education

(*a*) For the heavy patient it may be easier in the early stages for two physiotherapists to support the patient by having his arms round their shoulders. As the patient improves support can be given on either side, by the patient pushing down into the physiotherapist's hand.

(*b*) For a lighter patient one physiotherapist can support the patient from behind and transfer his weight from side to side as he walks while another physiotherapist kneels in front of the patient and assists in lifting his legs forward and blocking his knees. Assistance is reduced as soon as the patient begins to take over actively.

Practice in standing up and sitting down using the wall bars previously described.

Mat work can begin when the patient's condition allows and continues with the re-education of functional activities as previously described.

INTRACRANIAL ANEURYSMS

Intracranial aneurysms are balloon-like dilatations occurring at the bifurcation of vessels in the circulus arteriosus. The precipitating cause is thought to be a defect in the wall of the blood vessel of congenital origin. Aneurysms are also associated with arteriosclerosis and hypertension. The size varies from a pea to a plum and multiple aneurysms may be present.

Age groups most affected are individuals between thirty and fifty years of age.

Rupture of an aneurysm is the most common cause of spontaneous sub-arachnoid haemorrhage. Signs and symptoms from such a haemorrhage naturally depend on the severity and site of the bleeding. A minor leak from an aneurysm gives sudden severe neck pain, the pain then radiates up over the head and settles to a generalized headache and stiffness of the neck. Severe haemorrhage will cause increased intracranial pressure and loss of consciousness with various neurological deficiencies, depending upon the degree of damage from the haemorrhage.

Investigations to establish the diagnosis are:

1. *Lumbar puncture,* to establish the presence of blood in the cerebro-spinal fluid.
2. *Angiography,* to determine the exact site of the aneurysm.

SURGICAL TREATMENT

Unless an attempt is made surgically to deal with the aneurysm there is a constant danger of further haemorrhage which can be fatal.

To obtain a satisfactory result operative procedure is undertaken only if the patient is conscious and showing improvement from any neuro-logical deficits arising from the initial bleeding. All procedures are directed towards occluding the aneurysm:

1. By use of clips.
2. By a clip and wrapping the aneurysm in muslin gauze or muscle.
3. By clipping the feeding vessel intracranially to reduce the force of blood entering the aneurysm.

PHYSIOTHERAPY TREATMENT

1. Breathing exercises and teaching the patient to cough. If the level of consciousness is depressed suction may be necessary to remove secretions.

2. Passive movements if there are motor deficiencies.

3. Strengthening and maintenance of all muscles which are active and facilitation techniques to re-educate weak muscles.

If no complications occur as a result of operation the patient will be allowed to get out of bed approximately on the fifth day. Prior to getting up the head of the bed is slowly elevated until the patient can tolerate sitting up.

4. Balance re-education begins with the patient sitting on the edge of the bed with his feet supported. His blood pressure may require checking—a

significant rise or fall will necessitate his return to bed, otherwise he can progress to balance in standing, a short walk then return to bed.

5. Walking re-education will require minimum attention if no motor deficiencies were present after surgery. If a hemiparesis does exist re-education will be necessary.

Progression of Treatment

1. The patient is allowed up for progressively longer periods and gradually takes over his own personal care such as bathing, dressing, and going to the toilet.

2. His rehabilitation programme in both physiotherapy and occupational therapy departments is increased until he can cope with a full programme without undue fatigue, and demonstrate his ability to live independently.

Complications

Those most likely to occur are:

1. Further bleeding from the aneurysm while the surgeon is attempting to obliterate it. This may lead to further damage to the brain with a resultant increase in neurological defects.

2. Traction upon blood vessels in the field of surgery causing ischaemia of the brain area they supply, which may be severe enough to give rise to defects.

3. Oedema and thrombosis following surgery which may be severe enough to disturb the conscious level. These post-operative complications manifest themselves forty-eight hours after surgery and can completely alter the patient's prognosis.

The rehabilitation of a patient suffering from these complications may be:

1. As for the unconscious patient, or

2. as for a patient with hemiplegia or hemiparesis.

THE HEMIPLEGIC PATIENT

A complete loss of voluntary power or a partial loss which comprises a hemiparesis may be accompanied by:

(*a*) a sensory loss;

(*b*) a hemianopia;

(*c*) a speech defect with a right-sided voluntary power loss.

PHYSIOTHERAPY TREATMENT

1. Passive movements to the affected limbs to maintain full range joint

mobility. The patient is taught to do his own passive movements, which he must practise regularly.

2. Facilitation techniques to initiate contraction of the muscles of the hemiplegic limbs. After this has been achieved progressive development of muscle strength, range and co-ordination follows.

3. Functional activities and general strengthening exercises in bed.

4. Balance re-education in sitting when the patient is allowed to get up.

5. Walking re-education with the aid of two people in the initial stages progressing to one person and a tripod or walking stick as soon as possible. If the patient has a dropped foot when walking, a temporary toe raising spring may be necessary at first. A severe loss of voluntary power may make it necessary to have a caliper fitted for this purpose.

6. Stepping up and down from a step using the wall bars to steady the patient in the early stages, progressing to going up and down stairs which helps to strengthen weak leg muscles.

Progression of Treatment

As the patient is allowed up for longer periods his programme of treatment includes occupational therapy and he joins a class for general physiotherapy treatment which helps to retrain balance and strengthen the general musculature. It also serves to stimulate his interest in other people and helps him adjust to his disability.

Mat work is included as described for the rehabilitation of the unconscious patient, but more attention is devoted to balance re-education; the patient is placed in the various positions and balance re-education is given in each position.

LIGATION OF THE COMMON CAROTID ARTERY

This is carried out when certain aneurysms are difficult to approach by a direct method and only if the patient is neurologically intact, or nearly so. If there is an adequate cross circulation in the brain, the vessel is ligated in the neck under local anaesthetic. If cross circulation is not adequate a clamp is put on the vessel and the vessel occluded over a period of forty-eight hours, then finally ligated.

POST-OPERATIVE TREATMENT

The patient is nursed lying flat on the back with a thin pillow under the head and sandbags at either side to stop head movements. A constant check is kept on the blood pressure, pulse rate, conscious level, motor power and the reaction of the pupils to light, in case the patient's condition shows signs of deterioration

Forty-eight hours after occlusion of the artery the patient can be gradually elevated in bed. Side lying is allowed approximately on the third day. To minimize the risk of any thrombus formation (at the site of ligation) breaking off during turning, the patient holds his head in his hands, so effectively reducing neck movement.

The patient is allowed to get out of bed approximately on the seventh day. Prior to getting up he must be able to tolerate sitting erect in bed. His blood pressure must be checked before he is allowed to sit over the edge of the bed, when he achieves this position and when he returns to bed after being up. Any significant drop in blood pressure necessitates return to bed.

PHYSIOTHERAPY TREATMENT

The patient must be treated gently, to disturb him as little as possible; maintenance exercises which are practised hourly should be reduced to foot movements and static muscle contractions of the leg, abdominal and back muscles.

When the patient is ready to get up, balance re-education may be required in sitting up, then in standing, followed by walking.

Progression of Treatment

The patient is allowed to:

(a) get up and sit in a chair for increasing periods of time;

(b) walk increasing distances;

(c) go up and down stairs.

All progressions must be gently regulated, warning being given to the patient to change his position slowly as a rapid change causes dizziness; thus he must take his time when getting out of bed, standing up or turning round.

His stay in hospital is usually short and on discharge home he is instructed to continue with the slow, gradual resumption of normal activities.

INTRACRANIAL ANGIOMATOUS MALFORMATIONS (ARTERIOVENOUS ANOMALIES)

These malformations are congenital abnormalities of vascular development and occur on the surface of the brain or within the brain tissue, deriving a blood supply from one or both hemispheres, usually found in the younger age groups including children. Most of the lesions are arteriovenous malformations. The blood vessels of the malformation show degeneration of their walls, and direct communication between arteries and veins in some areas. If the malformation is small no diversion of blood from the capillary bed occurs, but a large one robs the brain of its blood supply.

SIGNS AND SYMPTOMS

These are variable but the following may occur:

1. Headaches of a migranous character.
2. Focal epilepsy.
3. Subarachnoid haemorrhage.
4. A spastic monoparesis or hemiparesis together with a sensory or visual loss.

INVESTIGATIONS

1. *Electroencephalography* may be used for diagnosing the cause of headaches and epilepsy.
2. *Angiography* will serve to display the malformation.

SURGICAL TREATMENT

A direct intracranial approach is made and the lesion excised (if it lies on the surface). Sometimes very complex lesions may be treated by occlusion of the feeding vessels.

PHYSIOTHERAPY TREATMENT

This follows the same course as previously described for aneurysms.

CAROTID ARTERY OCCLUSION

Arteriosclerosis with thrombus formation is the usual cause of common and internal carotid artery occlusion. The site of occlusion is most frequently at the origin of the internal carotid artery, occlusion may be complete or incomplete. The disease may be:

(a) of the ischaemic type, which cuts off the blood supply to the involved cerebral hemisphere. Any blood reaching the hemisphere is dependent upon a collateral circulation from the opposite side.

(b) of the multiple emboli type which continually shoots off small emboli from the site of the occlusion. Anticoagulants such as Dindevan and heparin are necessary for the management of this type.

SIGNS AND SYMPTOMS

A wide variety of symptoms and modes of onset can be produced by carotid artery occlusion.

1. *Hemiplegia*

(a) This may be profound and occurs suddenly, loss of consciousness usually accompanies this type of onset.

(b) Hemiparesis progressing to a hemiplegia.

(*c*) Transient motor weakness ('stuttering') usually affecting one extremity.

2. *Dysphasia, Sensory loss and various eye symptoms* are associated in some degree with the loss of voluntary power.

3. *Headache* behind the eye is often present.

Investigations

Angiography. By this means any occlusion is immediately revealed.

SURGICAL TREATMENT

In carefully selected cases surgery is of great value; contra-indications are:

1. Gross arteriosclerotic involvement of other cerebral vessels.
2. Loss of consciousness with the onset of symptoms carries a poor prognosis.

Surgical measures aim to:

(*a*) restore the normal blood flow;
(*b*) prevent further progression of the disease.

Endarterectomy

The arteriosclerotic portion of the artery and any thrombus is removed. If the arteriosclerotic area is too extensive a by-pass arterial graft is done.

PHYSIOTHERAPY TREATMENT

1. Immediate measures are required for the re-education of the hemiplegic limbs. Bearing in mind the likely sensory loss and field defects of the eyes the patient must be constantly reminded of the affected limbs. The position of the affected limbs should be checked regularly to reduce danger of

(*a*) damage to joints;
(*b*) circulatory obstruction.

Passive movements and facilitation techniques should be used to re-educate the affected muscles and the patient must be able to watch his limbs.

2. Balance and re-education in sitting aided by use of a mirror can begin when the patient is allowed to get up approximately between the fifth and seventh day.

3. Walking re-education is also aided by use of a mirror.

4. During mat work the patient must first be taught to adjust the position of his affected arm and leg before rolling and similar activities.

5. When sitting in a chair he must constantly be reminded to check the

position of his limbs. When walking unaided he must also be taught constantly to check that his foot is not catching on objects in his path and that he allows ample clearance going through doorways and when walking near a wall.

INTRACRANIAL ABSCESS

Infection causing an intracranial abscess can reach the brain by:

1. Spreading from a nearby source such as otitis media, mastoiditis or sinusitis.
2. Direct introduction from a stab wound which penetrates the skull.
3. Being blood borne from another source of infection in the body such as a lung abscess or chronic bronchitis.
4. From unknown sources.

The rate of growth of an abscess depends on the organism causing the infection. Many abscesses become encapsulated allowing the surgeon to drain them more easily or effect a complete removal.

SIGNS AND SYMPTOMS

These are very similar to those produced by cerebral tumours, that is headache and vomiting, but abscesses tend to give more intellectual upsets and the onset is more rapid; fever and meningitis also occur.

SURGICAL TREATMENT

(a) Complete removal where possible.

(b) Evacuation of pus from the abscess cavity. A drain is then inserted and antibiotics introduced. A check is kept on the size of the cavity by coating the walls with a radio-opaque solution and X-raying the area at two-day intervals.

Post-operative Treatment

The patient with an intracranial abscess is strictly barrier-nursed and not allowed to mix with other patients in the ward until the infection has been effectively controlled.

PHYSIOTHERAPY TREATMENT

The rate of progress will be governed by the patient's general condition. Any voluntary power loss will be re-educated by use of facilitation techniques.

A patient with no complications will be allowed to get up approximately

on the fifth post-operative day and can begin a full rehabilitation programme in the occupation and physiotherapy departments as soon as the
surgeon's permission is given.

INTRACRANIAL TUMOURS

Tumours found in and around the brain can be classified into:

1. *Primary Tumours*
   (a) Malignant of the glioma type. The malignancy of a tumour is
   judged upon its rate of growth and its tendency to infiltrate the brain
   tissue.
   (b) Benign, such as the meningiomas.
2. *Secondary Tumours*, which are blood-borne metastases from primary
tumours mainly in the lung and breast.

The rate of growth of a tumour is very variable depending on whether
it is malignant or benign. Tumours of the glioma type invade the brain
substance making complete removal difficult. Types like the meningioma
do not invade the brain, but present problems in view of their size and
extreme vascularity.

The location of a tumour is the most important factor irrespective of its
pathology, because it may involve the vital centres so directly threatening
the patient's life, or limiting surgical accessibility.

SIGNS AND SYMPTOMS

1. Some degree of raised intracranial pressure usually exists.
2. Focal signs develop pointing to the site of the tumour.

SURGICAL TREATMENT

1. This is undertaken where possible with a view to affecting a complete
removal of the tumour. Following an incomplete removal, the tumour may
recur. If the tumour is radio-sensitive a course of deep X-ray therapy will
follow surgery to shrink or destroy the remaining tumour cells, so increasing the patient's life expectancy.

2. Intrinsic tumours in the left tempero-parietal area are not usually
removed surgically as severe defects would result, namely dysphasia and
hemiplegia. Management may be as follows:
   (a) For a cystic type of tumour, the cyst is drained so relieving pressure
   in the area.
   (b) A minute part of the tumour is removed for biopsy, deep X-ray may
   then follow if the tumour is radio-sensitive, or injections of Epodyl
   which also destroys tumour cells.

(c) Bone can be removed to effect a decompression.

3. Tumours of the brain stem area are rare, but surgical intervention is often contra-indicated in view of the fatal damage which could result.

PHYSIOTHERAPY TREATMENT

A patient without complications is allowed to get up approximately the fifth day.

The patient with a hemiparesis or hemiplegia is treated as previously described.

CEREBELLAR TUMOURS

The majority of cerebellar tumours arise in or near the midline and may extend into one or both hemispheres, such as the medulloblastomas, astrocytomas, and are commoner in young people.

SIGNS AND SYMPTOMS

These differ considerably depending on the site of the tumour. The following occur in varying degrees:

1. Raised intracranial pressure.
2. Hypotonia.
3. Ataxia: this is probably most marked when the patient is walking. Ataxia is the result of the inability to stabilize the background activity essential for co-ordinated movement. Repeated movement tends to increase ataxia.
4. Giddiness.
5. Nystagmus.
6. Disturbance of function of some cranial nerves.
7. Sensory loss may occur but is the exception, not the rule.

SURGICAL TREATMENT

To excise this type of tumour a Cushing's cross-bow incision is used involving the arch of the atlas and a craniectomy of the occipital bone.

Post-operative Treatment

Due to (a) operative trauma, and (b) post-operative oedema, the ninth, tenth and eleventh cranial nerves may be temporarily out of action causing (1) loss of the cough reflex, (2) inability to swallow.

Nursing care is of importance. The patient must be nursed in side lying to prevent possible aspiration of vomit and mucus and artificially fed by Ryle's tube until he is able to swallow. This further reduces risk of aspiration of food or fluids.

PHYSIOTHERAPY TREATMENT

1. Breathing exercises must be practised by the patient. Suction may be necessary to remove secretions until the cough reflex returns. Even after return of the cough reflex suction may still be required, as the patient becomes quickly exhausted.

Other aims of treatment are:

(a) To strengthen the general musculature with particular attention to the neck muscles.

(b) To re-educate balance and co-ordination.

2. *Methods.* As the patient's condition improves post-operatively exercises can be given to strengthen the general musculature, particularly the back extensor muscles. Re-education of the neck muscles begins with static contractions approximately the seventh day and active exercises when sutures are removed about the tenth day.

3. Re-education of co-ordination begins in bed. The patient will find it easier to produce a co-ordinate movement against resistance, thus re-education can begin with

(a) resisted exercises for the ataxic limbs;

(b) holding a certain position against resistance from varying directions—this is termed stabilizing.

Balance re-education begins when the patient is allowed to get up usually between the fifth and seventh days. Balance is re-educated in sitting on the edge of the bed by means of the stabilizing technique already described.

Progression of Treatment

It must be emphasized that a patient with a cerebellar lesion fatigues quickly. He will probably have a history of vomiting for a variable period of time before operation leading to debility and dehydration. His programme of treatment in the physiotherapy and occupational therapy departments must be carefully graded to guard against exhaustion.

As his condition improves the following progressions will be made:

1. Mat work—as previously stated. Resisted exercises are more accurately carried out than free exercises, thus mat work begins with resisted activities such as rolling, hip raising. Stabilizing is done in each new position.

   Activities are progressed as previously described for mat work. Resisted crawling in all directions greatly helps balance and co-ordination.

2. Walking. Parallel bars and a mirror are of great value in the early

229

stages. Stabilizing in standing and resisted walking, walking forwards, backwards and sideways helps to regain the patient's self-confidence. Resistance against the head helps to steady a grossly ataxic patient.

If a walking aid is necessary to gain the patient's independence, elbow crutches or a reciprocal walking aid are more easily managed by the more ataxic patient. A stick may be adequate to support a less severely handicapped one.

ACOUSTIC NEURINOMA

This tumour arises from the sheath of the eighth cranial nerve.

Signs and symptoms

1. There is tinnitus at first then deafness as the tumour grows.
2. Vertigo is present.
3. A facial nerve lesion is produced as compression of the seventh nerve occurs.
4. Loss of (a) the corneal reflex, and (b) sensations of pain and temperature occur with compression of the fifth cranial nerve.
5. Ataxia of the limbs on the side of the tumour occurs with compression of the cerebellar hemisphere and cerebellar peduncles.

SURGICAL TREATMENT

The tumour can be completely excised which usually results in sacrificing the facial nerve.

Post-operative Treatment

The patient may have swallowing difficulties and loss of his cough reflex: this requires the same nursing care as for a cerebellar tumour. Because of the facial nerve palsy the patient will be unable to close his eye and an eye-glass is provided (a) to prevent damage to the cornea, and (b) to prevent infection. The nurse devotes special care to the eye until the patient's condition allows a tarsorrhaphy (this is a suturing together of the upper and lower lid). Vision of the eye is thus reduced which must be remembered during rehabilitation.

PHYSIOTHERAPY TREATMENT

1. Breathing exercises and attempts to cough. Suction may be necessary to remove secretions until the cough reflex has fully recovered. The patient practises his breathing exercises hourly.

2. The re-education of balance and co-ordination are as previously described for cerebellar ataxia. Progress can be more rapid as the patient does not fatigue so rapidly.

PARKINSONIAN SYNDROME

This syndrome results from lesions of the corpus striatum. The causes are:

1. Primary degeneration occurring mainly between fifty and sixty years of age. This condition is found more frequently in males.
2. Encephalitis lethargica develops in its chronic stage into Parkinsonism, affecting any age group and both sexes equally.
3. Cerebral arteriosclerosis can also produce this syndrome, occurring mainly in late middle and old age.

Parkinsonism is a progressive disease, the rate of progress being variable.

Signs and Symptoms

These may occur unilaterally or bilaterally and are as follows:

1. *Tremor*
   (*a*) occurring at rest and diminished by voluntary muscular effort.
   (*b*) aggravated by action;
   (*c*) a mixture of (*a*) and (*b*).

One or more limbs may be affected together with the face, eyelids, tongue, jaw and neck. Tremor is increased by tension, excitement and concentration. In company it is always worse and can be a great social nuisance.

2. *Rigidity*

This chiefly affects the limbs and is responsible for the loss of arm swinging when walking. In the face it appears as the classical mask with a fixed expression. The tongue, pharynx and vocal cords may be involved, causing speech impairment. Rigidity of the respiratory muscles predisposes the patient to complications of broncho-pneumonia.

3. Lack of initiation.
4. There may be difficulty in passing water or urgency of micturition.

Cases are selected for surgery usually with an upper age limit of sixty-five. A patient older than this is only considered if he is essentially unilaterally affected and has no physical or mental deterioration. The best results are obtained from the under sixty age group with a slowly progressive form of the disease.

Investigations and Assessments

1. X-ray. Plain films of the skull are taken.

2. Electro-encephalography.

3. Assessment by:

    (a) the pyschologist;

    (b) the speech therapist;

    (c) the occupational therapist;

    (d) the physiotherapist.

SURGICAL TREATMENT

Stereotaxic surgery is carried out under local anaesthetic in two stages, usually completed within the same day, or occasionally with a day of rest between.

The first stage consists of placing markers in the skull as a guide to the mid-sagittal plane of the brain.

The second stage consists of introducing Myodil into the lateral and third ventricle to outline the anterior and posterior commisures. An electrode is passed through an occipital burr hole to the thalamus. Coagulation is carried out in the ventro-lateral nucleus of the thalamus to reduce tremor and in the globus pallidus to reduce rigidity. (See Fig. 33.)

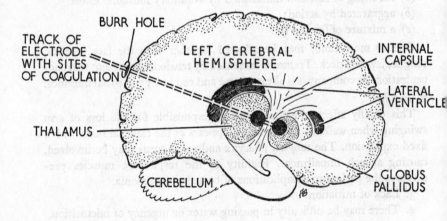

FIG. 33. DIAGRAM SHOWING POSITION OF BURR HOLE IN STEREOTAXIC SURGERY FOR PARKINSONISM

PHYSIOTHERAPY TREATMENT

1. Breathing exercises must be practised hourly by the patient to reduce the risk of broncho-pneumonia. Coughing may be difficult for the patient whose main symptom is rigidity.

2. The limbs freed from rigidity and tremor may require functional re-education. After loss of severe tremor the type of stabilizing exercises described for cerebellar ataxia help the patient to regain functional use of his limbs, particularly the upper one. Full range joint mobility is rapidly regained when symptoms have been relieved.

The patient is allowed to sit up in bed the day after operation and to get up the second post-operative day. Balance re-education is important for a patient with rigidity as the main symptom, and stabilization in sitting and standing is useful, the patient watching himself in a mirror. A patient with mainly tremor has little or no problem in regaining balance. Re-education of standing up and sitting down, walking, walking with arm swinging and turning round require patience and perseverance.

Standing up and sitting down especially if a low chair is being used is difficult for a Parkinsonian patient. He must be taught to tuck his feet well underneath him, then use his hands on the edge of the chair to push his weight forward over his feet then to straighten up. When sitting down he must be taught to feel for the chair and lower himself down gently.

Walking. To re-educate walking it must be impressed upon the patient to lift his feet and take a big step. Lifting the feet is over-emphasized at the outset, marking time on the spot prior to walking can be a useful preliminary followed by stepping over lines on the floor.

To re-educate arm-swinging while walking, poles are used, the patient holding one end of the pole in each hand, and the physiotherapist walking behind holding the other ends. Arm-swinging is done at first by the physiotherapist pushing the appropriate pole with the patient gradually taking over.

Turning. The great tendency is for the patient to jerk round suddenly when turning. He must be taught to do this slowly and lift his feet up. Re-education can begin with marking time on the spot, then turning round slowly still marking time.

Stairs. Apart from any difficulty with balance the Parkinsonian patient rarely has difficulty in going up or down stairs.

Progression of Treatment

Progress can be made rapidly in the physiotherapy and occupational therapy departments once the patient is allowed up. About the third day he will be able to participate in some class work to music to assist re-education of balance and mobility. The class work can be increased on successive days to a full programme which includes exercises in sitting, standing and on the mat. Mat work to retrain rolling, sitting up, standing up to lying down and vice versa and exercises on the mat to strengthen back extensor muscles are useful in that they help the patient regain his independence as he can then begin to move about in bed and get in and out of bed, activities which he will previously have found difficult.

INFANTILE HYDROCEPHALUS

This is an increase in the volume of the cerebrospinal fluid within the skull and is one of the congenital abnormalities found in babies. The increased volume of cerebrospinal fluid may be due to (*a*) an obstruction of the cerebrospinal fluid pathway, or (*b*) defects in the absorption mechanism.

Signs and Symptoms

1. Signs and symptoms of raised intracranial pressure.
2. Enlargement of the head. The anterior fontanelle bulges and the suture lines of the skull separate, scalp veins dilate, the eyeballs are displaced downwards.
3. Bizarre ocular movements occur.

HYDROCEPHALUS IN ADULTS

This can occur due to obstruction of the cerebrospinal fluid pathways; signs and symptoms are those of raised intracranial pressure.

SURGICAL TREATMENT

There are several methods of dealing with the problem, but the procedure which to date gives the most satisfactory result is drainage of the fluid from a ventricle to the right atrium of the heart, with a valve incorporated (see Fig. 34).

Physiotherapy Treatment

Only routine care is required.

EPILEPSY

Epilepsy can be described as a paroxysmal transitory disturbance of the functions of the brain which develops suddenly, ceases spontaneously, with a strong tendency to recurrence. Many varieties of epileptic attack exist, depending upon the site of origin, extent of spread and the nature of the disturbance of function.

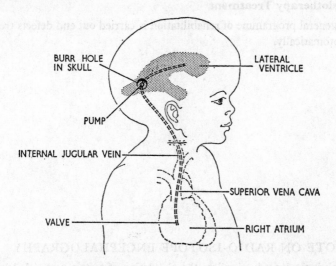

FIG. 34. THE DRAINAGE OF FLUID FROM A VENTRICLE TO THE RIGHT
ATRIUM OF THE HEART IN HYDROCEPHALUS

CAUSES

1. A local lesion in the brain, such as tumour or abscess, where epilepsy is the presenting feature.
2. Complication of a head injury due to a post traumatic scar.
3. Hereditary predisposition.
4. Unknown causes.

Investigations

1. *Electro-encephalography.* Recordings of the electrical activity of the brain can help to pinpoint the cause of epilepsy. If a focus can be determined, its nature can be investigated by other means.

2. Further appropriate measures: these will be selected according to the particular history of the patient.

SURGICAL TREATMENT

Surgery is only indicated for certain selected cases and is of value to a patient who has (*a*) epilepsy as the presenting feature of a brain lesion, or (*b*) a definite focus which gives rise to his epileptic attacks. Surgical procedures vary with the type of lesion to be excised. Temporal lobe epilepsy may be treated by lobectomy.

Physiotherapy Treatment

A general programme of rehabilitation is carried out and defects treated symptomatically.

A NOTE ON RADIO-ISOTOPE ENCEPHALOGRAPHY

This is the introduction into the circulation of certain materials labelled with radio-active isotopes, e.g. Mercury 197 and Technetium 99m. There is a selective uptake of these materials by most cerebral tumours and also to some extent by other cerebral lesions, e.g. infarcts, subdural haematomas, etc.

Scanning of the head by a suitable detection apparatus and recording the intensity and distribution of the radio-active material retained in the cerebrum and its coverings will locate most cerebral tumours accurately. The method is particularly effective with meningiomas and gliomas and can detect tumours 2 cm. in diameter upwards.

The method is safe, radiation dosage being less than with more conventional techniques and it sometimes enables more dangerous examinations, such as angiography and encephalography, to be dispensed with.

Physiotherapy treatment is unaffected by this procedure.

(For other **Special Investigations,** *see* pp. 198–205.)

Chapter XII

SURGICAL NEUROLOGY II

by M. C. BALFOUR, M.C.S.P.
Surgery of the Spinal Cord

ANATOMY AND PHYSIOLOGY

The spinal cord lies within the vertebral canal and extends from the foramen magnum to the lower border of the first lumbar vertebra. It is surrounded by meninges, as is the brain, and the cerebrospinal fluid circulates in the subarachnoid space between the pia mater and the arachnoid mater. This space descends as far as the second sacral vertebra. The blood supply is rich but complex and mainly derived from the posterior spinal arteries, the anterior spinal artery and segmental arteries which enter by the intervertebral foramina.

A pair of spinal nerves are given off at each segment of the cord but due to the cord being shorter than the vertebral canal the segments do not tally with the numerically corresponding vertebrae. In the cervical region the segments lie one vertebra higher, while in the lumbar region the fifth lumbar nerve root is given off at the level of the twelfth thoracic vertebra. The mass of lumbar and sacral nerve roots given off at the lower end of the spinal cord is termed the cauda equina (see Fig. 35).

Each nerve root consists of an anterior motor root and a posterior sensory root, which pass separately through the dura mater then unite. They then descend to the appropriate intervertebral foramen through which they issue. The course of these nerves is almost horizontal in the cervical region, but the lumbar nerves have a long vertical course before reaching their appropriate point of exit (see Fig. 35).

EFFECTS OF COMPRESSION ON THE SPINAL CORD

Any lesion in the region of the spinal cord which causes pressure affects the spinal cord and nerve roots in several ways:

237

1. Direct pressure interferes with conduction in the nerve roots and the spinal cord.
2. Pressure on the veins leads to oedema.
3. Pressure on the arteries leads to ischaemia.
4. Degeneration of nerve cells and fibres then takes place in the area.
5. The subarachnoid space becomes obstructed.

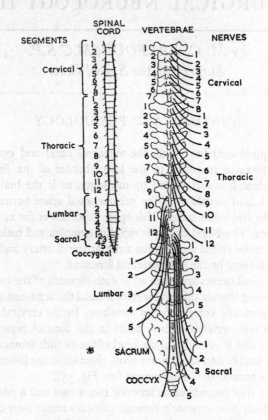

FIG. 35. DIAGRAM SHOWING SPINAL CORD AND SPINAL NERVES

Compression of the cord can occur anywhere throughout its length and affect one or several segments. The pressure may affect both sides if the lesion is central, or one side more than the other if the lesion is lateral· Pressure on one side of the cord can gradually displace the cord and the nerve roots towards the opposite side of the vertebral canal, thus involving the healthy side. Motor and sensory symptoms can arise on both sides of the body if the lesion is central but can give a Brown-Sequard type of syndrome if the lesion is confined to one side of the cord.

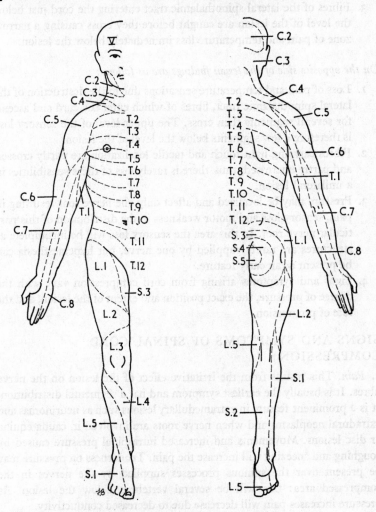

FIG. 36. DIAGRAM SHOWING THE INNERVATION OF THE SKIN

BROWN-SEQUARD SYNDROME

On the side of the lesion the following occur:

1. Loss of voluntary power due to the fact that the cerebrospinal tracts cross mainly in the medulla oblongata which lies well above the area of compression.

2. Loss of muscle and joint sense, vibratory sense and tactile discrimination due to involvement of the posterior column.
3. Fibres of the lateral spinothalamic tract entering the cord just below the level of the lesion are caught before they cross causing a narrow zone of pain and temperature loss immediately below the lesion.

On the opposite side of the lesion findings are as follows:

1. Loss of pain and temperature sensations due to the destruction of the lateral spinothalamic tract, fibres of which enter the cord and ascend for several segments then cross. The upper level of the sensory loss is therefore a few segments below the level of the lesion.
2. Fibres carrying light touch and tactile localization are partly crossed and partly uncrossed, thus there is rarely loss of these sensibilities in a unilateral lesion.
3. Pressure may be localized and affect only one nerve root resulting in pain, sensory loss and motor weakness in the distribution of this particular nerve root. In this area the sensory loss will be incomplete as structures are rarely supplied by one nerve, but hyperaesthesia can be present as an early feature.
4. Signs and symptoms arising from cord compression vary with the degree of pressure, the exact position and extent of the lesion, and the rate of progression.

SIGNS AND SYMPTOMS OF SPINAL CORD COMPRESSION

1. *Pain.* This results from the irritative effect of the lesion on the nerve fibres. It is usually the earliest symptom and has a segmental distribution. It is a prominent feature in extramedullary lesions such as neurinomas and extradural neoplasms and when nerve roots are involved in cauda equina or disc lesions. Movements and increased intraspinal pressure caused by coughing and sneezing will increase the pain. Tenderness on pressure may be present over the spinous processes supplied by the nerves in the compressed area: this will be several vertebrae below the lesion. As pressure increases pain will decrease due to decreased conductivity.

2. *Loss of motor power.* This usually follows the sensory disturbance and takes the form of a progressive weakness. The muscles affected are those supplied by the segments of the cord which are being compressed and those supplied by the segments below the lesion. If the lesion is unilateral the weakness is present on the same side of the body; with a central lesion both sides are involved, but one side is usually more affected than the other.

3. *Muscle tone.* At the level of the lesion, tone will be diminished or lost as this constitutes a lower motor neurone lesion. Below the level of the lesion there is an upper motor neurone lesion and tone will be increased as the pyramidal and extra pyramidal tracts are interrupted and the reflex arc is no longer inhibited by higher centres. In cauda equina lesions only a lower motor neurone lesion exists.

4. *Reflexes.* As with muscle tone reflexes are diminished at the level of the lesion and increased below the lesion.

5. *Sensation.* This is diminished or lost below the lesion. Types of sensation involved will depend upon the site of the lesion as previously described. Involvement of the posterior column will affect kinesthetic sensation, while the antero-lateral column will affect pain and temperature. In cauda equina lesions sensory loss of all types is likely in the root distribution.

6. *Sphincters.* These are not involved in the early stages but later precipitancy or difficulty with micturition develops and this may progress to retention of urine. Constipation is most usual with spinal neoplasms. Rectal incontinence rarely occurs.

7. *Autonomic disturbances.* Sweating does not occur below the level of the lesion. Vaso-motor disturbances occur resulting in impaired circulation.

8. *Cerebrospinal fluid.* If there is an obstruction of the subarachnoid space the chemical composition of this fluid changes. Its protein content is increased, which provides useful diagnostic information.

MODE OF ONSET

The onset of symptoms is usually gradual when due to a spinal neoplasm, but rapid in malignant disease involving the vertebral column.

To clarify the effects of spinal cord compression at different levels the following signs and symptoms will be found:

1. Compression at the fifth cervical segment

Muscle power and tone. Hypotonia and weakness will be present in the rhomboids, supra- and infra-spinatus, deltoid, biceps, brachialis and brachioradialis. Spasticity and loss of voluntary power occurs in the other muscles of the upper limbs supplied by segments below the level of the lesion and in the trunk and legs.

Reflexes. The biceps and brachioradialis jerks will be diminished or lost: the triceps jerks and those of the lower extremities will be exaggerated. An extensor plantar response will be elicited on stimulation of the sole of the foot and clonus may be present at the ankle and knee. Superficial abdominal reflexes are absent.

Sensation. Loss occurs in the upper limbs apart from the lateral aspect, and over the trunk and lower limbs.

Sphincters. The bladder and bowel functions are disturbed.

2. Compression of the cauda equina

Muscle power and tone. A flaccid paralysis occurs in muscles supplied by the compressed nerve roots. The muscles of the leg and foot are likely to be more involved than those of the hip and knee, due to the longer course within the vertebral canal of the nerves supplying them.

Reflexes. These are diminished according to the nerve roots involved. Compression of (*a*) the fourth lumbar nerve root will cause loss of the knee jerk, and (*b*) compression of the first sacral nerve root will cause loss of the ankle jerk.

Sensation. Some scattered loss occurs but it is not likely to be complete.

Sphincters. The bladder and bowel function will be disturbed.

SPECIAL INVESTIGATIONS

After careful clinical examination special investigations are carried out to establish the exact site, extent and nature of the lesion. The following are those most commonly used:

1. *X-rays.* Plain films are usually necessary.

2. *Lumbar puncture* is carried out to obtain specimens of cerebrospinal fluid for diagnostic purposes and to establish if there is a block of the subarachnoid space.

3. *Myelography.* Myodil or air, usually the former, is introduced via a lumbar puncture needle and guided to the appropriate region. Where a complete spinal block is present Myodil may be introduced via a cisternal

puncture into the cisterna magna and allowed to flow down to outline the upper level of the lesion. The Myodil is removed at the end of the examination as it tends to act as an irritant.

CONDITIONS SUITABLE FOR SURGERY

1. Neoplasms.

(a) Primary neoplasms arise from the cord, the meninges or the sheaths of the spinal nerves.

(b) Secondary neoplasms usually involve the vertebral bodies and may cause compression of the neural elements, that is the spinal cord and nerve roots.

2. Infections such as an epidural abscess which can only be dealt with by surgical intervention.

3. Protruded intervertebral discs.

4. Degenerative lesions such as cervical spondylosis where surgery is required to relieve existing symptoms and prevent further deterioration.

5. Intractable pain from lesions which may be outside the central nervous system.

6. Congenital deformities.

SPINAL NEOPLASMS

1. Neoplasms of the spinal cord

Spinal neoplasms occur in any age group but are rather more common between the ages of twenty and sixty years. The sexes are affected equally. They are classified:

(a) Extradural—those which lie outside the membranes surrounding the cord.

(b) Intradural—those which lie inside the membranes. This type is further classified into:

    (i) Extramedullary, which do not enter the spinal cord, such as the meningiomas and neurinomas.

    (ii) Intramedullary, which arise in the substance of the cord, such as the ependymomas.

The onset of symptoms with these neoplasms is usually very slow and may extend over a period of years.

2. Neoplasms of the vertebral column

The commonest type of neoplasm is a secondary carcinoma which usually attacks the vertebral body. The primary lesion is often the breast in women and the prostate gland and the lung in men. Sarcomas are examples of primary neoplasms. The secondary carcinomas grow very rapidly giving rise to acute spinal cord compression and require emergency treatment.

INFECTIONS OF THE SPINE

These include:

1. Epidural abscess.
2. Tuberculosis (Pott's paraplegia).

1. Epidural abscess

This can be caused by osteomyelitis of the vertebral column, infections in the body such as the lungs and peritoneal cavity, skin infections of the back and lumbar puncture. Tuberculosis of the spine may also produce a 'cold' abscess.

The size of the lesion can vary from a very small localized area to one involving the entire length of the cord. The onset of symptoms may be acute, sub-acute or chronic. If acute, emergency surgery will be required. Once pressure on the spinal cord has been relieved, antibiotics are introduced by means of a drain to control the infection.

2. Tuberculosis (Pott's paraplegia)

This usually occurs in children and young adults, but no age group is exempt. The infective process usually begins in the body of a vertebra and spreads to adjacent vertebral bodies which leads to their collapse, an angular deformity of the spine is thus produced. This deformity, an associated tuberculous abscess or interference with the vascular supply of subadjacent segments can disturb spinal cord function and a paraplegia may develop.

SURGICAL TREATMENT

To relieve compression of the spinal cord caused by neoplasms and abscesses a laminectomy is usually carried out at the appropriate levels. This decompresses the spinal cord without disturbing the stability of the vertebral column.

LAMINECTOMY

A fairly long midline incision is made, and the back muscles stripped from the spinous processes and the laminae which are then removed, the number removed depending on the extent of the lesion. Neoplasms of the extramedullary type are removed entirely or as far as possible. The intra-medullary type which invade the cord substance may not be removed entirely. The cord will be incised and as much material as possible re-moved, the dura being left open to effect a further decompression.

Post-operative Treatment

On return from theatre the patient is nursed in side lying with a pillow supporting his back, his underneath leg straight and the top leg flexed at hip and knee and supported by two pillows, one under the thigh and one under the leg. To prevent pressure sores two-hourly turns are essential, the patient going from side to front, from front to his other side. If there are signs of bladder involvement prior to operation a catheter will be draining the bladder which is maintained until bladder function returns, or an automatic bladder trained.

If there is loss of sensation the patient will be nursed on pillow packs to prevent the development of pressure sores. Great care must be taken to ensure that the coverings on the packs are kept unwrinkled. Positioning and turning procedures are as previously described. A bed cage is used to keep the weight of the bed clothes off the feet and a firm support placed at the bottom of the bed to maintain the feet at right angles thus preventing a foot drop.

For a lesion of the cervical spine, with loss of power and sensation in the upper limbs, careful positioning of the arms is necessary to ensure the elbows do not develop flexion contractures. A roll of Sorbo-rubber in the hand keeps the fingers in a functional position and the wrist is in slight extension. If necessary a pillow can be used to keep the upper arm away from the chest wall.

With an extensive laminectomy the patient may find back lying uncom-fortable until the tenth day, when sutures will be removed, or partly so, and the wound less tender.

GENERAL PHYSIOTHERAPY PRINCIPLES

Bearing in mind the principles outlined in the previous chapter, only specific points of post-operative physiotherapy treatment will follow each condition.

PHYSIOTHERAPY TREATMENT

1. Breathing exercises and coughing

When a lesion involves the intercostal and abdominal muscles, the dia-phragm is the only remaining muscle of respiration. The patient must be encouraged to practise breathing exercises regularly to reduce the danger of broncho-pneumonia. Coughing will be reduced in force and can be assisted by pushing up under the diaphragm with the hand. Where voluntary power allows, the patient is taught to do this for himself, if he is unable to do so the nurses are taught how to assist him.

2. Maintenance exercises

These are carried out where possible to maintain circulation. If no voluntary power is present passive movements are carried out twice daily.

3. Careful positioning and passive movements

These are necessary to prevent contractures. When the arms are involved it is important to retain full range shoulder movements, full extension of the elbow and prevent tightening of the wrist and finger flexors. Flexion and extension of the meta-carpal phalangeal joints and a full stretch on the web of the thumb are important. In the lower limb it is important to retain full extension of the hip and knee and the ability to get the feet to a right angle. Hamstring muscles should not be allowed to become tight. During the first few post-operative days no hamstring stretching should be given as it might produce pain due to stretching of the nerve roots and a pull of the meninges. After approximately one week gentle hamstring stretching can be commenced in a small range, gradually increasing until the leg, with the foot at 90 degrees to the leg, can be raised to a right angle to the body.

4. Return of function

This is encouraged by means of facilitation techniques.

5. Static abdominal contractions

These can begin immediately and static back muscle contractions begin approximately on the fifth day. Active abdominal work can begin when the sutures are removed and active back extension is begun approximately after one week.

6. Shoulder girdle strengthening

This may be started immediately with arm exercises. If the incision is a high one care must be taken that there is no pull on the wound. Spring resistance can be given if there is no danger of pulling on the wound, and can be commenced when the patient's back is comfortable. When there is gross loss of voluntary power in the lower limbs it is most important to develop the muscles of the shoulder girdle and latissimus dorsi as they will be required for lifting and when walking with crutches.

7. Balance re-education

This begins when the patient is allowed to get up, usually after the tenth day. It is advisable to get him to tolerate an upright position in bed before he gets up. Balance re-education can begin by sitting the patient over the edge of the bed with the feet supported on the floor or on a stool, then in a wheel chair. In the early stages a mirror is useful to help the patient regain his balance, especially if he has sensory loss. When he has gained balance in a wheel chair and on the edge of the bed, mat work can be started and balance in long sitting.

Mat work. The patient must practise sitting up, rolling from side to side and rolling on to his front, getting into a kneeling position and balancing in this position. He must practise moving across and up and down the mat using his arms to lift his buttocks. Hip raising and balancing in this position helps to regain stability. Back extension, hip extension and hamstring exercises can be given in prone lying. Crawling in all directions free and against resistance helps to strengthen hip muscles. Further balance re-education is done in kneeling and half-kneeling and practice in getting from this position on and off a chair or stool is the next progression.

Wheel chair. If the patient has a gross or permanent disability a wheel chair will be necessary to enable him to become independent. Each patient is measured and a chair and Sorbo-cushion is ordered to his specific requirements. The patient must be taught to control and manoeuvre his chair. When his balance and arm power are adequate the patient is taught to transfer himself from bed to wheel chair and from wheel chair to bed. Later he is taught to get from his chair to the mat and vice versa.

8. Re-education of walking

Re-education of walking commences with balance in standing. This usually begins with the patient between parallel bars with a mirror in front of him. When the patient can balance satisfactorily walking re-education is commenced. The ability to progress along these lines depends on the degree of voluntary power loss. When the patient is ready to stand various aids may be necessary. As a temporary measure plaster back slabs to keep the knees straight may be used. If gross muscle weakness persists calipers will be needed. The calipers are made to measure with a corset top, jointed at the knee and a toe-raising device if necessary. If weakness is only in the anterior tibial muscles, below-knee calipers may be needed.

The type of gait taught depends upon the level of the lesion. This may be four point if the lesion is at or below the tenth thoracic segment, or swing to, for lesions above this level. Once walking has become controlled in the parallel bars the patient can progress to using elbow crutches, beginning with one bar and one crutch, then balancing on both crutches, then to walking. A mirror can be used at the beginning of each progression until the patient gains the correct idea of balance and gait. If the patient uses a wheel chair he must be taught how to stand up and sit down using his crutches.

Stairs. The patient can be re-educated to use the stairs by using a banister rail and one elbow crutch. Going up the stairs the patient puts his crutch up on the step first then jumps his feet up. Coming down he swings his legs down one step then brings his crutch down.

When a patient has voluntary control of his hips and knees elbow crutches are not necessary. He can walk with the aid of quadruped or tripod sticks in initial stages, and may be progressed to walking sticks when his balance and confidence improve. When going upstairs he uses the banister rail and one stick—he puts his stick up first, then his right foot, the stick goes up to the next step, followed by his left foot. Coming down he puts his stick down first, then his right foot to the same step, his stick down to the next step followed by his left foot.

A patient with sensory loss. Measures taken to prevent pressure sores developing in the early stages of post-operative care have already been pointed out and nursing care has been directed to this end. If beds become wet they are immediately changed and the patient sponged and dried. Time must be taken to explain to the patient what this sensory loss means to him and he must be taught to look after his skin to prevent any sores developing. He should be instructed in the following points:

1. He must examine his skin carefully each day, using a mirror where necessary.
2. A hot-water bottle must never be used.
3. Special care must be taken when cutting toe- and finger-nails. If there is a tendency to ingrowing toe-nails the skin should be massaged away from the nail. If the nail does grow into the skin, suppuration may occur and the nail may need to be removed.
4. If thick hard skin develops on hands and feet it should be softened with cream or olive oil and removed.
5. Bath water must be checked for temperature before the patient gets

into the bath. A piece of sponge rubber in the bottom of the bath prevents the patient getting bruised. Cold water should be run into the bath first in case the heat of the bath itself causes a burn.

6. Warning should be given with regard to sitting near fires and radiators and in direct sunlight.

7. In cold weather the feet must be kept warm to prevent chilblains developing.

8. For patients with loss of sensation in the hands cups should have a protective covering or holder and a cigarette holder must be used if the patient smokes.

9. When sitting in his chair he must frequently lift his buttocks off the cushion to relieve pressure—this is taught immediately he starts using his wheel chair. If arm power is inadequate a physiotherapist, or nurse, must lift the patient regularly until his balance will allow him to move sufficiently from hip to hip to relieve pressure.

10. If the patient wishes to sit in an ordinary arm-chair he must make sure it has a soft seat.

11. Shoes must be chosen carefully to ensure they do not produce sores; soft leather with no toe-caps are advisable, and a half-size larger and a wider fitting than previously worn.

If a pressure sore develops the quickest way to heal this is to keep the patient in bed and nurse him in a position which will keep all pressure from the area. He should not be allowed to get up again until the sore is adequately healed.

INTERVERTEBRAL DISCS

Intervertebral discs are found between the bodies of the movable vertebrae and extend from the second cervical vertebra to the lumbosacral junction. In the lumbar region they are much thicker and shaped to the lumbar curve. Each vertebral body is covered with hyaline cartilage and the disc, consisting of an outer fibrocartilaginous annulus fibrosus and an inner gelatinous nucleus pulposus, is sandwiched between. The annulus fibrosus is weakest postero-laterally where it is inadequately supported by the spinous ligaments. This is where it becomes thinned as a result of trauma and may rupture completely if the initial trauma is sufficiently severe.

When the annulus fibrosus becomes thinned the results are as follows:

1. *The nucleus pulposus bulges* at the weakened point. The nerve root passing down the vertebral canal to emerge through the appropriate intervertebral foramen becomes stretched over this bulge. This causes pain due

to irritation with subsequent compression causing loss of sensation and motor power.

2. *The annulus fibrosus may rupture* and allow the nucleus to pass through the opening in the spinous ligaments to lie in the vertebral canal.

3. *Occasionally the nucleus pulposus may herniate* in the midline giving rise to symptoms similar to a spinal cord neoplasm in the cervical region and a cauda equina lesion in the lumbar region (see Fig. 37).

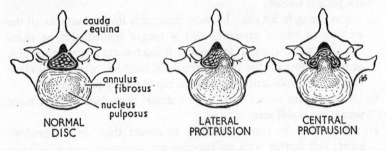

FIG. 37

LUMBAR DISC HERNIATIONS

The lumbar region is the commonest site of a disc herniation. The highest incidence is between the fourth and fifth lumbar and the fifth lumbar and the first sacral vertebrae.

General signs and symptoms of a lumbar disc herniation

1. Pain. Backache may be the presenting feature, but the patient usually complains of pain in the distribution of the sciatic nerve. Bending and straining will increase the pain.

2. The lumbar curve is obliterated and the paravertebral muscles are in spasm.

3. Scoliosis. Some degree of scoliosis may occur, usually away from the side of the lesion, which relieves pressure on the nerve root.

4. Straight leg-raising is decreased.

5. Sensory changes. These are usually found over the lateral aspect of the calf and heel.

6. Depressed tendon reflexes. The ankle jerk is diminished or lost if the first sacral nerve root is compressed. The knee jerk is diminished or lost if the fourth lumbar nerve root is compressed. These signs and symptoms are intermittent and will recur with any fresh trauma.

Syndrome of a disc protrusion between the fourth and fifth lumbar vertebrae

1. Pain, down the postero-lateral aspect of the thigh and lateral aspect of the leg, to the ankle.

2. Sensory changes, usually pins and needles, over the lateral aspect of the leg.

3. Motor weakness involving extensor hallucis longus first, but may eventually involve all the other dorsi-flexors.

Syndrome of a disc protrusion between the fifth lumbar and first sacral vertebrae

1. Pain, down the postero-lateral aspect of the thigh and lateral aspect of the leg extending to the outer border of the foot.

2. Sensory changes usually over the outer border of the foot and little toe, which may extend over the foot and involve the other toes.

3. The ankle jerk is depressed.

4. Motor weakness involving the plantar flexors.

CONSERVATIVE TREATMENT

1. Rest in bed until the symptoms abate. The patient must lie on a firm mattress or have fracture boards under the mattress to ensure his spine is adequately supported.

2. Continuous lumbar traction. This is to separate the vertebral bodies in the hope that the nucleus pulposus will return to its normal position.

3. Plaster jacket.

4. Physiotherapy.

INDICATIONS FOR SURGICAL TREATMENT

The relief of symptoms by surgical means becomes necessary:

1. When conservative treatment no longer affords relief.

2. When progressive nerve root involvement appears, namely weakness and sensory loss.

3. When there are signs of cauda equina compression and bladder involvement. Emergency surgery is required in this instance to prevent irreparable damage to the spinal cord.

Special Investigations

Myelogram. This is done only when there is any doubt about the diagnosis, but never as a routine measure.

SURGICAL TREATMENT

This treatment is aimed at the removal of the nucleus pulposus, or the ruptured part of the annulus fibrosus. The method of approach depends upon the site and size of the protrusion.

Several operative techniques can be used to remove a lumbar disc herniation, all requiring a fairly long midline incision, to expose the spinous processes and laminae. The following procedures can then be carried out:

1. *Fenestration.* At the site of the disc protrusion the ligament is removed between the laminae, then a small portion of the lamina of the vertebrae above and below the protrusion is removed and the nerve root retracted. The exposed protrusion is then incised and as much as possible of the nucleus pulposus gouged out.
2. *Laminectomy.* This procedure is used when both sides of the disc space requires exploration, usually in the case of a centrally protruded disc. The spinous process and both laminae are removed at the appropriate level and the disc protrusion dealt with as before.

POST-OPERATIVE TREATMENT

Nursing care is of paramount importance during the first few post-operative days. The patient is nursed in the side lying position previously described and turned two-hourly, going from side to front to his other side, all pillows being removed to facilitate turning. In the early post-operative period the patient uses a bed-pan in prone lying to avoid flexion of the spine.

PHYSIOTHERAPY TREATMENT

A wide variety of post-operative routines exists, each surgeon having his own ideas as to how the patient should be progressed. Each patient presents an individual problem and any routine must be adjusted to suit his capabilities. The general principles which apply to all routines are (a) to limit all exercises to the pain-free range of movement of the patient, and (b) when giving mobilizing exercises never force a particular movement.

Methods

1. Breathing exercises and coughing. The patient may require encouragement if his wound is painful. Firm pressure over the wound from the physiotherapist's hand and instructions to tighten his abdominal muscles as he coughs are helpful measures. Breathing exercises should be practised hourly.

2. Maintenance exercises confined to foot and knee movements are practised hourly by the patient. Hip movements in a small range of flexion and extension to the midline are delayed until the second day. Static abdominal work can be given. Abduction of the hip, and an increased range of flexion with extension beyond the midline and straight leg raising follow as progressions of hip movement.

3. Static contractions of back extensor muscles are usually commenced on the fourth day. At this stage the patient can begin lying on his back for short periods. Care must be taken with his posture so he is taught to appreciate when he is lying in a straight line. Active extension usually follows on the fifth day, the number of times the exercises are repeated and the strength of the exercises are gradually increased.

4. Any specific muscle weakness is re-educated by means of facilitation techniques.

5. The re-education of posture in lying is progressed to re-education of posture in standing. The surgeon decides when the patient should be allowed to get up, which will probably be about the fifth day. Before the patient gets up it is advisable to elevate the bed to allow him to adjust to a more upright position. It must be noted that the entire bed is elevated: the patient is not placed in a sitting position. The patient is taught to lie on his side at the edge of the bed, put his feet over the edge and sit up keeping his back straight. His posture is corrected as soon as he stands up and he is re-educated in walking when necessary. On returning to bed he sits on the edge of the bed and with his back straight lies down on his side, bringing his legs into bed as he does so. Some patients may find it easier to get out of bed from a prone lying position. To do this he moves himself into a diagonal position across the bed, when his feet touch the floor he then pushes himself into an upright position keeping his back straight. Getting into bed he keeps his back straight and lowers the top of his body by bending from the hips, then lifts his legs into bed. The patient is encouraged to get up for short periods and to walk about.

The following instructions should be given:

(a) A hard upright chair must be used and he must keep his back straight when sitting down and standing up. The sitting position should only be used at meal times and for short periods as it is usually an uncomfortable one.

(b) When picking objects up from the floor he should be taught to go down on one knee keeping his back straight.

(c) No lifting should be attempted.

(d) If his back becomes uncomfortable he should lie down and rest.

6. Mobilization of the spine begins after the sutures are removed, usually the tenth day. Side flexion, rotation and forward flexion are all encouraged. Hydrotherapy is a useful means by which mobility can be encouraged.

When the patient is ready for discharge home he should be given a scheme of exercises to practise daily and instructed to continue these exercises for an indefinite period. The surgeon will decide when the patient is able to assume his normal activities and if any change of employment is necessary.

CERVICAL DISC HERNIATIONS

Herniation of the nucleus pulposus in the cervical region is less common than in the lumbar region. The usual sites of herniation are between the fifth and sixth, and sixth and seventh cervical vertebrae. This is probably due to the greater stress at these levels, as they lie at the point where the free mobility of the cervical spine is changing to the relative immobility of the thoracic spine. Herniation can occur spontaneously or as a result of trauma. The protrusion is usually in a postero-lateral direction, but a central herniation can occur giving symptoms of spinal cord compression.

SIGNS AND SYMPTOMS

1. Pain occurs in the neck on movement and may be severe. Referred pain in the distribution of the compressed nerve root is also present.

2. There is rigidity of the neck muscles.

3. The head may be slightly flexed to the side of the lesion.

4. Muscle wasting occurs in the motor distribution of the compressed nerve root, but severe loss of muscle power is not usual.

5. Sensory changes may occur over the appropriate dermatome.

6. Tendon reflexes innervated by the compressed nerve are diminished or lost.

Conservative Treatment

Neck traction may be given to relieve pressure on the nerve root, and the neck immobilized by use of a collar.

Surgical Treatment

When conservative measures fail to relieve the symptoms surgical intervention is indicated. This will be described at the end of this section.

CERVICAL SPONDYLOSIS

Degeneration of the intervertebral discs with the formation of osteophytes, especially at the intervertebral joints, are the pathological changes giving rise to cervical spondylosis. These intervertebral joints are the articulations between the bodies of the cervical vertebrae, they lie at the lateral margins of the intervertebral discs and are sometimes known as the joints of Lushka.

Individuals most affected are those in the middle and older age groups. The most common site of the lesion is between the fifth and sixth and sixth and seventh vertebrae. Compression of the nerve roots can occur on one or both sides, at one or several levels.

The disease presents in two main patterns:

1. Cervical spondylosis with brachalgia, when the nerve roots are involved.
2. Cervical myelopathy when there is spinal cord involvement.

CERVICAL SPONDYLOSIS WITH BRACHALGIA

The history of symptoms is very variable and onset of radicular symptoms may be acute, sub-acute or insidious. An acute onset of symptoms which involves one nerve root closely resembles an acute cervical disc herniation. An insidious onset is characterized by burning and tingling sensations down the arm.

Signs and Symptoms

A general picture of the signs and symptoms is as follows:

1. Burning and tingling sensations often accompanied by pain radiating down the arm and into the fingers, the little and ring finger usually being involved. These symptoms tend to be worse at night.
2. The ability to appreciate light touch and pin prick is diminished in the dermatomes supplied by the compressed nerve roots.
3. There is localized tenderness of muscles supplied by the affected nerves.
4. Kinesthetic sensation is impaired.
5. Slight muscle wasting and hypotonia are present in the muscles supplied by the compressed nerve roots.
6. Tendon reflexes are diminished or lost.
7. Neck movements are limited but relatively pain free.
8. Local tenderness in the neck is elicited on pressure.

Conservative Treatment

1. Immobilization by use of a collar.
2. Physiotherapy, including traction, heat, massage, and exercises.

CERVICAL MYELOPATHY

SIGNS AND SYMPTOMS

The patient presents with a progressive, spastic paraparesis with variable sensory loss, which cannot be differentiated from the signs and symptoms of a spinal cord neoplasm. Findings therefore are as for cervical cord compression.

SURGICAL MANAGEMENT

This is designed to relieve nerve roots and spinal cord compression by the degenerated disc and osteophyte formation. The anterior approach is superseding the posterior approach but both will be mentioned.

1. If the lesion is lateral and the nerve root only is involved, a posterior approach with a hemilaminectomy is usually undertaken.
2. If myelopathy is present two alternative approaches are possible:
    (a) a wide decompression of the spinal cord by means of a laminectomy, or
    (b) an anterior cervical decompression and fusion.

Post-operative Treatment following hemilaminectomy or laminectomy.

The patient is nursed in side lying, until his neck wound becomes less tender and he can tolerate back lying.

PHYSIOTHERAPY TREATMENT

Following Hemilaminectomy

If this involves one level only the patient will be allowed to get up between the fifth and seventh days. Static neck exercises particularly for the neck extensor muscles may begin about the same time. Active neck and shoulder exercises follow when sutures are removed approximately on the tenth day. Any muscle weakness is re-educated by facilitation techniques.

Following Laminectomy

If several laminae have been removed the patient will remain in bed until the tenth day. Static neck exercises can begin on the seventh day. Some surgeons prefer a leather collar to be fitted before the patient is allowed to get up and he continues to wear it for a variable period of time. Once sutures have been removed gentle neck and shoulder exercises may be done without the collar and particular attention must be paid to the patient's head and shoulder posture.

ANTERIOR CERVICAL DECOMPRESSION AND FUSION

This operation has been found to be more effective than a laminectomy.

The anatomy of the cervical region is such that a posterior approach by means of a laminectomy requires retraction of the spinal cord in order to reach the disc protrusion and the osteophytes. Manipulation of the spinal cord may upset its blood supply with disastrous results. The posterior approach can also weaken the neck muscles and subluxation may occur as a post-operative complication.

The anterior approach is a much safer procedure. Discs and osteophytes can be completely excised and the spine fused to prevent further osteophyte formation. Indications for operation are:

1. Disease of the cervical discs when conservative measures have failed to relieve the symptoms.
2. Certain types of injury to the cervical spine due to hyperextension and hyperflexion of the neck.
3. Certain neoplasms and infective processes such as tuberculosis of the cervical spine.

SURGICAL PROCEDURE

The patient lies supine with 25 pounds head traction. An incision is made in a skin crease in the right carotid triangle exposing the anterior aspect of the spinal column from the second cervical to the first thoracic vertebral body. At the appropriate level a hole, half an inch in diameter is drilled through the disc and adjacent vertebral bodies until the posterior longitudinal ligament is reached. The debris of disc material and osteophytes is removed and a plug of bone, usually from the left iliac crest, inserted in the hole.

Post-operative Treatment

The patient returns from theatre in a supine position with a thin ring of Sorbo-rubber under his head. The ring has the centre removed and so serves to relieve pressure on the back of the head. Sandbags are placed at either side of the head to prevent movement; the patient being kept in this position for ten days. After the third day the bed is elevated to an angle of 45 degrees for variable periods. To aid venous return from the lower limbs the patient is tipped head down for thirty minutes every two hours during his period of bed rest.

On the tenth day, when the patient is allowed to get up, a leather collar is put on before he is permitted to sit upright, prior to getting out of bed. This collar is made to measure before operation and fitted to ensure it is comfortable. The collar is then worn for ten to fourteen days if only one or two disc spaces have been fused, and for a month if three discs have been treated.

POST-OPERATIVE PHYSIOTHERAPY

1. Breathing exercises and coughing. The patient practises his breathing exercises hourly.

2. Maintenance exercises. Particular attention is given to the left lower limb, especially hip movements. The patient needs encouragement to begin hip movements and quadriceps contractions, as the hip area is stiff and painful following the removal of bone from the ileum. Gentle full-range movements of the shoulder joints must be encouraged. Maintenance exercises must be practised hourly.

3. Re-education of any muscle weakness is carried out by means of facilitation techniques.

4. Walking re-education is often necessary, especially if the lower limbs were spastic due to spinal cord compression. Walking between parallel bars with the aid of a mirror helps the patient to appreciate where to place his feet. Later some type of walking aid may be necessary to make him independent.

Care of the patient's neck

Aims
1. To strengthen neck and shoulder muscles.
2. To regain mobility.

Methods
1. Static contractions of neck and shoulder muscles are begun approximately on the seventh day with the patient in a supine position. When he is out of bed wearing a collar he is encouraged to practise these static contractions at regular intervals.

2. When the collar is removed between three to six weeks from the date of operation active neck and shoulder exercises are given.

INTRACTABLE PAIN

Intractable pain describes a chronic severe pain which persists after the primary lesion has been treated. This type of pain serves no useful purpose and the patient's suffering can be relieved only by constant narcotic therapy. This becomes progressively less effective and there is a constant danger of addiction to the drugs used.

Intractable Pain

Pain cannot be measured and has different characteristics depending on its origin. Innumerable factors can influence it, among the most important are the patient's personality, intelligence and emotional maturity. A careful assessment is thus essential before surgical measures are undertaken to relieve pain. When surgery is used for this purpose it is an indication that no further treatment is possible for the original disease.

Lesions giving rise to intractable pain are largely carcinomas outside the central nervous system. Herpes zoster, operational scars, amputation stump, neuromas, phantom limb pain, and some cord lesions are non-malignant causes.

SURGICAL TREATMENT
Posterior Rhizotomy

The appropriate posterior spinal nerve roots are sectioned between the spinal cord and the posterior spinal ganglion, on the same side of the body as the intractable pain is appreciated. Due to the overlap of the sensory supply from one dermatome to another, it is necessary to section at least two sensory roots above and below the area in which pain is localized by the patient. This operation is carried out for post-herpetic pain and painful scars, but after a period of time the intractable pain tends to recur. It is of no use for limb pain, as it destroys muscle and joint sensation, which would give rise to a severe disability.

Spinothalamic Cordotomy

Fibres of the lateral spinothalamic tract are divided on the opposite side of the body to that on which the pain is appreciated. To achieve a permanent result this procedure must be done several segments higher than the localization of pain, to allow for the fact that (a) fibres carrying sensations of pain and temperature enter the spinal cord and ascend for several segments before crossing the midline to join the lateral spino-thalamic tract; (b) no matter how deep the incision made at operation, the level of sensory loss always descends during the first post-operative week.

The patient is so anaesthetized during this type of operation that he can be roused when the surgeon is ready to divide the lateral spinothalamic tract. The patient co-operates by telling the surgeon the level of his sensory loss and when an adequate level is reached he is re-anaesthetized and the operation completed.

Spinothalamic cordotomies are used to relieve pain from malignant disease especially those affecting the pelvic region. A bilateral cordotomy may be necessary for a patient who suffers from bilateral symptoms, but this procedure can produce motor weakness below the level of the surgical lesion. Bladder and bowel function are often permanently disturbed, accompanied by the loss of sexual function in the male. High cervical cordotomy may damage the respiratory pathway, innervating the diaphragm and intercostal muscles, producing an ipsilateral paralysis.

PHYSIOTHERAPY TREATMENT

Following cordotomy in the thoracic region static contractions of the back extensor muscles can begin about the seventh post-operative day, and active extension exercises when sutures are removed, approximately the tenth day.

Following a high cervical cordotomy neck extensor muscles require retraining; static contractions can begin about the seventh post-operative day, and gentle neck mobilization when sutures are removed, approximately the tenth day. Chest care is most important if there is a diaphragmatic and intercostal muscle paralysis.

The patient should be allowed to get up between the seventh and tenth day if his general condition is satisfactory. It is important to teach him how to look after the area of pain and temperature loss. A patient with a unilateral loss should be reminded to use his normal side for testing the temperature of bath water. He must look after his affected side in the manner previously described for the paraplegic patient.

Further advances

Percutaneous cordotomy is gradually replacing open procedures, while stereotaxic cordotomy is now being developed to bring greater accuracy to lesion making. Obvious advantages of percutaneous procedures are that the patient only requires a local anaesthetic, there is no longer a painful wound, so earlier mobilization is therefore possible.

If for any reason a high cervical cordotomy is contra-indicated a stereotaxic lesion can be made in a portion of the thalamic nucleus, and is often successful in relieving pain. Certain patients whose pain may not have been adequately relieved by a surgical lesion at a lower level may derive great benefit from a thalamotomy.

SPINA BIFIDA

This is a congenital abnormality due to incomplete closure of the vertebral canal and may be associated with an abnormality of the spinal cord. There are varying degrees of severity of this defect as follows:

1. Spina bifida occulta

This may be marked by a dimple in the skin, or a tuft of hair overlying

Spina Bifida

a fatty mass in the lumbo-sacral region. Nerve roots of the cauda equina may be matted together at the level of the bony defect. Mild symptoms of saddle hypalgesia and intermittent urinary disturbances may occur. Surgery may be undertaken in carefully selected cases. The majority of patients with spina bifida occulta have no symptoms and no treatment is necessary.

2. Meningocele

Over the bony defect a sac, containing meninges and cerebrospinal fluid, bulges out on the surface of the back. This type of abnormality can occur in any part of the spinal column.

3. Meningomyelocele

The sac in this case also contains nerve roots and portions of the spinal cord.

4. Syringomyelocele

The portions of spinal cord in the sac cause pressure on the central canal of the spinal cord.

5. Myelocele

The spinal cord completely fills the sac.

Defects of the meningocele type and those of increasing severity require immediate surgery, to prevent a cerebrospinal fluid leak developing which could give rise to infection, and to prevent further neural damage. The contents of the sac are buried beneath the surface and covered by muscle and skin to form some measure of protection. Hydrocephalus frequently accompanies this type of deformity and may require surgery, as previously described, following repair of the spinal defect. Partial or total paresis may occur as a result of these deformities, a partial paresis may give rise to contractures and deformities which will require surgery when the baby is about nine months old.

PHYSIOTHERAPY TREATMENT

Routine chest care is required. Passive movements of the lower limbs and attempts to stimulate the baby to move his legs voluntarily are required, to maintain circulation and prevent contractures.

Chapter XIII

PERIPHERAL NERVE INJURIES

by B. SUTCLIFFE, M.C.S.P.

STRUCTURE

A peripheral nerve is composed of motor, sensory, and autonomic fibres. The motor and sensory fibres are myelinated. A neurone consists of a nerve cell and its processes, the dendrites, and the axon or nerve fibre. The nutrition of the axon and the preservation of its structure depend on its intact connection with the cell body. The nerve fibre is the long process of a neurone, and its function is to conduct the nerve impulse.

A myelinated nerve fibre consists of a central core of semi-fluid axoplasm, which is thought to flow from the cell body to the periphery.

The axoplasm contains a fibrillar component running parallel to the axis of the fibre. Around this is the cell membrane, the axolemma, then a myelin sheath consisting of Schwann cells. The sheath is interrupted at intervals by the nodes of Ranvier and is surrounded by the outermost covering, the neurilemma.

The myelin sheath acts as an insulator. In myelinated nerves, the nerve impulse travels at greater speed than in unmyelinated ones. The impulse leaps from node to node. This process is known as saltatory conduction (*saltare*, Latin, to leap), and this method is the most economical in energy expenditure.

In peripheral nerve trunks the neurilemma is surrounded by a thin layer of reticular fibres forming the endoneurium. Bundles of nerve fibres are enclosed in a connective tissue capsule, the perineurium, and bundles of them are further surrounded by connective tissue called the epineurium.

The motor unit consists of one anterior horn cell, its peripheral axon and many muscle fibres, the number varying inversely with the precision of the muscle concerned. The sensory fibres convey impulses from the skin, muscles, joints, and other deep structures, to the posterior root ganglia and then to the spinal cord. The sympathetic fibres of the autonomic nervous system are post-ganglionic from the sympathetic ganglia. These fibres innervate involuntary structures such as blood vessels, sweat and sebaceous glands.

CAUSES OF INJURY

Peripheral nerves are frequently injured by laceration. The median and ulnar nerves may be cut at the wrist by knives or by glass. They may be injured by direct pressure, e.g. the radial nerve can be damaged by a fracture of the humerus, or a blow on the upper arm, or pressure from callus. Pressure may lead to ischaemia, as when the median nerve is compressed in the carpal tunnel by proliferation of the synovial sheaths. A delayed (i.e. a tardy) paralysis may affect the ulnar nerve as it is stretched by an increasing cubitus valgus deformity following elbow injuries. They may also be injured by forced traction, as in brachial plexus lesions associated with motor cycle accidents. The victim grips the handlebars of the machine while the head is forcibly side-flexed or as the shoulder is depressed by striking the ground at the same time as the head is side-flexed to the opposite side.

Pressure from a tourniquet, or badly applied plaster may be another cause of injury.

Industrial and traffic accidents and gunshot wounds may cause peripheral nerve injury in addition to widespread damage to other tissue.

TYPES

Sir Herbert Seddon has described three types of nerve injury, and classified them according to the amount of damage sustained. These are known as neurapraxia, axonotmesis and neurotmesis.

1. *Neurapraxia* can be defined as a non-degenerative lesion, although electrical tests often show there is some slight evidence of degeneration. Electrical stimulation above the block does not cause contraction of the muscles supplied but it may be possible to stimulate the nerve with a very high current.

Motor paralysis is usually complete but sensory loss is unusual. Recovery is complete in a few weeks.

2. *Axonotmesis* is a degenerative lesion in which the axon degenerates but

the supporting tissues are intact. The nerve fibres can therefore regenerate to reach their original end organs. Provided the muscles, joints and skin have been maintained in good condition, recovery should be almost perfect.

3. In *neurotmesis* the axon and nerve sheath are severed. Suture must be carried out so that the axons may grow down a tunnel to the peripheral end organs. There is bound to be some scarring at the site of the repair and this may cause obstruction or misdirection of the nerve fibres. Motor and sensory fibres do not necessarily return to their original end organs and there will be incomplete restoration of power and faulty localization of sensory stimuli. In these cases re-education of function is essential. The three types of nerve damage can be found in one injury.

DEGENERATION

When a nerve is severed retrograde degeneration occurs for 2–3 cm. in the central stump and changes occur in the nerve distal to the site of injury. This process is known as Wallerian degeneration. Initially the axis cylinder breaks up, and, rather more slowly, the myelin sheath becomes oily droplets. This debris is cleared away by macrophage activity and within three months Schwann cells fill the endoneurial tubes. Progressive changes occur in the muscle fibres and the coarse striation becomes less obvious: the muscles are gradually replaced by fibrous tissue. There is complete fibrosis after two years if reinnervation has not occurred.

REGENERATION

Regeneration occurs by the growth of fibres from the central axon. Many fibres may grow down one endoneurial tube if the nerve ends are in apposition. After two or three weeks all but one degenerates, and this one grows down to the periphery. Myelin sheaths begin to develop in about fifteen days and follow the course of the growing fibrils. When the axon reaches the nerve ending it may establish a connection but the end plate formed depends on the function of the parent cell and is not necessarily appropriate to the structure innervated.

The time taken for recovery depends upon the distance which the regenerating nerve fibres have to travel from the site of injury to their destination. The average rate of motor recovery is 1.5 mm. per day in the early stages, but slows later.

EFFECTS OF PERIPHERAL NERVE INJURIES

These injuries affect the motor, sensory and autonomic nerves.

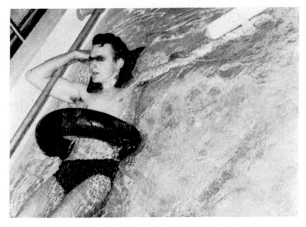

VI. Photograph showing patient with a brachial plexus palsy exercising in a pool with a float (*see* p. 271)

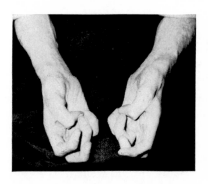

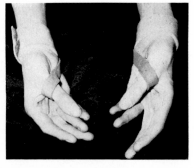

VII. (*a*) Bilateral abductor pollicis brevis paralysis
(*see* p. 272)

VII. (*b*) Photograph of another patient with the same disability but showing thumb position corrected with a lively splint

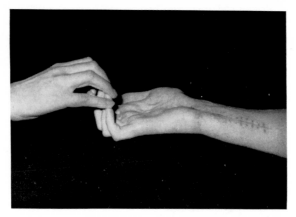

VIII. Photograph showing patient with flexion of the proximal interphalangeal joints when wrist extended due to adherent flexor sublimis digitorum at the wrist joint (*see* p. 273)

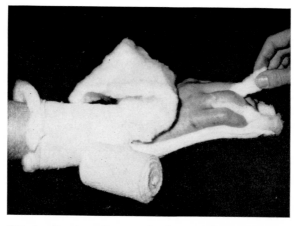

IX. Application of a stretch plaster. The cotton wool is placed under and over the hand and wrist and between the fingers to prevent trauma on anaesthetic areas (*see* p. 273)

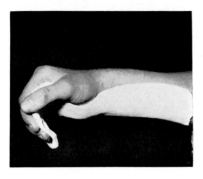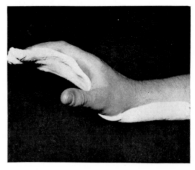

X. (*a*) Plaster made for patient with ulnar nerve lesion

X. (*b*) Photograph showing position gained one month later

(*see* p. 273)

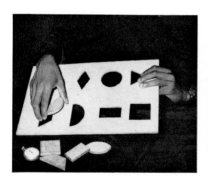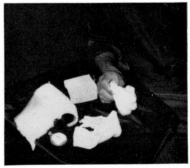

XI. (*a*) The use of simple wooden shapes for sensory re-education

XI. (*b*) The use of contrasting textures for sensory re-education

(*see* p. 273)

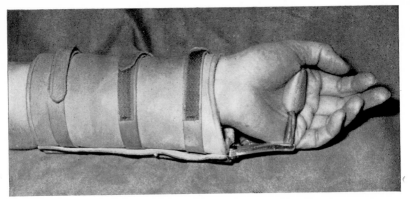

XII. Radial lively splint (*see* p. 274)

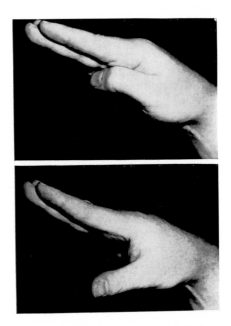

XIII. Trick extension of the thumb in a complete radial nerve lesion. The patient is using abductor pollicis brevis to extend the proximal interphalangeal joint (*see* p. 274)

1. Motor Nerves

Interruption of the motor nerve leads to a lower motor neurone paralysis and there is loss of active movement in the muscles it supplies.

Muscle atrophy progresses rapidly over the first three months and it is important that patients are made aware of this or they may attribute the decreasing size of the limb to the physiotherapist's efforts. Deformities are caused by the unopposed action of the antagonist muscles, e.g., when the radial nerve is injured the wrist is held in flexion by gravity and the action of the unaffected wrist flexors.

2. Sensory Nerves

Division of a sensory nerve causes complete loss of skin sensation over the area it exclusively supplies. This area decreases as adjacent nerves take over sensation at the periphery. There is atrophy of the soft tissues, and the circumference of the limb is lessened.

3. Autonomic Nerves (Vasomotor, sudomotor and trophic)

The effects of these injuries are not fully understood but may be due to interruption of efferent sympathetic fibres concerned in vaso-constriction. These disturbances are most marked in injuries involving the median, ulnar and sciatic nerves. The skin over the anaesthetic area becomes smooth, shiny and scaly. There is loss of sweating and the nails are brittle.

The skin is liable to burns and pressure sores, particularly in the early stages, when the patient has not become accustomed to protecting the anaesthetic areas. Once trophic lesions have occurred these are slow to heal and liable to become infected. The limb takes the temperature of its surroundings and for this reason it is very important to protect the hand and foot from excessive cold by wearing warm gloves and socks. The limb becomes oedematous when dependent. Adhesions between tendons and their sheaths and fibrous changes in muscles and joints are complications of the nerve injury owing to lack of movements. They are not a direct result of the nerve injury and can be prevented by maintaining the circulation and the full range of joint movements.

TREATMENT

Non-operative Treatment

The aim is to keep the limb in the best possible condition until the nerve regenerates. Recovery of the nerve will be useless if the joints have become stiff and contractures have occurred in the muscles. A combination of well-directed physiotherapy, occupational therapy and lively splintage are necessary to achieve this. The lively splints should be designed to correct deformity and to encourage function. The splint allows the patient to make use of compensatory movements, and this will help to keep the pattern of movement in the patient's mind during the months of paralysis and will encourage him to use the limb more and thus maintain the circulation.

Operative Treatment

If a nerve is completely divided suture must be performed. Nerve suture is usually delayed for at least three weeks after injury unless the wound is clean and operative conditions are ideal. The nerve ends are approximated and secured at the initial operation, to prevent retraction of the stumps.

At the secondary operation the nerve ends are resected until unscarred tissue is reached and an end to end suture is performed. It is found that the nerve sheath thickens after division and will hold the sutures better a few weeks after injury.

After suture it is necessary to position the adjacent joints to avoid tension on the nerve ends, but acute flexion must be avoided, as subsequent mobilization will stretch and separate the nerve ends. Tension can be avoided sometimes by extensive resection or by transposition—for example, when the ulnar nerve is transferred to the anterior aspect of the elbow joint.

Extensive gaps can be bridged by a nerve graft. The sural or medial cutaneous nerve of the forearm is used.

When the sutured nerve is predominantly motor and concerned with power, for example, the radial nerve, then post-operative function is good. It is less satisfactory when fine co-ordination is involved as in lesions of facial or ulnar nerves. It is in these cases that intensive re-education is vital, to retrain muscles which may be re-innervated by axons which have grown down to different end organs.

When a nerve is compressed by surrounding scar tissue, then neurolysis is performed to free it.

When nerve repair is not feasible, then reconstructive surgery of tendons and joints is considered.

For example to provide power of opposition to the thumb in a median nerve lesion, the tendon of flexor sublimis digitorum from the ring finger can be re-routed into the base of the proximal phalanx of the thumb to restore opposition.

In the hand, grip and opposition are useful only if there is sensation.

Treatment

In permanent sensory loss of the median nerve distribution, neurovascular skin island transfers have been made from the ulnar side. To provide sensation, the area of skin plus its nerve and blood supply is transferred from the ring finger. For precision grip, sensation is needed on the palmar aspect of the thumb and on the lateral parts of the fingers opposing the thumb.

PHYSIOTHERAPY TREATMENT

The treatment of peripheral nerve injuries involves a team led by the orthopaedic surgeon or physical medicine specialist and backed by the skill and enthusiasm of the physiotherapists and occupational therapists. It has been found that a short period of planned treatment involving physiotherapy and occupational therapy four times each day is much more effective and economical than treatment given three times weekly and extended over a much longer period.

The doctor and the therapists should see the patient together to integrate the treatment and to see that the physiotherapy and occupational therapy are complementary.

There are two stages of treatment: these are the stage of paralysis and the stage of recovery. The principles of treatment in the first stage are as follows:

1. To maintain or obtain full movement.
2. To maintain and improve the circulation.
3. To correct deformity.
4. To encourage function.
5. To increase the strength of the unaffected muscles.

Prior to treatment, an assessment should be made. When treating the upper limb, it is easy to be confused by trick movements and variations in nerve supply. One person in five has an anomalous nerve supply in the hand. This can be confirmed by electrical stimulation. If in a median nerve lesion the muscles of the thenar eminence are unaffected, it may be a partial lesion, or the muscles may be supplied by the ulnar nerve. Stimulation of the ulnar nerve at the elbow or wrist may show that it innervates all the intrinsic hand muscles.

The range of movement is measured with a goniometer. Extension and flexion of each joint are recorded to indicate deformity. These measurements should be repeated each week. Muscle power is measured using the 0–5 Medical Research Council scale. This assessment is valuable to show that the regime is effective and to encourage the patient to continue the treatment away from the department. First priority must be given to the removal of oedema, or fibrin is deposited and the tissues become bound together and permanent stiffness will result. Early elevation will prevent this. The upper limb should be supported in a sling to hold the hand near the opposite shoulder and allow free finger movements. Until oedema is under control the limb should be elevated at night. If a drip stand can be obtained, a sling or roller towel can be fixed to it and the arm elevated in this. In lower limb injuries the patient should sleep with the foot of the bed raised on blocks and during the day have the support of an elastic Scott-Curwen bandage, or Tubigrip, and a well-fitting shoe. If there are associated injuries, such as open wounds and fractures, considerable ingenuity may be needed to devise methods of elevating the affected limb, but oedema must be removed as soon as possible.

Massage is given, in elevation, to reduce the swelling, and with olive oil to improve the dry scaly skin. Any form of heat should be applied with special care, as burns can occur so easily over the anaesthetic areas. Wax baths are useful for the hand and foot, if the temperature of the wax is not above 115°F. (45°C.). Alternatively warm water soaks are effective, safe and simple. Saline soaks are used if there are unhealed areas.

Active movements are encouraged where possible, or joints must be moved passively to maintain and increase the range of movement. When passive movements are given the joint mobility should be compared with the sound side so that joints are not over-stretched.

Proprioceptive neuro-muscular facilitation techniques are used to maintain and to increase muscle power, and are also valuable to emphasize what the patient can achieve and to keep the pattern of movement in his mind. Trick movements are taught and encouraged and tend to disappear just before an active contraction is detected.

As has already been explained, early provision of a lively splint encourages functional use of the limb as well as correcting any deformity due to unopposed muscular action.

During the stage of recovery, motor and sensory re-education are needed.

As re-innervation proceeds, it will be found that a muscle will first contract as a synergist prior to prime mover action. Muscle work should be encouraged in many different forms, P.N.F. springs, weights, hydrotherapy, games, and occupational therapy.

Details of sensory re-education will be given under the treatment of a median nerve injury.

An assessment of the patient's ability to work may be carried out in the occupational therapy department and results of this will be valuable in planning future employment.

Treatment

PHYSIOTHERAPY IN SOME SPECIFIC NERVE INJURIES

The aims and methods already outlined apply to the following nerve injuries but specific points will be discussed.

Brachial Plexus Lesions

Injuries to the brachial plexus may be complete or partial and upper trunk lesions are the most frequent. The lesions may combine the three types of nerve injury, neurapraxia, axonotmesis and neurotmesis.

The plexus may be injured by traction as in motor-cycle accidents or it may be damaged by stabs and gunshot wounds, by fractures of the clavicle and dislocation of the shoulder joint. The motor and sensory changes will depend on the site of the lesion.

There are two tests which indicate if the site of the lesion is proximal or distal to the posterior root ganglia.

1. *The axon reflex test.* When the nerve roots are avulsed, axon reflexes will still be obtained in the skin of the arm because the peripheral axons of the posterior root have not been interrupted and are connected with their nutrient cells in the posterior root ganglia.

2. *The sensory conduction test.* This test is carried out by electromyography and if a sensory action potential is obtained from a digital nerve, the peripheral axons are connected with the posterior root ganglion.

It is usual to wait ten to fourteen days after the injury before performing these tests, to give time for Wallerian degeneration to occur. Tests carried out within a day or two of the injury may give inaccurate results.

If the results of the test are positive it can be inferred that the lesion is pre-ganglionic, but if the result is negative this may infer one of two things, either that the lesion is pre-ganglionic or that it is both pre- and post-ganglionic. Myelograms can be performed to show if there has been a pre-ganglionic lesion. It will be clear that if the lesion is pre-ganglionic then hopes of recovery are negligible and early amputation may be advisable.

If the first thoracic nerve is involved then pre-ganglionic fibres to the head and neck will be affected causing a Horner's syndrome. The pupil is constricted as the sphincter pupillae, supplied by parasympathetic fibres running in the occulomotor nerve, are unopposed. The eyelid droops (ptosis) and sweating is lost over the face on the side of the lesion.

Causalgia

Causalgia means heat pain and applies to the persistent burning pain which sometimes follows nerve injuries and occasionally occurs in brachial plexus lesions, more often in partial injuries than complete ones. Intense pain radiates down the limb and may be precipitated by a sudden noise or shock. The pain can be very distressing but usually improves slowly over two to three months. Analgesics are rarely helpful for this type of pain and drugs such as chlorpromazine (Largactil), which have an effect on the cerebral cortex are used. The patient is then aware of the pain but not disturbed by it.

In complete lesions all the muscles of the upper limb are paralysed except trapezius and there is complete anaesthesia apart from a small area on the medial side of the upper arm, which is supplied by the intercosto-brachial nerve. The limb hangs limply from the shoulder in medial rotation, the humerus may subluxate, the elbow is extended and the forearm pronated. The hand loses its normal contour and becomes blue and swollen if dependent.

Partial lesions involving the upper trunk will affect the muscles around the shoulder and the elbow flexors. Lesions of the lower trunk will affect the small muscles of the hand.

SURGICAL TREATMENT

In complete lesions the arm may be amputated above the elbow and the shoulder joint arthrodesed. Physiotherapy will be required to gain compensatory mobility and power in the scapula and shoulder girdle.

In a partial lesion to regain elbow flexion Clark's pectoral transplant may be used. In this operation the sternal origin of pectoralis major is mobilized and transplanted into the biceps tendon at the elbow.

When the wrist flexors are normal but the wrist and finger extensors are paralysed an arthrodesis of the wrist will assist functional use of the hand.

In partial lesions a combination of lively splintage and reconstructive surgery will often restore function. When the elbow flexors are paralysed function of the shoulder and hand can be facilitated by a splint incorporating a spring to encourage elbow flexion. If the injury is recovering, the strength of the spring can be reduced as the power of the muscle increases. A stop hinge (see Plates XIV and XV) can be fitted at the elbow, instead of a spring, if both flexors and extensors are affected so that the elbow may be held in a number of different positions to facilitate use of the shoulder and hand.

PHYSIOTHERAPY

Passive movements to the affected joints should begin as soon as possible. Delay may be unavoidable if there are un-united fractures. A full range of movement of all joints is given twice daily. Mobility must be

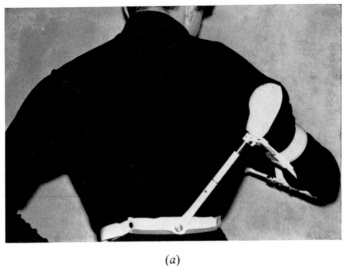

(*a*)

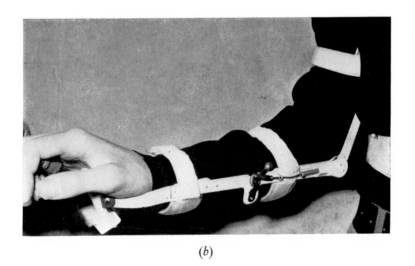

(*b*)

XIV. Two views of the flail arm appliance for use with partial or complete brachial plexus lesions (*see* p. 270).

This splint and the one illustrated in Plate XV were designed by Mr. D. W. Collins as a result of a joint project between The Royal National Orthopaedic Hospital, London and Queen Mary's Hospital, Roehampton. They are manufactured by Hugh Steeper Ltd.

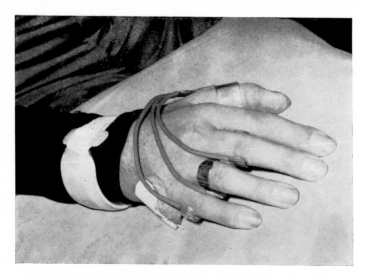

XV. A lively splint supporting the fingers in extension. It can be worn with the flail arm appliance shown in Plate XIV (*see* p. 270).

maintained in lateral rotation of the shoulder joint, elbow flexion and extension and flexion and extension of the metacarpophalangeal joints and full mobility of the thumb. The thumb web and metacarpophalangeal joints soon become stiff if they are not frequently moved. Stiffness once it has occurred, will take weeks of intensive treatment to correct. The more intelligent patient can be taught to maintain the joint range himself. He should be advised to move the shoulder in a lying position and the elbow and hand sitting at a table. If time is taken to explain why this is so important his co-operation will be gained more readily. Movements in hydrotherapy are helpful and floats can be used to support the arm (see Plate VI).

Compensatory movements are encouraged and it is possible to re-educate shoulder abduction when infraspinatus and biceps are contracting. If the shoulder is in full lateral rotation with the elbow flexed to a right angle, then the long head of biceps and triceps assisted by infraspinatus can abduct the shoulder to 90 degrees. Above this the clavicular head of pectoralis major and serratus anterior complete the movement. Elevation of the shoulder girdle must be prevented as abduction is attempted. This compensatory movement is only possible if the shoulder is fully mobile and then strong abduction can be restored.

CIRCUMFLEX NERVE INJURY

The circumflex nerve supplies deltoid and teres minor, and may be injured in fractures of the surgical neck of the humerus, and in dislocations of the shoulder joint. The patient is unable to abduct the arm and there is marked flattening of the contour of the shoulder.

If compensatory movements are taught, powerful abduction can be restored. Some patients readily teach themselves this movement, whilst in others it may take several weeks of intensive re-education. The normal movement is completely restored as re-innervation of deltoid takes place.

ULNAR AND MEDIAN NERVE INJURY

The ulnar and median nerves may be cut at the wrist as a result of putting the hand through a window. Tendons and arteries are usually cut at the same time. The tendon of palmaris longus and flexor pollicis longus and flexor sublimis are cut with the median nerve, and flexor carpi ulnaris and the ulnar artery with the ulnar nerve. It is usual for primary tendon suture to be performed.

Both nerves may be involved in elbow injuries. Fractures of the medial epicondyle often involve the ulnar nerve. The median nerve may be compressed in the carpal tunnel by pressure from proliferation of the synovial sheaths of the flexor tendons. This can be relieved by surgical division of the flexor retinaculum.

The deformity in ulnar nerve lesions is known as the claw hand. There is hyperextension of the metacarpophalangeal joints of annularis and minimus, due to overaction of extensor digitorum, unopposed by the paralysed medial two lumbricals. If the lesion is at the elbow, there will be paralysis of flexor profundus digitorum to these two fingers.

The deformity can be corrected by an ulnar lively splint. This prevents hyperextension of the metacarpophalangeal joints, and extensor digitorum can act as an extensor of the fingers, as the metacarpophalangeal joints are stabilized.

The sensory loss does not severely impair the patient's function, although burns are liable to occur on the affected fingers and ulnar border of the hand.

The deformity in a median nerve lesion is known as the monkey hand. The thumb is held alongside the index finger by extensor pollicis longus, unopposed by the paralysed abductor pollicis brevis and opponens pollicis. The thenar eminence is flattened, as there is atrophy of abductor pollicis brevis, opponens pollicis and the superficial head of flexor pollicis brevis (see Plate VII).

The sensory loss is a severe disability as sensation is lacking over most of the palm and over the index and middle fingers and the thumb, therefore the patient is unable to recognize objects in his hand or to judge the pressure exerted by his thumb and fingers.

Progression of Treatment following Secondary Suture of Median and Ulnar Nerves

If the suture is at the wrist, this joint is usually immobilized in flexion by a plaster splint for three weeks. If it is at the elbow and extensive resection has been necessary, then a turn-buckle plaster may be applied to maintain the elbow in flexion. After three weeks the elbow is gradually extended by the use of the turn-buckle until full movement is regained, usually in three to five weeks. The turn-buckle is designed to allow movement into elbow flexion but controls extension.

One to three weeks. Active movements are encouraged for the unaffected joints of the upper limb.

Three to five weeks. The daily treatment follows the routine for a peripheral nerve injury avoiding tension on the sutured nerve ends. It should be remembered that a little stiffness in the joints of the hand can be a

Treatment

major disability. The nails should be cut by the physiotherapist to prevent the patient damaging his insensitive skin. If there are unhealed areas, or if trophic lesions have occurred, then saline soaks are used and the wounds cleaned with half-strength eusol.

Treatment should be repeated three to four times daily and alternate with periods of occupational therapy.

Six to eight weeks. Deeper massage with lanolin is given to free adherent scars.

In these cases it is essential to appreciate the difference between deformities caused by over-action of the antagonists, joint stiffness, and those caused by tendon adherence, due to associated injuries. In the contracture following laceration of the flexor aspect of the wrist, flexor sublimis digitorum may become adherent and then the proximal interphalangeal joints are held at 90° flexion (see Plate VIII). This deformity disappears as the wrist and metacarpophalangeal joints are flexed and tension on flexor sublimis digitorum is released, and re-appears as the wrist and metacarpophalangeal joints are extended.

Proprioceptive neuromuscular facilitation techniques are used. The flexion abduction pattern encourages extension of the wrist and fingers. Strengthening and relaxation techniques are employed in unilateral and bilateral patterns.

Games are useful and can include those with cards, matches and tiddlywinks. Games such as volleyball, in which forcible wrist and finger extension might occur, are not suitable.

When full passive mobility has been restored lively splints are needed.

Eight to ten weeks. Now more vigorous resisted exercises can be introduced. If full mobility has not been restored, then passive stretching is required. The stretch should be slow and steady and combined with relaxation techniques to avoid stimulating the stretch reflex. Stubborn cases are treated by making serial stretch plasters, which is a skilled technique and must be applied with care and under medical supervision (see Plates IX and X).

When movements are full the patient should continue the treatment at home and whenever possible return to work. He is seen by the doctor at intervals throughout this period and treatment is resumed when re-innervation takes place. As soon as there are signs of sensation in the palm and fingers sensory re-education begins so that the patient may use the altered sensation to train stereognosis.

Large, easily held blocks of wood of varying weights, shaped as cylinders, cubes, or hexagons, may be used. Some sides are covered in materials of contrasting texture, such as sandpaper and velvet (see Plate XI). The patient is blindfolded and is asked to assess the difference in weight, describe the size, the material from which it is made and name the object. It is important that the object is not seen beforehand. Similar assessments are made, using everyday articles and coins. By this method the mental picture can be associated with the actual one and with practice the objects be visualized through the hand. This regime should be continued at home daily.

Training can be given in localization of sensation, which, owing to cross innervation, will be faulty.

The first muscle to recover following ulnar nerve suture at the wrist is abductor minimi digiti (between 80 to 100 days), and a contraction can be elicited first in opposition of the thumb to the little finger. It is easy to be misled by contraction of flexor carpi ulnaris pulling on an adherent wrist scar.

In a median nerve lesion the first sign of recovery is an improvement of the thumb position, before a contraction can be felt in abductor pollicis brevis. Intensive re-education is essential. This must include functional activities as well as individual and group re-education of the recovering muscles.

RADIAL NERVE INJURY

The radial nerve is most frequently injured where it winds round the humerus, as a result of fractures or by pressure from the callus formation. It may also be damaged in the axilla by pressure from an axillary crutch.

Complete interruption of the nerve in or above the axilla causes paralysis of the elbow, wrist and finger extensors. If the injury is below the axilla the triceps will not be affected. Though there is inability to extend the wrist or metacarpophalangeal joints, the interphalangeal joints can be extended by the interossei and lumbricals and the thumb by abductor pollicis brevis, as it has an insertion into the extensor expansion of the thumb (see Plate XIII).

The simplest and most functional lively splint consists of parallel forearm bars within a leather gauntlet, a horizontal palmar bar just proximal to the metacarpophalangeal joints of the fingers and a spring hinge at the wrist so arranged to enable the patient to flex the wrist and fingers against it and it will then return the wrist to a functional position in extension (see Plate XII). The interphalangeal joints are free and the thumb rests in a good position. A light splint may be required at night to support the wrist in extension with a leather or fibre-glass gauntlet.

During the stage of recovery, triceps is re-educated using slings and hydrotherapy. Movements should also be given with the arm elevated to prevent trick action by the depressors of the shoulder.

PERIPHERAL NERVE INJURY TO THE LOWER LIMB

The sciatic nerve may be stretched when the hip is dislocated, or severed by wounds of the pelvis or thigh. The lateral popliteal division is damaged by fractures of the neck of the fibula or by pressure from strapping or plaster.

After complete interruption of the sciatic nerve there is paralysis of the hamstrings and all the muscles distal to the knee. In lateral popliteal injuries foot-drop occurs as there is paralysis of the anterior tibial and peroneal muscles. The foot falls into equino-varus and drops at each step due to gravity and the unopposed pull of the calf muscles. The sensory loss is over the dorsum of the foot and lateral side of the leg.

The deformity can be corrected by a toe-raising spring or a foot-drop device fitted into the heel of the shoe.

A night splint should be made to support the foot at 90° dorsiflexion and in the mid-position between inversion and eversion. This will help to prevent contracture of the calf muscles and clawing of the toes. The splint should extend for an inch distal to the toes to keep the weight of the bed-clothes off the foot.

Passive movements should be given daily. The patient can stretch the tendo Achillis by standing with the affected foot on a low step and pushing his body-weight over the flexed knee, with the sole of the foot resting firmly on the step.

Contractures can be stretched with the patient in prone lying; this is also the easiest position in which to make stretch plasters to correct stubborn contractures.

Walking and postural re-education are essential with the patient wearing a foot-drop spring. Without a toe-raising device there is usually a tendency to exaggerated hip and knee flexion as the patient tries to prevent the toes touching the ground.

During the stage of recovery proprioceptive facilitation techniques are used, the flexion adduction pattern with the knee flexed being useful to encourage tibialis anterior to contract synergistically.

The peronei and anterior tibials can both be stimulated by using balance reactions. A balance board is also used to re-educate these muscles. A balance board is a large piece of wood under which is fastened a rounded shape which allows it to roll in all directions.

The support from the toe-raising spring is reduced as the strength of the dorsiflexors increases.

In all lower limb injuries postural re-education and the correction of gait should be included in treatment.

A triple arthrodesis may be performed for irreparable lateral popliteal lesions.

Lesions of the medial popliteal division of the sciatic nerve may occur in supracondylar fractures of the femur. There is paralysis of the calf, posterior tibial and plantar muscles. Contractures of the plantar fascia may occur following paralysis of the interossei and lumbricals.

Trophic lesions are liable to occur on the sole of the foot, due to the lack of sensation and vasomotor changes.

It is essential that shoes fit well. A sponge rubber insole is useful to prevent trophic lesions.

Hyperaesthesia can be severe. This may be relieved by encouraging the patient to walk on his bare feet on different surfaces such as linoleum, rubber, carpet and tiles.

The femoral and obturator nerves are rarely injured. Division of the femoral nerve causes paralysis of the quadriceps and the knee tends to give way in walking and the body cannot be raised on stairs.

Patients learn to compensate for this loss in walking by hyper-extending the knee and can achieve a surprisingly good walk.

ELECTRICAL STIMULATION

It is believed by some eminent authorities that electrical stimulation of denervated muscles is essential for recovery. It has been proved that muscle bulk is preserved by daily stimulation but as far as is known it has not been proved that bulk and function are necessarily related. If full-time intensive treatment is given as described above, there appears to be no detrimental effect from not stimulating the denervated muscles electrically. Patients with complete brachial plexus lesions, who have not received electrical treatment, have been seen with worthwhile recovery in the hand two to three years after injury, and recovery of independent interosseous action has also been observed following suture of the ulnar nerve at the wrist. Electrical stimulation may be useful during the recovery stage as an aid to re-education.

Chapter XIV

RECENT INJURIES

Violence, mild or severe, may damage any of the tissues of the body. The skin may be broken or deeper tissues may be injured while the skin remains intact. If the skin is unbroken there is less danger of infection since the skin forms a barrier to the entry of bacteria and debris into the wound.

The changes in the tissues after injury

Whatever the injury, whether it is of skin and superficial tissue only, or of muscle, tendon, ligament or bone, the changes which follow are basically the same since their purpose is to remove the debris and prepare the way for repair.

The immediate change is an outpouring of blood and lymph into the tissues from the ruptured vessels. This may spread widely if the tissues are torn and lax or may be retained in a small area if fascial bands and membranes are intact. Very rapidly the changes of inflammation begin. Inflammatory exudate is added to the blood and lymph, the area becomes packed with inflammatory cells and small vessels become blocked by thrombus formation. Phagocytic cells begin the process of liquefaction of solid debris. If the injury involves secreting surfaces such as synovial or mucous membranes increased secretions are added to the exudate.

The tension within the tissues resulting from these changes is not readily relieved because drainage is impaired by the damage and blocking of the small veins and lymphatics and by the slowing of the circulation which results from decreased movement of the injured region. Most injured areas show considerable oedema which is a feature of inflammatory response.

REPAIR

The changes of inflammation gradually merge into those of repair and again these are fundamentally the same whatever the tissue.

The first step in repair is the clotting of the blood and exudate. The clot acts as an irritant and multiplication of cells and capillaries in the surrounding tissue is therefore stimulated. These cells and capillaries grow into the clot which is gradually converted into granulation tissue.

The subsequent steps vary with the tissue which has been damaged. Cells which have become specialized often lose the power of reproduction and tissues such as muscle and nerve cannot, therefore, be replaced by similar tissue. Other tissues such as skin and bone are able to regenerate. Those which are unable to reproduce themselves complete their repair by the formation of scar tissue. The fibroblasts of the granulation tissue form fine fibrils which radiate in any direction through the tissue. Gradually the fibrils thicken and over the course of weeks those bundles which lie in anatomical orientation coarsen and take the normal strains thrown on the region, while those placed in other directions are absorbed. As the fibres thicken and contract the capillaries are obliterated and the cells flattened. Eventually white fibrous tissue remains. This gives a firm repair, but unfortunately it has a tendency to contract unless kept supple by constant movement. Contracture may lead to deformity and interference with function. Alternately if this tissue is subjected to repeated stretching it will gradually lengthen. If this occurs in the repair of muscle or tendon, the muscle will be lengthened and its power, therefore, reduced.

In tissues such as skin and bone, which retain the power of reproduction, the granulation tissue is replaced by the multiplication of the specialized cells instead of by the production of fibrous tissue. Thus in skin the cells of the epidermis are able to multiply and so, when the superficial surface of the skin is broken, the cells multiply and slide sideways to cover the wound.

These processes of repair may occur in sites remote from the damaged area. Blood and exudate can seep into surrounding healthy tissue, particularly under the influence of gravity. If not rapidly absorbed it will clot and organize. Here the new tissue can only be a nuisance because it thickens the area, and mats fibres together. Thus function is impaired.

Rate of repair

Many factors influence the rate at which repair of body tissues takes place. *The greater the gap* in the tissues the longer will repair take and sometimes repair can be speeded up by suturing the tissues and so lessening the gap.

The amount of movement which occurs at the site of injury is also an important factor. Excess movement tends to delay repair and increase the amount of fibrous tissue formed. If, for example, movement occurs between the bone ends following fracture, granulation tissue will be constantly broken down and fibrous tissue will form instead of bone. For this reason damaged tissues are usually protected until repair is complete. A ruptured tendon will be sutured and then immobilized for several weeks; a fractured bone, if movement of the bone ends is likely, will be splinted until consolidation is reached; a stretched ligament will be protected from further stretching until it is healed.

The degree of vascularity of the damaged tissues will affect the rate of repair. A good blood supply is necessary to provide the nutrition for the growing tissue, but some tissues such as tendon and ligament have a naturally poor blood supply and are, therefore, slow to heal. Occasionally the blood supply is seriously impaired as a result of the injury and repair will then be delayed. This is so in some fractures of the scaphoid in which the proximal fragment with little periosteum and no muscle attachments is cut off from its nutrition.

The blood supply of the injured tissues is also impaired by the accumulation of fluid resulting from bleeding and inflammation, and by lack of movement. The oedema should, therefore, be dispersed as rapidly as possible; this can often be achieved by elevation of the part, firm bandaging, muscle contractions and movements, if permitted.

Protection from infection. The presence of harmful organisms delays healing because more destruction of tissue occurs and consequently there is eventually more to be replaced. Longer time is needed for repair and more scar tissue is formed.If there is an established infection, a wide incision may be made and careful excision of all dead tissue together with chemotherapy should be carried out.

There are, of course, other factors which influence rate of repair such as age, general health and size of bone, but these are not influenced to any extent by treatment.

Physiotherapy in relation to repair

Any means which helps to disperse oedema and stimulate the circulation will aid repair provided that it does not produce excessive movement at the site of injury. Elevation of an injured part and rhythmic muscle contractions are nearly always valuable. Massage is useful, but cannot be given over a fracture site immediately after the injury or over an open wound.

If there is an open wound care must be taken to prevent infection and when the wound begins to heal it is important not to break down granulations by careless handling of dressings since this will delay healing. Heat and ultra-violet therapy will often help to clean wounds and stimulate repair processes.

Early active movements are useful to prevent organization of exudate which has spread into undamaged tissues, but these must be used with care to avoid delaying healing of the damaged tissues. Often the damaged tissues are immobilized and movements can safely be given to joints not included in the splints. In fractures of the shafts of the tibia and fibula, for example, some surgeons like ankle and knee movements to be given at once while the bone ends are protected by a short splint or internal fixation; later when the joints are free and exudate absorbed full immobilization is carried out.

SIGNS AND SYMPTOMS OF RECENT INJURIES OF SOFT TISSUES

Whatever the injury there is always pain, tenderness, swelling and muscle spasm, though these vary in their intensity. If the damaged area is sufficiently superficial, heat and redness will develop and in most injuries bruising will appear later. There are also the characteristic signs of the particular tissue which has been damaged. Often the radiograph will confirm the diagnosis.

Synovitis is usually recognized by its characteristic swelling. This is an effusion, the irritation of the synovial membrane resulting in an outpouring of synovial fluid into the joint cavity. It does not develop fully for six to eight hours after the injury and it moves on palpation unless the capsule is too fully distended. Since it is contained within the capsule it does not seep into the surrounding tissues and so it follows the outline of the synovial membrane and fills up the hollows around the joint.

The pain in this lesion is more in the nature of a feeling of tension and is increased by movement of the joint. The joint is held in the position of ease with contraction of one group of muscles and inhibition of its antagonists.

In tenosynovitis the effusion is within the tendon sheath and the swelling is soft and 'sausage-shaped'. Movement of the tendon within the sheath is painful, therefore active contraction of the muscle and passive movement in the opposite direction are both uncomfortable. If the injury is chronic the swelling feels firmer and there is often crepitus when the tendon moves in the roughened sheath.

Signs and Symptoms of Recent Injuries of Soft Tissues

Bursitis shows an isolated soft fluctuating swelling within the confines of the bursa. The amount of pain varies with the bursa affected. If the swollen bursa is in such a position that it is pressed on then pain will be present. Thus an olecranon bursitis is not often painful, but an acute subacromial bursitis is exceedingly painful on the slightest movement of the shoulder. A chronic bursitis in which the walls of the bursa are adherent will usually hamper movement since the purpose of the bursa is to give ease of movement.

In ligamentous injuries the swelling is more diffuse since it is not within the capsule. These injuries are characterized by tenderness over the site of damage and pain when the ligament is stretched. If the ligament is completely ruptured, there will be an abnormal range of movement and instability of the joint when the acute symptoms have subsided.

Contusion and rupture of muscles. In these injuries there is usually much bleeding since muscles are very vascular, especially in athletes. There is, therefore, considerable swelling with great tension and later much bruising often extending well away from the site of injury. Temporarily the elasticity, extensibility and contractility of the muscle are reduced and it is difficult and painful to produce even a weak contraction.

If the muscle is completely ruptured it will not be possible to contract it. Once swelling and pain have subsided there will be an obvious gap between the ends and the belly of the muscle will be seen at a higher level. An abnormally wide range of movement in the opposite direction is also a feature. Power will gradually return, but the full power will not be restored unless the muscle is sutured, since the gap will be filled with fibrous tissue, which will, with repeated movements, gradually lengthen.

Rupture of a tendon can be recognized by the immediate loss of function. Rupture of the extensor pollicis longus tendon, for example, is usually followed by inability to extend the terminal joint of the thumb and a tendency for the tip of the thumb to remain in flexion. The tendon can no longer be seen or palpated. There is not usually much swelling unless the tendon is a large one and the force also ruptured the soft tissues around. The belly of the muscle retracts after the rupture and a gap results so that healing does not usually occur unless the tendon is sutured.

Dislocations are often recognized by obvious deformity of the joint and sometimes the bones can be felt to be in an abnormal relationship towards one another. Movement is usually grossly restricted or impossible and pain is severe at first due to the tearing of the soft tissues and pressure of the dislocated bone on other structures. The dislocation can readily be confirmed by the radiograph if it has not been immediately reduced.

TREATMENT OF RECENT INJURIES OF SOFT TISSUES

Methods of treatment vary with the different types of injury, but there is one principle in every injury from a mild contusion to a severe fracture or dislocation. This is the restoration of the patient as rapidly as possible to his pre-accident condition or even in a few cases to a state better than before the accident. This is what is meant by the term rehabilitation. As a member of the rehabilitation team the physiotherapist plays a part mainly in the direction of strengthening muscles, increasing joint range and helping the patient to gain confidence. To do this effectively she should know as much as possible of the work the patient has to do and visits to the factories in the district are an important part of her preparation to become a valuable member of the rehabilitation team.

The main principles of physiotherapy for each type of injury will be set out below, but it is essential to realize that a force which stretches or ruptures one tissue nearly always damages others at the same time and it is not possible to treat one tissue separately.

Principles of treatment of damaged Synovial membrane

The synovial membrane of a joint may be injured by sudden twists and strains or occasionally by a direct blow over the joint. It reacts to injury by inflammation and the outpouring of synovial fluid resulting in an effusion in the joint. If the effusion is considerable the joint will be held in the position in which the capsule and ligaments are relaxed; there will be, therefore, increased tone in one group of muscles and decreased tone or complete inhibition in its antagonists. Muscle atrophy is, as a consequence, likely to develop.

The first principle of treatment, therefore, is *to gain quick absorption of the effusion and prevent any further damage* which would increase it. If, therefore, the effusion is considerable the joint is aspirated and in any case a firm pressure bandage is applied. This supports the joint and limits the amount of fluid. It also helps to ensure the rest which is necessary for the first twenty-four to forty-eight hours.

The second principle is to *prevent muscle atrophy* by overcoming inhibition and exercising all muscles round the joint. Once effusion begins to absorb, discomfort becomes less and provided there is no other injury the patient will relax the muscles which hold the joint in the position of ease.

Treatment of Recent Injuries of Soft Tissues

As soon as the pressure bandage is applied rhythmic contractions of those muscles showing inhibition or decreased tone must be taught. In some patients this is difficult, but by explanation of 'what and why' and by demonstration on the uninjured side it can usually be obtained. If contraction cannot be obtained in this way, it can often be initiated by electrical stimulation.

Once the rhythmic contractions can be done exercises using the muscles statically are added, for example, in a synovitis of knee quadriceps contractions are followed by leg exercises keeping the knee straight.

When this particular group of muscles is working well, contractions of other muscles controlling the joint are added.

The third principle is to ensure that *no limitation of range develops*. This rarely occurs in a simple synovitis since the synovial fluid has anticoagulant properties. If the synovitis is complicated by haemarthrosis or damage to other joint structures the joint may become stiff. In a simple synovitis movements of the joint are started when the effusion is subsiding. They are used mainly so that the muscles can be strengthened and should be given without weight until the effusion has practically disappeared and the muscles are strong enough to control the joint against gravity. If the injury is more complicated movements may not be begun until later.

The fourth principle is to *regain full confidence in the limb* and so full normal use. Usually in a simple synovitis the effusion has subsided in seven to ten days and by this time the range is full and the muscles working well; it remains only to see that the joint is being used normally. The activities which the patient usually undertakes should be checked and practised as far as possible. In weight-bearing joints this involves walking, running, climbing stairs, jumping and for some patients vigorous games and activities.

Principles of treatment of Bursitis

An *acute* traumatic bursitis is the result of a blow on the bursa such as a fall on the knee or shoulder. If the inflamed bursa is not subjected to pressure it rarely causes much trouble and little, if any, treatment is required. If, like the subacromial bursa, any movement causes pain, treatment is required because the joint will be held still in the most comfortable position and muscle atrophy will result. The principles of treatment are, therefore, similar to those for synovitis.

A *chronic* bursitis is more common than an acute condition. It is due to repeated minor irritation usually from pressure and is characterized by thickening of the bursal walls which later goes on to atrophy. The two layers of the bursa often become adherent and the ease of movement which the bursa should provide is lost. Movement is therefore limited and it is often painful at the point at which pressure is brought to bear on the bursa. The first principle of treatment is, therefore, to *prevent pressure* and the patient should be taught to avoid the movement which causes pain.

An attempt may be made to *reduce the adherence of the bursal walls.* Some authorities advocate the use of deep transverse frictions to move one layer of the bursa over the other, others prefer to stimulate the circulation by using some form of deep heat such as ultrasonic or short-wave therapy.

It is important to see that the *muscles are restored to normal strength* and that *limitation of range does not develop.* Free and resisted exercises are taught, but care must be taken in their selection. Range must be obtained without causing pressure on the bursa.

Principles of treatment of Tenosynovitis

Inflammation of a tendon sheath may be acute or chronic. The *acute* tenosynovitis is usually the result of sudden wrench or direct blow over the tendon and the principles of treatment are again similar to those for synovitis. Rest and support usually result in rapid resolution of the inflammation and absorption of the effusion and no further treatment is required. But if there is any limitation of movement after thirty-six to forty-eight hours short-wave diathermy and exercises will help to promote resolution and full recovery.

A *chronic* tenosynovitis is the result of over-use of the tendon in a new occupation or one which is resumed after a period of rest. It is characterized by thickening of the synovial sheath and the formation of tiny fibrinoid nodules known as melon-seed bodies. Movement of the tendon within the thickened and roughened sheath is, therefore, painful and difficult and function is impaired.

The object of the treatment therefore is *to make movement easier.* This may be done by prolonged rest by means of splinting so that the tendon cannot be moved, or by trying to improve the blood supply to the sheath so that the unnecessary tissue is absorbed. This is done by the use of heat or by deep transverse frictions applied directly over the thickened area. These soften and stretch the fibrous thickenings and produce a local hyperaemia. Some surgeons prefer to incise the sheath or to excise a section and this is followed by active movements so that adhesions do not form.

Principles of treatment of Muscular and Tendinous Injuries

Injuries may be simple contusions, strains or ruptures. They are common injuries, particularly in athletes and professional footballers at the beginning of the season.

A *contusion* is a crushing injury, the result of a blow or kick, and is characterized by rupture of blood and lymph vessels in the connective tissue framework of the muscle with inflammation of the muscle fibres. Temporarily tone is diminished and there is loss of the properties of extensibility and contractility. If untreated, organization of blood and exudate will result in scarring within the muscle and this together with diminished use will cause atrophy.

A *strain* occurs when a muscle has been unable to resist a sudden stretching force; the connective tissue is stretched and a few fibres of the muscle may be ruptured. The muscle is lengthened and for the time being is not capable of contracting to its full extent. The same lesion may occur in the tendon or at the teno-periostial junction. The muscles in which this lesion is most likely to occur are those in which there has been previous injury or those with poor elasticity, not capable of normal lengthening.

Rupture may occur in the belly of the muscle, at the musculo-tendinous junction, in the tendon or at its attachment to bone. The cause may be an inco-ordinated contraction, forcibly stretching when the muscle is actively contracting or a blow on a contracted muscle. Immediate spasm of the muscle retracts the proximal part and a gap appears which is rapidly filled with blood and inflammatory exudate. Much blood also seeps among the surrounding undamaged fibres. If untreated, organization rapidly occurs with scarring and repair of the rupture by fibrous tissue. With repeated movement this tissue will stretch and the muscle, therefore, will gradually lengthen. For this reason the immediate treatment is *suture so that a gap does not develop* and lengthening does not occur. This is followed by immobilization until repair is sound. The period of immobilization for a muscle rupture is not necessarily long, often not more than ten days to three weeks, because muscle heals rapidly since its vascularity is good. It is, however, usually longer for the less vascular tendon.

In all muscle injuries the most important principle is the *prevention of scar tissue formation*. The extravasated blood and lymph tends to clot and organize. The fibrous tissue so formed mats the muscle fibres together interfering with their contraction and may sometimes bind them to the underlying bone if the contusion or strain is deep-seated. This tendency is marked because the muscle is painful and the patient tends to avoid its use, the circulation is therefore slowed and the fibres do not move over

Recent Injuries

each other. If the patient is a trained athlete there are far more patent blood vessels in the muscle and bleeding is greater following injury.

It is, therefore, very important to keep the bleeding as slight as possible and to hasten the absorption of the exudate while at the same time keeping the muscle fibres moving so that the sticky exudate does not have a chance to clot. This is best done by encouraging muscle contractions and non-weight-bearing exercises at once though sometimes strapping is used to give support and protection and in all cases competitive sport is avoided. Heat should be avoided for the first few days because by producing vaso-dilation it increases bleeding. The use of ultrasonic therapy is often most successful because it produces a fine vibration of the tissues and so prevents organization and promotes rapid absorption. It may also be possible to limit bleeding by firm pressure over the site of injury or by stretching the muscle, so causing pressure on the fibres by its fascial framework and leaving no room for blood to accumulate. Thus a footballer who sustains a crush or strain of quadriceps may be encouraged to squat on his heels immediately following the injury.

Atrophy of the damaged muscle will be prevented by the immediate use of contractions and exercises, but perhaps the most important thing of all is *to restore the patient's confidence in his limb.* This particularly applies to the man who earns his living by sport or very heavy work. He may know that the muscle is back to normal, but he may find it difficult to trust it, and, therefore, cannot put out his best in his particular occupation. Thus early use of the limb, quickly progressed exercises, and almost immediate return to his sport, provided he does not enter into competitive activity, is important.

If the muscle or tendon is ruptured it cannot be exercised until repair is sound; contractions and exercises are, therefore, delayed, but in the meanwhile joints not immobilized should be exercised in order to stimulate the circulation, and the limb should be used as normally as possible. When the surgeon permits use of the muscle graded exercises are commenced. Strongly resisted work for the muscle is avoided for several weeks.

In spite of careful planning and treatment fibrous tissue scars do sometimes form. If these can be maintained supple they may not cause any trouble, consequently if there is thickening in the muscle or tendon, the object is *to try to soften and stretch the fibrous tissue;* this can be done by deep transverse friction across the thickened area or by the use of localized measures to improve the blood supply, followed by deep massage and vigorous movements.

Treatment of Recent Injuries of Soft Tissues

Principles of treatment of Ligamentous Injuries

Ligaments are damaged by a sudden force applied to a joint which, taking the muscle unawares, carries the joint beyond its normal range. The ligament may be slightly stretched if the force is not too great, a few of its blood and lymph vessels will be ruptured and a small amount of bleeding and inflammatory exudate will occur. If the force is greater some of its fibres may be torn and there will then be more bleeding, especially as the loose connective tissue and often the tendon sheaths will also be damaged. The force may be great enough to rupture the ligament completely, usually tearing it from one of its bony attachments and sometimes as it is torn off it takes with it a flake of bone.

In the first two injuries there will be pain, tenderness and swelling, but the stability of the joint is not impaired; if, however, the ligament is avulsed the joint will be unstable and once pain and swelling have subsided abnormal movement is usually possible. Treatment of the two types of injury, therefore, differs.

If the injury is not a complete rupture the chief trouble lies in the danger of organization of the exudate so that the ligament becomes bound down to the bones between its attachments. This will limit movement and when early signs of the injury have gone there will remain some tenderness and pain on the extremes of movement. The main principle of treatment, therefore, is to *prevent the formation of excess fibrous tissue and adherence of the ligament*. To do this the amount of bleeding and exudate should be kept to a minimum by preventing further damage to the ligament, while at the same time organization of exudate, except that necessary for repair, must be prevented. These two aims can be fulfilled by giving rest and support to the ligament, by strapping or firm bandaging, while moving the joint within the limits of the support and exercising all other joints of the limb. The patient contracts the muscles against the elastic support of the strapping and so there is a pumping effect on the exudate. If a bandage is worn it can be removed so that ultrasonic therapy or Galvanism and massage can be applied with the limb elevated to disperse the swelling. Transverse frictions across the damaged part of the ligament will also help to prevent adherence.

At the same time that the ligament was stretched some stretching will have been applied to the muscles and tendons on that aspect of the limb. *Exercises for the muscles* should, therefore, be given; these will also have the effect of strengthening the muscles to compensate for the temporary weakening of the ligament. Thus in a sprained ankle exercises for the peronei are important if the lateral ligament is stretched.

287

Recent Injuries

If the ligament has been completely ruptured it is essential that adequate time should be given for repair as the stability of the joint is so important. The *first principle is, therefore, to obtain healing of the ligament.* Ligaments are constructed of white fibrous and elastic tissue whose vascularity is poor and healing powers slow. Immobilization is, therefore, required for a lengthy period, usually for eight to ten weeks though this can sometimes be reduced by surgical repair of the ligament. In spite of long immobilization the ligament is often permanently weakened and the *second principle of treatment is to hypertrophy the muscles* which normally act with the ligament so that they are stronger than normal to compensate for the weakened ligament. Thus if the medial ligament of the knee is ruptured the quadriceps, particularly vastus medialis, should be developed. During the period of immobilization only rhythmic contractions and static or synergic work can be done, but as soon as the splint is removed concentric and eccentric work can be added. Since the complete rupture will be accompanied by much bleeding, thickening and adhesion formation are very likely and *these should be lessened as far as possible by exercise of all joints not immobilized*, and as soon as the splint is removed any that have formed may be softened by heat and deep massage and stretched by active exercises.

In both types of injury encouragement to full normal use of the joint, as soon as the ligament has healed, is essential.

Principles of treatment of Dislocations

A dislocation is a condition in which there is displacement of one of the bone ends entering into the formation of a joint, so that the articular surfaces are no longer in contact with one another. If they lie partly in contact, but not in normal apposition, they are said to be subluxated; if they are completely apart, they are dislocated. Any joint may suffer dislocation if the violence is sufficient, but those which are most likely to suffer are those, such as the shoulder joint, which have the least natural stability. The actual damage produced at the time of dislocation is primarily of soft tissue, though sometimes articular cartilage and cartilaginous discs and rims are affected. In addition, the dislocation may be complicated by fracture of adjacent bony processes and by damage to nerves and blood vessels.

It is almost inevitable that, as one bone is displaced, the capsule of the joint is torn. For example, if the forearm bones are dislocated backwards at the elbow, the lower attachments of the capsule will be torn; while a rent will appear in the patellar retinacula if the patella is dislocated. Accessory ligaments may also be stretched or torn according to the direction taken by the bone end. Much areolar connective tissue will be affected and many tiny blood vessels in the capsule and areolar tissue will be ruptured, and

288

haemorrhage into this and neighbouring tissue results. Displacement of bone cannot occur without a considerable strain on muscles and tendons. As the stretch is put on the attachment of the muscle to the bone end there is danger of elevating the periosteum away from the underlying bone and damaging the blood vessels which pass from the deep layer of the periosteum into the bone. Bleeding then occurs between the periosteum and the bone and a sub-periosteal haematoma may develop. Dislocation must usually be accompanied by a synovitis, since the synovial membrane will be damaged by the tearing of the capsule and by the strain as the bone moves out of the normal position.

Treatment is mainly directed towards the recovery of full function. The first principle is, therefore, *reduction*. The articular surfaces must be brought into normal alignment as soon as possible so that further damage to the ligaments, muscles, blood vessels and nerves does not take place. The surgeon, therefore, reduces the dislocation as soon as it is diagnosed, if the patient's condition is suitable. The longer the bone is out of place, the more difficult it is to reduce, since the rent in the capsule, through which the bone must be passed, quickly repairs and adhesions rapidly form.

The second principle is the *prevention of further damage* so that the inflammatory exudate is kept to a minimal quantity and torn capsule, ligaments and labrum can heal. Rest is, therefore, indicated. Opinions vary as to whether immobilization is required, but since tearing of the capsule and ligaments has occurred, stability is likely to be affected and many surgeons, therefore, use fixation by bandages, slings, traction or plaster until ligaments have had a chance to heal.

Since oedema is to be expected as a result of the vasodilatation and damage to veins and lymphatic vessels, a third principle is the *promotion of absorption* of the exudate before it has time to organize into adhesions. This may be carried out while the joint is being rested, by the use of heat and massage proximal to the area of injury and by rhythmic contractions of the muscles acting on the joint. In some cases early active movements may be allowed. All active movements of joints not immobilized will help to stimulate the circulation, aid drainage and speed absorption of traumatic exudate.

Since joints become stiff not only due to adhesion formation, but also as the result of muscle weakness and lack of use, a fourth principle is the *prevention of muscle atrophy*. This is important, also, because the muscles are the first line of defence of the joint, and, if the muscles are weak, the joint is later liable to be subjected to repeated strains and stresses which cause osteo-arthritic changes. Weak muscles are rarely liable to lead to re-dislocation, though subluxation sometimes occurs. For example, if the muscles round the shoulder joint are atrophied, the head of the humerus tends to drop in the glenoid cavity and movement is weakened and impaired. Muscle atrophy is lessened by rhythmic muscle contractions and by early active movements if these are possible.

Strength may not be gained quickly and graded resisted exercises are essential. These may be given as soon as movements are allowed, at first manually and in a small range, but quickly progressed in range and strength. If exercises are commenced in the supine position, they should also be given in sitting, so that they are performed against the force of gravity.

Since nerve lesions and myositis ossificans are possible complications, it is important to be on the *watch for evidence of either of these*. Whatever the dislocation may be, a check should be carried out daily on all the movements of all joints below the level of the lesion. For example, in patients who have suffered a dislocation in the region of the elbow, great care should be taken to test the movements of the fingers. In addition the cutaneous sensation should be compared with that of the opposite side to ensure that no nerve lesion is present.

If there is tenderness and spasm of muscle near a joint and movement is decreasing in range, myositis ossificans may be suspected. If either nerve involvement or myositis ossificans is suspected, a report should be made at once to the surgeon so that treatment for the complication may be instituted (see Chapter XIII and pp. 301 and 302).

As in all other injuries, the final object is the *restoration of normal function* and full confidence in the limb. Consequently co-ordination work, games and occupational activities should be added to the scheme of treatment as soon as pain and muscle spasm have subsided and strength and range are improving.

FRACTURES

A fracture is a solution or break in the continuity of bone, and, being an event which occurs suddenly, it is usually accompanied by a certain amount of shock. The force which is enough to break the bone must also damage other tissues. Muscles, blood vessels, fascia and skin may also be involved. Sometimes nerves are affected.

The actual damage to the bone consists in a break in its continuity, associated with tearing of the intra-osseous vessels, and usually some degree of laceration of the periosteum, which may also be stripped from the bone for some distance from the fracture. When this happens, the haematoma formed by bleeding from the bone ends is allowed to escape into the surrounding tissues. In most instances this is of no importance, but at times displaced bone-forming cells come to lie in the muscles and predispose to myositis ossificans traumatica.

The surrounding soft tissues will also be damaged; some muscle fibres will be torn; much tearing of fascia and other connective tissue will occur; many blood vessels will be ruptured, and considerable extravasation of blood will take place. There will be a tendency for this blood to seep into surrounding tissues, possibly even reaching the deep surface of the skin, so that bruising becomes obvious.

The presence of tissue debris and blood clot acts as a stimulus to the production of a reaction comparable to that seen in an acute inflammation; indeed, apart from the absence of bacteria, it is indistinguishable. Neighbouring small vessels dilate and hyperaemia results, and the area is invaded by multinuclear cells. The bone shows an interesting reaction to this hyperaemia; the bone salts are absorbed and decalcification of the fractured bone ends takes place. The excess calcium is found in the blood and in the tissue exudate round the lesion. This then is the actual damage, and may be complicated by injury to nerves, large blood vessels, viscera or skin.

REPAIR

The fundamental basis of repair to any tissue, including bone, is by the formation of granulation tissue.

The final result is, however, different for two main reasons. In the first place bone-forming cells are available in the periosteum, endosteum and bone marrow, and, in the second place, when there is hyperaemia round bone, calcium is absorbed from the bone and is in high concentration in the surrounding fluid. Thus two main essentials for bone formation, bone-forming cells and calcium, are available.

Repair progresses through three stages: granulation tissue, callus and consolidation.

Granulation Tissue Formation

At the time of the injury, bleeding occurs between the stripped-up periosteum and the bone, between the fractured bone ends, and in the damaged soft tissues. The blood clots, and a haematoma is formed in these areas. The haematoma and damaged tissues stimulate the formation of granulation tissue, but the speed of its formation varies in different areas. Around the bone ends beneath the periosteum and in the soft tissues granulation tissue will have formed in seven to ten days, but it cannot be so rapidly formed between the bone ends in regions of dense cortical bone owing to their less plentiful blood supply. By the time three weeks have passed, however, the whole area of the fracture should be filled with highly vascular granulations.

Callus Formation

Granulation tissue beneath the periosteum and between the bone ends will be invaded by bone-forming cells from the periosteum, endosteum and bone marrow. These cells will form fibrous tissue or bone, depending on what happens at the fracture site. If strains and stresses are prevented and compression of the bone ends is encouraged, trabeculae of soft bone will be laid down around the blood vessels. If movement is allowed, fibrous tissue will form and lead to non-union.

With immobility and compression, the granulation tissue becomes permeated by soft bone. Gradually calcium salts are deposited and the mass becomes increasingly firm and hard. This 'callus', as it is now called, develops first beneath the periosteum where it acts as a temporary splint, ensuring that the bone ends remain in apposition, although some movement may occur in an angular direction. This thin sheath of callus has further layers applied to its deep surface, and as this occurs, its restraining effect on the bone increases, until even angulation is prevented.

When no movement can be felt, and there is no tenderness on pressure, union is said to be sound, and the fracture can be expected to stand up to gentle use, although weight-bearing may not yet be advisable.

Even though the initial haematoma may spread into the muscle planes, it is uncommon for bone formation to do so. The reason for this limitation is not known. Instead the granulation tissue gradually becomes organized into avascular fibrous tissue.

Consolidation

The callus which has been forming has no definite lamellar arrangement, and is formed in excess of that finally required. Over a period of months, it is gradually absorbed and replaced between the bone ends by bone of a definite pattern, trabeculae being laid down to withstand the normal strains and stresses. When this has occurred, and the callus round the bone ends and in the medullary cavity has been absorbed, the bone architecture appears normal, and consolidation is said to be complete.

RATE OF REPAIR

If the previous explanation has been followed, it will be realized that the time taken to gain sound repair of bone depends on many factors. Some of these factors will be local ones, others general.

Repair

The presence of a haematoma is to some extent helpful, since the fibrin of the clotted blood provides a framework on which the granulations can grow. Thus infection, which leads to liquefaction of the clot, and damage to delicate growing capillaries will diminish the rate of union. It also explains why dense cortical bone, which is relatively avascular, heals more slowly than does cancellous bone with its plentiful supply. Similarly an oblique or spiral fracture involves a greater area of cancellous bone than does a transverse lesion, and therefore tends to heal more rapidly. The same reasoning does not always hold good for comminuted fractures, however, since some of the fragments may have their blood supply cut off, and are thus unable to throw out callus. Their cells die, and it is not until they become revascularized and new osteoblasts develop that they can take an active part in the healing process.

The pattern of blood supply to the bone involved is of the greatest importance. The ends of all long bones contain a larger proportion of cancellous bone, are adjacent to the vascular anastomosis which is present round joints, and are close to fleshy origins of muscles, and for these reasons the blood supply is greater. Thus a fracture at the end of a bone can be expected to unite more rapidly than a lesion of the shaft.

Loss or diminished stimulus for repair will lead to delay in union. This is particularly so in the formation of callus between the bone ends. Separation of the bone ends by excessive traction or interposition of soft parts will often be enough to suppress completely any radiological evidence of repair.

If one of two parallel bones is fractured, impingement of one bone end on the other is difficult to obtain, or the same thing may happen if one unites more rapidly than the other. It is most important for the physiotherapist to remember this, because she can do much to encourage union. If the fracture is well immobilized by a carefully applied plaster, active use of all joints left free, and frequent contraction and relaxation of muscles controlling the immobilized joints will maintain a good local circulation, thus ensuring removal of metabolites and plentiful supply of minerals and protein necessary for healing. In addition intramuscular and intra-articular adhesions will be reduced, and recovery of function will be quicker when the plaster is removed.

Absolute immobility is impossible to achieve, even by internal fixation, but fortunately the pattern of the early deposition of callus compensates for this defect. Nevertheless, immobilization within fine limits is required to promote union in most fractures, and this can be provided by conventional methods.

The rate of repair therefore varies considerably depending on local factors, but is also dependent on the general condition, age, and state of nutrition of the patient. Children, with their more active metabolism, will show union earlier than adults, but in patients of comparable age, it is often difficult to pinpoint a definite cause for delay. Special diets, extra calcium and supplementary sunlight appear to have little effect on the rate of union unless the deficiency is gross.

Physiotherapy in relation to Repair

When granulation tissue is growing between the bone ends, compression and absence of strain are essential factors, if the tissue is to be converted into callus. In some fractures these are naturally assured; the bone ends may be firmly impacted or they may be held together by muscle action, or the violence which caused the fracture may not have caused displacement. In other cases the essentials can only be obtained by rigid immobilization. The importance of active movements to help natural repair is related to the fact that blood and inflammatory exudate seep not only among the damaged soft tissues, but also into the undamaged surrounding areas. In both sites it tends to clot and organize into fibrous tissue. In this way fibrosis can occur in neighbouring joint capsules and fibrous tissues may form between healthy muscle fibres and tendons and surrounding tissues. Soft tissues thus become thickened and matted together, and their pliability is lost, while joints become stiff and limited in range.

It is tempting in a fracture impacted in an acceptable position to leave the limb free in the early stages in order to carry out active exercises, and thus to encourage early absorption of traumatic exudate. But if one remembers the osteoporosis which follows traumatic hyperaemia, one can see that subsequent disimpaction is likely, and the original position may be difficult to regain. For this reason it is customary to apply the appropriate method of immobilization and to encourage activity of all joints left free, and to practise isometric movements of all muscle groups covering immobilized articulations.

CAUSES OF FRACTURES

The exact cause of the fracture will vary. Considerable violence is needed to break a healthy bone, but, if the structure of the bone is altered, a very small force may produce a fracture.

PATHOLOGICAL FRACTURES

If one considers the development and activity of bone, it is reasonable to suppose that alterations in bone formation and bone absorption may so change the bone that it becomes unduly predisposed or susceptible to fracture, which may then occur after only slight violence. Osteoporosis is usually the result, either of infective processes which cause hyperaemic decalcification, or of diminished function or old age. Obviously the activity of any tissue depends on the function of that part. If, for example, there is extensive paralysis of the muscles of a limb, then the limb cannot be used normally and osteoporosis of its bones occurs. Again, long immobilization of fractures without muscular exercises will lead to osteoporosis and a spontaneous fracture has been known to complicate matters when splintage has been removed. Again, bone formation may be defective because sufficient calcium is not available and the bone formed is soft, consequently bending under weight. Therefore cracks tend to appear on the convex side of the curve. This is seen in rickets and in the adult form, osteomalacia. Again, in some cases, there are congenital defects. Mature bone cannot then be produced by osteoblasts and the bones are therefore delicate and fragile —this explains the multiple fractures in osteogenesis imperfecta (fragilitas ossium). In other cases, the parathyroids are over-active and bone absorption much outpaces bone formation, so that the bones become fibrous and show cystic cavities, as is seen in osteitis fibrosa cystica. Sometimes bone destruction occurs because bone tumours or cysts are developing (see Plate XVI), and then there is much more likelihood of fractures occurring. Many other examples could be quoted, but these serve to give some idea of the reason for the pathological fracture.

FRACTURES CAUSED BY VIOLENCE WHEN THE BONE IS NORMAL

There are many ways in which violence can be applied. Direct violence usually causes a transverse fracture at the level of the blow, whereas indirect force leads to an oblique lesion. One variety of indirect force is a rotational strain, which produces a spiral fracture when applied to a single bone, and is therefore only seen in the thigh or the arm. The level of an oblique fracture depends on the anatomy of the part, since the supporting effect of ligaments, aponeuroses, etc., will protect some parts of the adjacent bone. A common example of this phenomenon is the combination of fractures in the distal third of the tibia and neck of fibula produced by a rotation strain applied to the foot.

Another way in which a fracture may be caused is by a force which pulls the bone apart, and is occasionally seen when a teenager trips, forcibly flexing the knee when the quadriceps are strongly contracting, so avulsing the epiphysis of the tibial tubercle. The commonly quoted transverse fracture of the patella is not an example of this mechanism, because there is also the element of leverage provided by the femoral condyles acting as a fulcrum.

CLASSIFICATION OF FRACTURES

Fractures may be classified into two main groups—simple and compound. Simple fractures are those in which the skin is not broken. Compound are those in which the skin is broken, and these may well prove more serious since the way is open for infection to reach the soft tissues or the bone ends. Both simple and compound fractures may have other terms applied to them. Thus the bone ends may be driven into each other, and they are then known as impacted fractures. Sometimes there is a crack only without separation. This is an incomplete fracture, and is often known as a fissured fracture.

DISPLACEMENT

When a bone is broken, provided that the ends are not driven into each other, considerable alteration of the position of the fragments may occur. This is due to the type and direction of violence, and to the muscle spasm which will follow the injury. Movement of fractured bone ends is painful, hence surrounding muscles contract to hold the fragments immobile. The result of this spasm depends on the strength and number of muscles, their attachments and particular direction of pull. Sometimes displacement is negligible, but it may also be very extensive. Extensive displacement may cause trouble, not only because malunion would occur, if it is unreduced, but also because important structures may be pressed on, or damaged. Displacement is well illustrated in fractures of the shaft of the radius and ulna above the level of the insertion of pronator teres. In this case, supinator and biceps are attached to the upper fragment, which is therefore supinated, while both pronators pronate the lower fragment. Again in subtrochanteric fractures of the femur, the powerful ilio-psoas muscle will flex the upper fragment which is also abducted by the gluteus medius and minimus, pulling on their attachments on the great trochanter.

The importance of displacement depends on several factors. Union will occur even if the fracture is left unreduced, provided that there is some compression of the granulation tissue between the bone ends but there may be such displacement that the fracture will unite with so much deformity that the normal use of the limb will be impaired. This is known as malunion. Malunion is relatively unimportant in children because cellular activity is great and remodelling of bone occurs easily, so that alignment is rapibly improved. Malunion in the shaft of a long bone, if it is the result of rotational displacement or angulation, may be serious because it might upset the mechanics of the joint distal to the fracture. As long muscles retract the lower fragment, union may occur with overlapping. This would be serious in lower extremity fractures because it would result in shortening of the limb; in the upper extremity, obviously, this would be less important. Lateral displacement would, on the other hand, make little difference to function in either extremity.

It will be seen from this that it may or may not be necessary to reduce fractures. If bone fragments have few or no muscular attachments, as, for example, in the case of a fractured scaphoid, displacement would be negligible and reduction unnecessary. Where there are many attachments, particularly if the muscles are long-bellied and powerful, then displacement may require reduction.

MAIN SIGNS AND SYMPTOMS OF FRACTURES

The main symptoms found in the majority of fractures are pain, swelling and loss of function, although it must be appreciated that one or more of these may be absent in a particular case.

Signs include swelling, deformity, abnormal mobility and crepitus and they may all be present. Bruising is variable, and depends on the type of tissue covering the fracture. It may not appear for several days after the injury, and then often at a site remote from the lesion because of the influence of gravity.

Deformity may be a feature, but this depends on the displacement and on the amount of swelling which, if considerable, may mask the deformity. Deformity is very obvious in many cases of fracture of the lower end of the radius, or of the shafts of radius and ulna, or in fractures of the shaft of the tibia since, in these cases, displacement is likely and there is little soft tissue bulk covering the bone. On the other hand there will be no deformity when the head of the radius or the scaphoid is fractured. In many cases there is a characteristic attitude. In fractures of the clavicle the buttress of the shoulder is lost and the arm tends to drop and fall forward. The patient therefore presents himself, supporting the elbow and holding the head to the affected side. In fractures of the supracondylar area of the humerus with backward displacement, the arm is supported but is held in some degrees of extension. Again in fractures of the neck of the femur, the leg lies in adduction and lateral rotation.

Active movement is usually absent since movement, if the bone is broken, would produce pain and is therefore prevented by muscle spasm. In any case even if the fragments are impacted, there is so much soft tissue damage that the patient is unwilling to move the part.

The patient usually complains of pain—this is severe at the moment of fracture and is often accompanied by a feeling of sickness. It tends to occur in waves, particularly if slight jarring occurs. Tenderness will be readily elicited by palpation over the site of fracture, while muscle spasm will be seen and felt.

COMPLICATIONS OF FRACTURES

There are many possible complications of fractures, some of which can be dealt with by the physiotherapist, and these latter will be discussed here at rather greater length.

STIFF JOINTS

Stiff joints may develop for a variety of reasons. Perkins lists these as: synovial adhesions, shrinkage of the capsule, inextensibility of muscles, incongruity of joint surfaces and organization of traumatic exudate. To these might be added one or two factors which relate to individual joints such as the adherence of the quadriceps or the patella to the bone in fractures of the femur, or the fibrosis or calcification of the capsule in supracondylar fractures of the humerus.

Synovial adhesions may occur because the synovial membrane not only lines the capsule but is reflected on to the non-articular parts of the bone within the capsule. Certain parts of the membrane are, therefore, normally in contact and would tend to adhere to one another if it were not for the presence of the synovial fluid. When joint movement is absent the circulation of the fluid is reduced, adhesions therefore tend to form and painful limited movement results.

Fibrous tissues have a natural tendency to shorten, normal length being maintained by constant movement. If joint movement is diminished the capsule and accessory ligaments tend to shrink and full range movement then becomes impossible. Still greater shrinkage occurs, if as a result of circulatory stasis, sero-fibrinous exudate soaks the capsule and organizes into fibrous tissue.

Extensibility is the ability possessed by all voluntary muscles to shorten and lengthen. This property is lost if it is not repeatedly used. If a patient persistently holds the arm to the side the adductors are never lengthened and their power to lengthen is diminished. When prolonged immobilization of a joint is necessary one group of muscles is likely to remain in its shortened position and its antagonist is correspondingly lengthened. The stiff knee which sometimes follows a fracture of the shaft of the femur is often due to the fact that the quadriceps muscle has remained so long in its shortened position that it has lost the ability to lengthen.

This loss of extensibility does not occur if the muscle is encouraged to relax completely from time to time during the period of immobilization. Thus during the period of immobility, if the hamstring muscles are made to contract against resistance, the quadriceps will relax and their ability to lengthen will be maintained.

If a fracture involves one of the articular surfaces of a joint with even slight displacement it may prove impossible to obtain perfect smoothness and 'fit' of this surface, however careful the reduction. Gradually arthritic changes then develop. This is the reason why many surgeons do not immobilize such fractures but, having obtained the best possible reduction, insist on immediate movements so that the surface is moulded into the shape of the opposing undamaged surface.

Following a fracture blood and inflammatory exudate seep into all the neighbouring tissues, and because its absorption is delayed as a result of damage to veins and lymphatics, it *organizes into fibrous tissue*. This tissue will bind down muscles and tendons, and will invade the ligaments of the joints. If this organization is allowed to occur joint stiffness inevitably results.

The stiffness may also be due to less specific causes. The patient may be frightened to move joints not encased in plaster, especially if traumatic oedema has gravitated into the area.

Sometimes the joint stiffness is the result of general trophic changes in the limb when the patient fails to use the part, and the effect is as if the brain has discarded the limb. This phenomenon has never been satisfactorily explained, but one commonly accepted theory is that central connections are lost through disuse. With suitable and long-continued physiotherapy, mainly Faradic stimulation and proprioceptive neuromuscular facilitation, control is regained, but the process usually takes several months.

Sometimes, when the splint is removed, the joints appear stiff and the range does not progress as desired. The patient then tries to increase the range by force. This results in stretching of the ligaments, which irritates them and results in a sero-fibrinous exudate with more adhesion formation.

Again, if a rigid splint has been worn for a lengthy period, the tone of the soft tissues must inevitably be lowered. When the support is removed and the limb is allowed to hang dependent, the blood vessels, which should be supported by the tone of the muscles and the firmness of the fascia, no longer receive this support and will dilate. Increased filtration of blood plasma takes place from the dilated vessels. This clots, organizes and forms dense thickening which, together with much fluid, hampers movement.

Obviously much can be done to prevent these events and this is where physiotherapy is of such value, both during and after the period of rest.

VASCULAR DISTURBANCES

Considerable damage may be done to blood vessels both by the violence causing the fracture and by the fractured bone ends. This damage may result in irreparable harm to the other tissues. Simple contusion of an artery or vein may lead to thrombus formation. This in itself is not serious since impairment of flow in the main vessel means failure to remove metabolites in the area, resulting in dilatation of collateral vessels and consequently, after quite a short time, sufficient blood will enter the limb through these vessels. Sometimes however the presence of a thrombus may act as an irritant to the autonomic nerves of the vessels and vaso-spasm results.

Vaso-spasm may be the result not only of a thrombus but also of direct irritation of the sympathetic network which lies in the same sheath as the vessels. In either case it means spasm of all vessels distal to the damage and sometimes of those proximal, since it is probable that messages reach the sympathetic trunk and bring about reflex spasm of all vessels of the limb. The effect of vaso-spasm depends on how widespread it is and how prolonged. In less severe cases, it causes fibrous infiltration, because the capillaries dilate, and the endothelium becomes more permeable, venous blood regurgitates, increased filtration occurs and excess tissue fluid organizes. Fibrous tissue contracts and the limb may, if not treated adequately, show deformity and impaired function. In more severe or prolonged lesions, serious ischaemia causes necrosis of muscle and nerve. Necrotic muscular tissue is replaced by fibrous tissue which has not the function of muscles, and tends to contract. Necrotic nerve tissue undergoes Wallerian degeneration and paralysis and lost sensation results. It is possible, of course, for ischaemia to be so great that gangrene occurs.

Though it is rare, almost complete obstruction of arterial inflow and venous and lymphatic drainage may be the result of intense swelling or over-tight bandages and splints.

The onset of severe ischaemia can usually be recognized. Pallor and pulselessness are invariably early signs and pain is also a common feature. Should the condition persist the area becomes swollen, cyanosed and cold. Numbness and paraesthesiae also occur. It usually falls to the physiotherapist to recognize these warnings and report them, since she is likely to see the patient daily, at least in the early days of his treatment when vascular disturbances are most likely to be manifest.

Complications of Fractures

NERVE LESIONS

Nerve tissues can be damaged at the time of accident or much later. Tissue may be lacerated, destroyed, pressed on by haemorrhage, or be deprived of its blood supply through thrombosis of its vessels. The brain or spinal cord may be damaged in fractures of the skull or fracture-dislocations of the vertebral column. Peripheral nerves may be contused, severed or stretched so that their conductivity is impaired or lost. The blow, which fractures the head of the fibula, may contuse the lateral popliteal nerve, so that it temporarily ceases to function. The backward displacement of the lower fragment in a supracondylar fracture of the humerus, may stretch the median nerve so that it loses its conductivity. The radial nerve, as it lies in the radial groove, might be lacerated in transverse fractures of the shaft of the humerus. Many such illustrations can be given. The majority of the lesions are examples of neurapraxia, as it is not often that severance of axons or of the whole nerve takes place, and consequently recovery is usually rapid, but the more quickly the lesion is detected the earlier can treatment, designed to maintain the condition of joints, skin, bone and muscles, be instituted, and the more likelihood there is of achieving a perfect result. Recognition is not difficult if a careful check is kept on all movements not prevented by splintage and on the sensibility of the part. Hence, for example, in a fracture of the surgical neck of the humerus, in which the circumflex nerve is very occasionally damaged, it is important to test daily the patient's ability to contract the deltoid muscle.

Later, nerves may be irritated by repeated friction when, as a result of fracture, bony grooves have been roughened, or compressed in scar tissue, or stretched by increasing deformity.

DEVELOPMENT OF DEFORMITIES

Reflex inhibition of muscles often occurs where there is pain; muscles atrophy because they cannot function fully when splints are worn; patients are unwilling to move because they fear pain, and consequently weakened power is often seen when the fracture is firmly united. Weakened muscles mean the development of deformities—this is one of the causes of the clawed toes so often seen following fractures of the tibia and fibula treated in plaster (see Chapter XXI), and of the flat foot which complicates an abduction fracture-dislocation of the ankle. The weak vastus medialis following fractures of the thigh, or round the knee, may lead to knock knee. Such complications are avoidable if muscle tone and strength is maintained at the highest level possible while immobilization is necessary and is rapidly built up to normal when movement is allowed. This again is the duty of the physiotherapist.

MYOSITIS OSSIFICANS TRAUMATICA

New bone may be formed beneath the periosteum or in muscle and this may hamper movement (see Plate XVII). Particularly in those fractures which are accompanied by subluxation or dislocation of joints, the periosteum may be elevated by muscle or ligamentous pull, as is sometimes seen in a fracture of the tibia and malleoli with backward displacement of the foot, when the anterior ligament of the joint elevates the periosteum just in front of the articular surface. Unless the periosteum is replaced immediately, a clot of blood from the ruptured vessels forms between it and the bone. This haematoma will undergo organization, but, since it is in the region of bone cells, it will be converted into bone. Whether or not this matters, depends on the exact site and size of the haematoma. A large, bony outgrowth on the anterior aspect of the trochlea of the talus might impede dorsiflexion; whereas a small, ossified, haematoma between the periosteum and coronoid of the ulna would probably not impede flexion of the elbow. Presence of this complication will be recognized by tenderness over the site, spasm of muscles in the region, and increasing pain on movement with decreasing range. It is important that it should be detected, since vigorous active or passive movements will increase the bone formation, but more important still is avoidance of those things which might start its formation. After reduction of bone and joint, the periosteum will fall back into place and a haematoma should not develop. Gentle active movements will not re-displace it, but passive movements or too vigorous active movements might well elevate it again. Where this complication is likely these measures should be avoided.

Occasionally bone actually forms in muscle. If the periosteum is elevated and torn at the same time as muscle fibres are ruptured, some bone cells may escape into the muscle and may lay down bone which will hamper the muscle's action.

INJURY TO MUSCLES AND TENDONS

Some muscle fibres will inevitably be torn in fractures, especially where there is displacement. These, however, heal easily by scar tissue, which, if kept supple by movement, does not interfere with contraction and relaxation to any considerable extent. Sometimes, however, muscles may become inflamed and adherent to underlying bone and adjacent structures. Tendons are occasionally lacerated by sharp bone-edges or are torn from their insertion and require suture. A late complication of a Colles' fracture is a rupture of the long extensor tendon of the thumb, due to roughening of the groove on the posterior aspect of the radius, in which the tendon lies. Such ruptures can be detected at once because of inability to perform the movement normally produced by the tendon, and the taking up of a special position. For example, in the rupture of extensor pollicis longus, the terminal phalanx of the thumb drops.

ALTERATIONS IN GAIT

In lower limb fractures a limp often occurs when the patient begins to take weight either in the plaster or without splints. When a weight-bearing plaster is in use it is customary to find patients walking with a lateral rotation twist on the 'heel' and an abduction swing of the whole leg if the knee is included in the plaster. This should never be allowed since wrong walking in the plaster is not only a strain on muscles and joints, but will also result in a limp when the plaster is removed. Every patient must be taught to stand correctly and only then should he be taught to walk well in the plaster, avoiding the abduction swing by hip updrawing and the lateral rotation by rocking forward on the 'heel' or rocker sole.

When the plaster is removed, a limp tends to develop because the patient is afraid to take the full weight on the injured leg. There may also be pain. Pain is not usually felt at the site of fracture but in the sole of the foot. The normal pattern of walking includes strong contraction of the long flexors of the toes to give a powerful thrust off and to support the medial longitudinal arch of the foot. If the patient has been walking for some time in a plaster splint the long flexors are not used and proprioceptive impulses from these muscles no longer reach the cerebrum. When the patient starts to walk without the plaster, as the heel is lifted the long flexors no longer adequately support the arch and pain results. Inhibition of the calf muscles follows and there is therefore a limp. Normal heel-toe gait may also be difficult because of limited range of movement in the foot and ankle, and limited strength in the calf muscles. Co-ordination between the two legs will also be impaired, since weak muscles do not react as rapidly as strong ones. Thus one may see the patient walking with steps of unequal length and uneven rhythm, taking a longer stride with the injured limb and only bringing the other up to it, hurrying to transfer the weight on to the uninjured side and leaning over to this side, to save his injured limb from weight-bearing as much as possible.

Limping is harmful as it will rapidly become a habit. It puts muscles and ligaments in faulty positions predisposing towards deformity, and straining joints and muscles not only of the affected leg, but also of the other leg and the trunk.

Alterations in gait must, therefore, be watched for and prevented by the physiotherapist.

Recent Injuries

LOSS OF FUNCTION

Occasionally a limb is seen in which union is sound and in perfect alignment, but the general condition is poor, the skin is atrophied and inelastic, muscles are wasted, and joints are stiff. This is usually because the patient has not been encouraged to use the limb during the period of immobilization or protection, and has tended to forget about it, so that the brain has discarded it as a useful part of the body. In such a case, in-coming nerve impulses are ignored, so they are not sent out, and the result is severe trophic change. This could have been avoided by functional use of the part.

Many other complications do arise, but they are less common. Pulmonary embolism may be the result of venous thrombosis due to damage to veins, or may be due to the release of a particle of fat from the bone marrow. Shock is always present to some extent. This should be remembered when patients suffering from fractures are sent, the same or the succeeding day to the physiotherapy department. Sepsis may occur and may delay union by causing a break up of the fracture-haematoma. Malunion may occur, and may or may not be important. Delayed union and non-union do occasionally occur, but these can rarely be affected in any way by physiotherapy, though one point might be borne in mind—union will be slow if the bone ends are not in apposition. This may occur, for example, if one of two parallel bones is fractured when the uninjured bone will prevent the fractured ends from impinging on one another. Help may be given in such a case by training strong contractions of the long muscles passing over the site of fracture so that, by their contraction, they pull the bone ends together to provide the stimulus for union.

Growth is occasionally impaired if a fracture line passes through an epiphysis, and deformity then results. Thus, for example, if growth is impaired on the lateral side of the humerus in a fracture of the lateral condyle in the child, then, as the medial side grows at its normal rate, an increase in the carrying angle will result.

Principles of treatment of Fractures

The object of all fracture treatment is the restoration of the patient to the pre-accident condition or to a state as near this as possible. To achieve this three things are necessary: sound union of the bone ends in a position which does not upset the mechanics of the limb; the absence of stiff joints and atrophied muscles; and full restoration of function and confidence in the part.

Treatment falls, therefore, into two main sections, the treatment of the bone injury and the treatment of the soft tissues, but both should be taking place at the same time.

TREATMENT OF THE BONE INJURY

This may involve reduction, immobilization and protection though often these are not needed.

Reduction is necessary only when displacement of the bone ends would be harmful to the final result. There may be, for example, overlap in bones of the lower extremity which would cause shortening of the leg. There might be complete separation of the fragments so that compression is impossible or one fragment may be angulated or rotated in such a way as to upset the mechanics of the limb. There may also be interposition of soft tissues between the ends, making union impossible.

If reduction is necessary it is carried out under anaesthesia so that muscles are relaxed and further damage to soft tissues is avoided. It is achieved either by closed manipulation, traction or open operation.

Immobilization is not always necessary, but if necessary it is used for one of three purposes: to obtain compression between the bone ends and prevent harmful stresses; to prevent displacement of the bone ends, which would result in malunion; and to prevent pain.

Compression. If there is no compression between the fragments and continual stress is applied to the granulation tissue, union will be by fibrous tissue, not bone. In many fractures compression is obtained either because there is already impaction or because the tone of the muscles tends to draw the fragments together. There are only a few fractures, therefore, in which immobilization is required for the purpose of compression. These are fractures in which there is soft tissue between the fragments, or the bone ends are separated by muscle action, or the distal fragment has no muscle attachments so that it is not pulled towards the proximal bone end.

In these few cases immobilization is essential until there is consolidation, that is until the bone ends are joined by bone, therefore prolonged fixation is necessary. During this time harmful stresses must be avoided, consequently the splint must be rigid and must be kept on without interruption. To prevent strains it is necessary to fix the joints above and below the fracture site. For example, if the shafts of the radius and ulna are fractured pronation and supination of the forearm would cause rotational stress on the granulation tissue, both wrist and elbow joints must, therefore, be fixed. Splints which embody these principles have been called by Perkins.

Pure Splints—P standing for prolonged, U for uninterrupted, R for rigid, and E for extensive.

Displacement. If the violence which caused the fracture did not produce displacement, movements following the injury are not likely to produce later displacement. If the displacement which did occur was not considered sufficiently harmful to need reduction, splinting will not be necessary. There are, however, some occasions when displacement might occur after reduction, as for example in spiral and oblique fractures of the shafts of long bones when muscle spasm may pull up the distal fragment. In such cases immobilization is necessary, but it is only necessary until union has occurred and the bone ends move as one, and it need not be continued until there is consolidation. Since its purpose is only to prevent displacement it need not be so extensive. Perkins calls this type of splint a Simple Splint.

Pain. There may be no need for fixation to control the fragments, but a splint may still be applied. Experience has proved that if a part is painful and is not supported the patient will keep it rigid with his own muscles and in spite of instructions will not move it. If there is much damage to soft tissues there will be considerable oedema and without movement this will rapidly organize and a stiff useless part will develop. This is possibly the basis of the condition known as Sudeck's atrophy which occasionally develops following injuries of hand or foot. Such injuries are better supported until the pain subsides even though the actual fracture does not require immobilization. This seems to apply particularly to crush injuries of the hand in which the metacarpals or phalanges are fractured.

Certain fractures round the ankle which do not interfere with the stability of the joint, and do not, therefore, require immobilization may be treated in a below-knee plaster because pain is lessened and the patient, therefore, walks better.

Duration of Immobilization. It follows from what has been said that splints are retained a varying length of time according to their purpose. For relief of pain only it will be a matter of two or three weeks; if to prevent displacement, then they are retained until there is union; if to prevent harmful stress, until there is consolidation. While no certain length of time can be given at which each bone will be united or consolidated a general idea can be given. Upper limb bones heal about twice as quickly as those of the lower limb. Transverse fractures, with less raw area from which granulation tissue can grow, take twice as long as spiral or oblique fractures.

Consolidation also takes twice as long as union. A glance at the table given by Perkins will prove helpful.

	UPPER LIMB		LOWER LIMB	
	Union	*Consolidation*	*Union*	*Consolidation*
Spiral Fractures	3 weeks	6 weeks	6 weeks	12 weeks
Transverse Fractures	6 weeks	12 weeks	12 weeks	24 weeks

Sometimes when splinting is only required until union is complete some further form of protection is still required. It may be that there is considerable strain because the joint above or below is stiff. This is clearly illustrated in a fracture of the shaft of the femur. Here where there are long powerful muscles, compression is naturally obtained, but splinting is required to prevent overlapping or rotational displacement. The splint can, therefore, be removed when there is union, but the femur has to withstand the whole body weight and though it is now safe to move the leg freely it would not be safe to stand on it. Protection must therefore be given in ambulation either by using crutches and not taking weight on the leg or by means of a weight-relieving caliper.

Fixation, whether pure or simple, may be obtained by external splints of plaster, metal, plastic material or traction or it may be in the form of internal fixation by pins, nails, screws or plates. Often both methods are combined. The surgeon has to take many points into consideration in making his choice. Internal fixation often reduces the length of time that joints have to be immobilized or the patient has to remain in bed, but it means an operation and not all patients are willing or suitable to undergo surgery. It has in the end to be the patient's choice.

TREATMENT OF SOFT TISSUES AFTER FRACTURES

Since this is largely the province of the physiotherapist it is essential that she should have a clear understanding of what the damage is and what part she can play in its treatment. It has already been pointed out that soft tissue damage will occur at the time of the accident, but further damage may occur during the period of fixation, particularly if immobilization has to be complete and prolonged.

Bruising and oedema are common features immediately following the injury, while, later, it is not unusual to note muscle atrophy, stiff joints, disturbed circulation and gross impairment of function.

Recent Injuries

Haemorrhage occurs as a result of the rupture of blood vessels. The blood will clot and, if not rapidly absorbed, it will result in fibrous tissue which will hamper the action of muscles and the movement of joints.

Oedema is inevitable. The normal reaction to irritation is vasodilatation with consequent hyperaemia, rise in hydrostatic pressure and increased filtration. In addition, damage to the veins and lymphatics will impair tissue drainage so that swelling must occur. There is also likely to be oedema due to impairment of vasomotor control.

Later oedema will occur if movement of joints not immobilized is not encouraged, since immobility means a slowing of blood flow and congestion, with increased formation of tissue fluid.

Damage to muscles will occur at the time of injury, as some fibres are torn, but, during the period of immobilization, damage will continue unless great care is taken. The formation of fibrous tissue will not only repair the torn fibres, but will also occur between undamaged fibres binding them together and consequently hampering action. A certain degree of atrophy will occur because the size of the fibres depends on the maintenance of normal function and, although the muscles can be exercised within the support, they cannot work as fully as they should. This atrophy inevitably means diminished power.

Again muscles, whose joints are enclosed within splints, are unable to lengthen fully, and, if they do not do so over a period of time, they gradually lose this power. Consequently, when the fixation is removed and movement is commenced, full range cannot be obtained.

Loss of cerebral control over the part. In considering damage to soft tissue one very important factor to be remembered is the effect of the loss of cerebral control over the limb. A painful limb is kept still, and the brain rapidly discards it as a useful member, consequently ignoring nerve impulses coming to it from the limb. All parts of the limb are directly or indirectly controlled by the brain, largely as a result of incoming nerve impulses, and if these are ignored, messages are not sent out. The blood vessels no longer receive constrictor impulses from the vasomotor centre and consequently their tone decreases. They dilate and congestion and stagnation occur. Marked trophic changes then take place affecting all structures. Bones show excessive decalcification, muscles become grossly atrophied, joints become stiff, and oedema occurs. The skin too shows the effects of diminished activity and nutrition in its thin shiny condition, the absence of sweat and hairs, the dryness and a tendency to break down and to heal slowly or not at all.

THE PART PLAYED BY PHYSIOTHERAPY IN THE TREATMENT OF THE SOFT TISSUES

Though complete immobility may be necessary even for many weeks, severe effects on soft tissue such as have been described are not necessary if suitable measures are taken to prevent them.

Haemorrhage and oedema. Active movement is the best way of dispersing blood before it clots and organizes, and of promoting absorption of oedema or of lessening its formation. Even if a limb is encased in plaster some joints will be free and if these are moved vigorously the general circulation of the limb will be stimulated. Often areas outside a plaster are swollen, such as the oedematous fingers following a Colles' fracture and these can be freely exercised. To be effective these movements must be in full range, strong and often repeated. The majority of patients, particularly in the early days following a fracture, are frightened of movement, partly because it may be a little uncomfortable, and partly because they fear that it will harm the broken bone. They need, therefore, definite explanation of the effect of keeping the joints still and of the value of movement, together with instruction in what movements to do, how these should be done, and how often exercise should be carried out. Not only should an explanation be given, but supervision is essential until there is absolute certainty that oedema has subsided, joint movement is full and the patient can be trusted to continue on his own.

It is not essential to perform full-range movements to prevent organization of blood and tissue fluid. A slight movement of muscle fibres, a mild contraction causing movement of a tendon within its sheath, is enough to prevent the structures being 'stuck' together. If a patient is, therefore, taught, in addition to movements of joints not immobilized, to contract and relax the muscles within the plaster, additional effect will be gained.

Damage to muscular tissue. As has already been seen, unnecessary formation of scar tissue within muscle from organization of blood clot can be avoided by contraction of muscles within splints and movement of joints not included in the support.

Atrophy cannot be completely prevented if full function is impossible, but it can be lessened by the same active contractions, provided they are practised often enough—five minutes of every hour for the exercises should be the instructions given to every patient. The small amount of atrophy then present should be capable of rapid restoration to normal when the apparatus is removed. On many occasions, actual resisted work can be given, even when extensive plasters are being worn. Attempts to move joints against the resistance of the plaster illustrate such resisted work.

Loss of elasticity and ability to lengthen can also be minimized. It will be recalled that when a group of muscles contracts to perform a movement, its antagonistic group 'lets go' gradually, acting as a graded resistance to help make the movement smooth. If, on the other hand, the movement is a resisted one, this control is no longer needed, and the antagonistic muscles, therefore, relax. To maintain this ability to relax and so keep elasticity and length of muscle, resisted work is essential and it is an important part of the treatment that the patient should be taught movements which are against the resistance of the plaster. No matter what the fracture, if it is perfectly immobilized, resisted work by muscles within the plaster is free from danger, and is always beneficial.

Stiff joints. Much can be done to prevent the development of stiff joints. Synovial adhesions can be prevented by movement of joints if they are not immobilized and by attempted movements of those enclosed in splints. Extensibility of muscle is maintained by encouraging such movements as will lengthen all muscles, where this is possible, or by movements attempted against the resistance of the plaster in the cases of fractures treated by fixation. Incongruity of joint surfaces is lessened by early active movements, while organization of exudate is prevented by rhythmic muscle contractions and relaxations, movement of all joints not immobilized, and normal use of the limb as far as possible.

Loss of connection between brain and limb. This can be avoided if the brain is not allowed to forget the limb. By far the best way to achieve this object is to encourage as normal use of the part as possible. It must always be borne in mind that, over the course of years, patterns of movement develop in the cerebral cortex. These patterns differ in different people according to the work they do, and the hobbies and activities they follow. The best way to maintain connection between limb and brain is to continue the normal activities, provided that this is possible, and if it is not possible, to practise something which is near the normal. For example, in the case of a housewife who is wearing a plaster applied to immobilize a Colles' fracture, she is encouraged to continue her duties about the house, avoiding only those which would actually damage the splint. The patient who has sustained a fracture-dislocation of the ankle, except in severe cases, can safely walk, if his plaster splint is satisfactory. In this way it is impossible for the brain to discard the limb. The factory worker with a fracture of the shaft of radius, enclosed in a plaster splint from upper arm to metacarpal heads, can still use his fingers and thumb fully, and should practise, not only simple finger bending and stretching and parting and closing, but movements similar if possible to those of his job in the factory. It is necessary, therefore, for the physiotherapist to find out the movements, and it is desirable for her, if she has many such cases, to visit the factory and see the job for herself noting what processes it entails.

In conclusion it will be noted that active work is the predominant feature and that this is possible while complete immobility of the bone ends is being maintained. If it is carried out, much damage is avoided and many weeks of treatment, following immobilization, are not required.

There are occasions when actual splintage is not used. If it is not required, then the surgeon is satisfied that correct apposition is secured in spite of freedom, and the physiotherapist can rest assured that active movement is still safe if carried out on the lines indicated. In cases where splints are not worn, there is, of course, the possibility of using other physical measures as adjuncts, but great care should be taken not to allow them to replace activity. Inductothermy proximal to the site of fracture will stimulate drainage, and, later, applied over the site, will promote softening of such exudate as has organized. Novocain ionization may lessen vasodilatation by its analgesic effect on nerve endings. Effleurage and squeezing kneading will stimulate the circulation and aid drainage, but should be applied in early cases proximal to the site of fracture. Electrical stimulation may help the patient to learn to do active work in the very early days of injury, but should not be continued when power to work actively has returned. Nevertheless it must be repeated once more that these are only adjuncts and voluntary activity is the essential.

Chapter XV

INJURIES OF THE UPPER
EXTREMITY

INJURIES ROUND THE SHOULDER
AND FRACTURES OF THE SHAFT OF THE HUMERUS

The great characteristic of the shoulder joint is its *wide range of movement*. This has been estimated at about 120 degrees during elevation of the arm to the vertical position. To achieve this wide range the structure of the joint has been adapted to give mobility at the expense of stability. This is clearly seen in the size and shape of the articular surfaces and in the arrangements of the capsule and ligaments.

The articular surface of the head of the humerus is considerably larger than that of the glenoid cavity so that only a small part of the surface is in contact with the cavity at any one time. The glenoid (Gk. glene=shallow) cavity, as its name implies, is also very shallow and the head of the humerus cannot fit into it. Nor are the two surfaces held firmly together by the capsule since, except at its upper part, the capsule is loose and has little in the way of reinforcing ligamentous bands.

Such strength and stability as the joint possesses is dependent upon the muscles. These may be divided into two main groups: those which are mainly responsible for the movements of the humerus and those which steady the head of the humerus during these movements. To the latter group the term 'rotator cuff' has been applied. These are short muscles which pass from the scapula to a point just distal to the anatomical neck of the humerus. Their insertions are continuous and they blend, as they pass across the joint, with the capsule from which they cannot be detached. Three of these short muscles, the subscapularis, infraspinatus and teres minor, rotate the humerus, the fourth, supraspinatus, lying above the joint is an abductor (see Fig. 38, p. 313). The cuff has two important functions other than that of rotation: it holds the head of the humerus firmly against the glenoid cavity so that as the arm is moved it does not slide in the cavity; it depresses the head in the cavity as the arm is raised, lessening pressure by the coraco-acromial arch on the structures at the top of the shoulder. This action counteracts that of deltoid which, because of the direction of its fibres, tends to pull the humerus vertically upwards as it

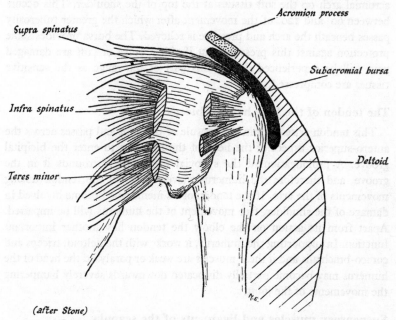

(after Stone)

FIG. 38. POSTERIOR ASPECT OF THE RIGHT SHOULDER JOINT

contracts. This part of the functions of the cuff was at one time thought to be entirely the work of supraspinatus, but it is now known that the whole cuff contracts when deltoid is brought into action. The cuff and deltoid work smoothly together from the beginning of raising the arm throughout the movement.

The Subacromial Bursa

A bursa lies between the superior aspect of the shoulder joint and the under surface of the coraco-acromial arch. Its floor blends with the supra-spinatus and greater tuberosity of the humerus, its roof is attached to the under surface of the arch, the anterior and posterior borders are free. The two layers are in contact with one another, but slide easily due to lubrication by the synovial fluid. Thus the floor and roof move over one another in every movement at the humero-scapular joint. It might well be said that the bursa forms an additional articular cavity between the top of the shoulder joint and the inferior aspect of the arch. Changes in the bursa leading to atrophy, roughening of its walls or adherence of the roof and floor will inevitably result in diminished movement of the shoulder joint. Every time the arm is abducted some pressure is exerted by the coraco-acromial arch on the soft tissues at the top of the shoulder. This occurs between 60° and 120° of the movement after which the greater tuberosity passes beneath the arch and pressure is relieved. The bursa provides some protection against this pressure, but if either bursa or cuff are damaged pain will be experienced during this part of the range as the sensitive tissues are compressed.

The tendon of the long head of biceps

This tendon arises within the capsule of the joint and passes across the antero-superior aspect of the head of the humerus to enter the bicipital groove. A prolongation of the synovial membrane surrounds it in the groove, and therefore the humerus moves easily on the tendon during movements of the arm. If the tendon or its membrane become involved in damage of the shoulder, free movement of the humerus will be impaired. Apart from its action on the elbow the tendon has another important function. In supporting the humerus, it works with the deltoid, triceps and coraco-brachialis and if these muscles are weak or paralysed the head of the humerus may become partially dislocated downwards severely hampering the movements of the joint.

Suspensory muscles and ligaments of the scapula

These are necessary because the scapula does not articulate with the chest wall other than indirectly through the clavicle. Trapezius, levator scapulae, and the rhomboids all prevent the scapula from dropping downwards while the coraco-clavicular ligament ties the scapula firmly to the clavicle and dislocation downwards of the scapula at the acromio-clavicular joint cannot occur without rupture of this ligament. If this ligament is ruptured by such an injury as a fall on the point of the shoulder hypertrophy of the suspensory muscles is important to compensate for the weakened ligament.

Movements of the shoulder

Raising the arm from the side to the vertical position involves movement not only at the shoulder joint, but also in the sterno-clavicular and acromio-clavicular joints. Throughout the whole range of the movement all three joints are involved and the smooth co-ordination of these joints has been called by Codman 'Scapulo-humeral rhythm'. As the arm is raised through the first few degrees the main movement is in the humero-scapular joint. The rotator cuff steadies the head of the humerus and prevents the upward pull of deltoid while deltoid lifts the arm. Almost immediately, the scapula begins to move both upward and round the chest wall so that the glenoid cavity faces increasingly upward and the point of the shoulder is raised. This makes movement of the humerus easier and adds to its range. During the upward movement of the scapula depression of the sternal end of the clavicle occurs at the sterno-clavicular joint and during rotation, movement takes place at the acromio-clavicular joint. Pain or stiffness of any one of these three joints interferes with the co-ordination of the movement and upsets the scapulo-humeral rhythm. Probably one of the commonest causes of this disturbance is trouble in the subacromial bursa or rotator cuff. In this case as soon as an attempt is made to raise the arm pain results in inhibition of the cuff, the deltoid therefore fails to lift the arm, only pulling the humerus vertically upwards beneath the coraco-acromial arch. The arm is raised sideways by excessive rotation of the scapula and elevation of the point of the shoulder, and only if the arm reaches the horizontal can abduction in the shoulder joint occur. This alteration of the normal rhythm is spoken of as 'reversed scapulo-humeral rhythm' (see Plate XIX).

Rotation of the arm

Rotation of the arm is a very important movement and without lateral rotation full elevation cannot be obtained. If the arm is raised sideways it is also laterally rotated, this results in a larger area of the articular surface of the head of the humerus being available and so ensures a wider range of movement, in addition it takes the greater tuberosity on to a posterior plane whence it can pass beneath the wider part of the coraco-acromial arch avoiding pressure on the soft tissues at the top of the shoulder. If the arm is raised forwards this lateral rotation is unnecessary. A check on the movements and on the actual bones will verify these facts. It is essential for full use of the arm that these movements should be retained and in all shoulder injuries, almost without exception, even if nothing else is possible, medial and lateral rotation with the arm by the side should be practised from the time of injury. If the rotator cuff, capsule or bursa is damaged this movement will prevent the two layers of the bursa becoming adherent and the shoulder joint is unlikely to become stiff provided these two remain free.

The painful arc of movement

This is a term often used when the structures of the shoulder joint have been damaged. It usually refers to pain during abduction of the arm between 60° and 120° of movement, movement being painless before and after these points are reached. It is explained by the fact that, as the arm is moved through these degrees, sensitive structures, supraspinatus and the subacromial bursa, impinge against and are compressed by the coraco-acromial arch. When the arm is lowered the same painful arc appears. Another explanation has been offered. It appears that supraspinatus reaches its maximum contraction between 80° and 120° of elevation, therefore if the tendon is damaged or inflamed most pain would be present at this point. It is probable that both reasons are present in many lesions of the shoulder.

PHYSIOTHERAPY IN INJURIES ROUND THE SHOULDER

Although the exact method of carrying out treatment may vary with the different injuries the principles underlying the treatment are the same.

In most injuries there is a tendency for the shoulder joint to become stiff

The movements which are most limited are abduction and lateral rotation. This is partly due to the fact that the position of ease, in which the capsule and ligaments are relaxed, is with the arm by the side in the position of adduction and medial rotation. This position is also most often used if the limb is immobilized. The anterior part of the capsule, the sub-scapularis, pectoralis major and latissimus dorsi all tend to shorten in this position. Stiffness also tends to develop because there is often considerable exudate and bleeding and these, particularly in middle-aged and elderly patients, are slow to absorb, consequently organizing with the formation of adhesions and fibrous thickenings. In many injuries, particularly those affecting the rotator cuff, the floor and roof of the subacromial bursa tend to become adherent with reduction in the range of shoulder movement. In addition the patient with a painful shoulder rapidly develops inco-ordinate movement raising the arm by scapular rotation and avoiding use of the shoulder joint with consequent loss of range in this joint.

For these reasons measures must be taken early to prevent loss of range. These measures are a combination of rest and exercise. *Rest* is gained by the use of a large arm sling for a few days. This allows the inflammatory reaction and pain to subside, but it is removed for exercise and discarded as soon as the arm is comfortable without it. Immobilization may be used for ten days to three weeks in some dislocations of the shoulder and acro-mio-clavicular joints, and unimpacted fractures of the surgical neck of the humerus in young people.

Exercises except in the injuries noted above should be begun at once, but must be carried out with as little pain as possible and with care to ensure normal scapulo-humeral rhythm (see below). In all injuries, but especially those in which immobilization is necessary, rhythmic contractions of all muscles around the joint will diminish stiffness, because as the muscles contract, they squeeze the exudate out of the tissue spaces. The contraction and relaxation has a pumping effect on the blood and lymph vessels stimulating absorption and diminishing organization.

Injuries round the shoulder joint tend to be followed by atrophy and weakness of the muscles

This occurs particularly in the abductors and lateral rotators and upsets muscle balance leading to inco-ordinated movement. These particular groups are affected because of the tendency to hold the painful arm to the side. If the cuff is damaged it fails to contract as the arm is lifted and elevation is produced by rotation of the scapula with lack of use of the flexors and abductors as well as the cuff. Lack of normal use of the shoulder also causes atrophy of biceps, triceps and coraco-brachialis and this results in downward drop of the head of the humerus in the glenoid cavity. Exercises to strengthen all the muscles are, therefore, necessary.

If the arm is not immobilized resistance to prevent loss of strength can be started immediately after the injury, using gravity and gentle manual resistance. If the patient tries arm elevation in lying or arm abduction in side lying the resistance of gravity is immediately brought into the movement. In addition slight manual resistance given at the elbow will ensure a stronger muscular contraction. Resistance may later be given by weights, balls and poles. The exercises must be progressive and against sufficient resistance.

Though all muscles should be exercised, especial attention must be given to the rotator cuff, deltoid and biceps and triceps. Thus lateral rotation, elbow flexion and extension, forearm supination and shoulder abduction require particular stress. If any of these are prevented by the method of immobilization, rhythmic contractions of the muscles must be substituted.

Most shoulder injuries are painful either immediately after the injury or within a few hours

The injury itself damages the nerve endings and sets up painful stimuli and later traumatic exudate produces tension and, therefore, pain. Pain is increased at first by movement and there is therefore muscle spasm which serves only to increase pain as fatigue products accumulate in the hypertonic muscles. If early movement to prevent stiffness and atrophy are to be obtained pain and spasm must be relieved before the movements are attempted. In most injuries the use of infra-red rays will have a sedative effect. Massage is often valuable because it will also have a sedative effect on nerve endings and in addition will help to disperse the oedema and so reduce tension. A careful watch should be kept when heat is used because in certain lesions it may increase the pain. This is so in acute bursal or rotator cuff injuries in which nocturnal pain is a feature. Certainly deep heat should not be used in these cases.

In addition to heat and massage, training the patient to relax the muscles is important while gentle resistance to movements will bring about reciprocal relaxation of antagonists. Later if pain is due to tight muscles the 'hold-relax' and 'contract-relax' techniques are useful.

In the later stages of treatment of shoulder injuries, pain may occur on movement due to contracture of the capsule and tendons and fibrous tissue formation or adherence of the walls of the bursa or the tendon of biceps in its groove. These can be dealt with by deep heating and deep transverse frictions, but they should, as far as is possible, be prevented rather than treated once they have developed.

Pain limiting movement can often be avoided by suitable choice of starting positions (see below).

One of the most important objects in the treatment of shoulder injuries is to *ensure that the patient co-operates and carries out his treatment many times a day*. This can only be done if the patient understands why the exercises are valuable and what will happen if he fails to do them. A careful explanation is given and as each exercise is taught its purpose is explained. The exercises are clearly written out with a note how many times each exercise should be done and how often during the day. When the patient returns for treatment he should be taken through the exercises to see if he knows them and is doing them correctly. If the patient is elderly much encouragement will be needed and only a few essential exercises should be given. Instructions on dressing and washing himself and carrying out simple tasks in the house will probably take precedence over set home exercises.

Some points in the choice of exercises and their performance

Starting position. In all injuries, but particularly in those around the shoulder, the starting position in which the exercise is carried out is very important.

The lying position is useful because the patient is fully supported and will more easily relax the muscles. All movements will, therefore, be preceded by fuller relaxation. In this position the arm is more stable since it is supported by the plinth, lateral rotation is easier therefore and there is no obstruction to the full range of movement. In lying it is easier to apply traction and for many of the movements the force of gravity is eliminated. There are, however, two disadvantages. Elderly people do not like to lie flat and are rarely comfortable in this position; this can be overcome by raising the head and shoulders slightly. The arm tends to fall back in lying and this not only causes pain, but means that movements tend to be carried out in the plane of the body rather than that of the scapula; the best way to deal with this problem is to support the arm on pillows or sandbags. Full range of medial rotation and extension are not obtainable in this position.

Side lying is a useful position in which to practise abduction if the rotator cuff or bursa is the source of trouble. In side lying the deltoid starts to contract in its most stretched and, therefore, most strong position, but as movement continues it becomes less effective and the resistance of gravity becomes less, consequently its vertical pull on the humerus is lessened and pressure on the damaged tissues is reduced; the movement is, therefore, more comfortable. The side-lying position is also useful if strengthening work for the lateral rotators is required.

Sitting is a good position because the back can be supported while movements are carried out against gravity and with auto-assisted or resisted pulleys. Elderly patients are more comfortable in this position and the arm can be moved in the plane of the scapula. It is a good position both for pendulum swinging movements if the patient leans forward and for assisted or resisted pulley work for the rotators. If the patient leans slightly sideways on the chair full extension can be obtained (see Plate XX).

Stoop Stride Standing is an excellent position from which to begin arm elevation and lateral rotation if there is a painful arc of movement. If the patient first takes a lax stoop standing position and then allows his arms to hang loosely it will then be seen that, quite passively, the arms are already nearly in the reach position. The patient next carries them forward as far as he can within the limit of pain; this movement does not involve work against gravity, therefore deltoid does not contract strongly and pressure on the upper part of the shoulder is avoided. The next step is to hold the arms in this position and bring the trunk to the erect position; movement of the arm can usually then be completed without pain since the painful arc has been passed. The arms are then lowered sideways and if there is pain the patient drops forward and then relaxes the arm, thus the painful 'catch' on the downward movement is avoided.

In the same way, in the lax stoop standing position, the hands can be placed behind the neck and the elbows gently pressed back; the patient holding this arm position then returns to the erect posture and it will be seen that there is good lateral rotation.

This position is also useful for pendular arm-swinging exercises in younger patients. It is usually modified to stoop walking standing, and the unaffected hand is placed on the forward knee to provide stability.

Standing may be useful for such exercises as trying to reach higher points on shelves or the wall bars. It is a good position for home practice of lateral rotation when if the patient stands back to the wall, the arm is stabilized and he can aim at touching the wall with the back of the forearm. If he moves the feet forward and presses the elbows back against the wall, so pushing the trunk forward, there is strong resistance for the extensor muscles. The position should not be used unnecessarily for elderly people as it is tiring and requires considerable muscle work to maintain. It is, however, necessary for many games and activities.

Types of Exercises

Exercises selected should be active and preferably only using such equipment as can be made available at home. The patient can then practise them at regular intervals throughout the day. If, however, a workshop is available machinery should be used. This should, as far as possible, be similar to that used by the patient in his work, but may be adapted in such a way that it calls for the particular movement in which the patient requires practice. In this case the patient will probably attend for the day and practice at home can be confined to the carrying-out of a few set exercises.

The exercises chosen must include every movement of which the joints are capable, especially lateral rotation of the shoulder, and care must be taken that the normal scapulo-humeral rhythm is used. This is helped by using a mirror and by training the patient to press the shoulder down and lift the elbow out as he raises the arm, and by doing bilateral exercises to prevent tilting of the trunk.

Active exercises will include assisted, free and resisted work.

Assisted exercises include movements in which the weight of the arm is taken either manually, by slings, or by self-assistance as when the hands are clasped and the arms raised. The auto-assisted pulleys are extremely valuable both for elevation and lateral rotation.

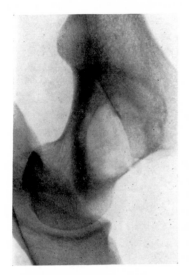 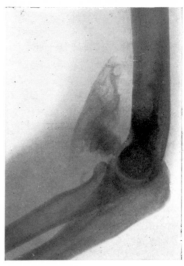

XVI. Pathological fracture through area of the cyst in the neck of the femur (*see* p. 295)

XVII. Myositis ossificans (*see* p. 302)

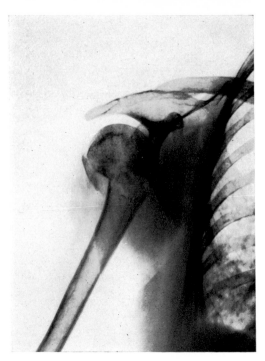

XVIII. Abduction fracture of surgical neck of humerus with fracture of greater tuberosity (*see* pp. 324, 327)

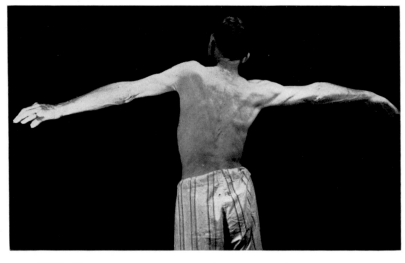

XIX. Showing reversed scapulo-humeral rhythm (*see* p. 315)

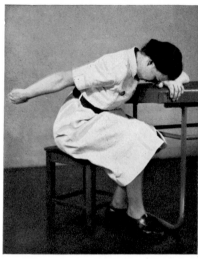
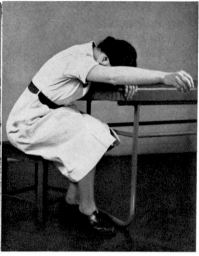

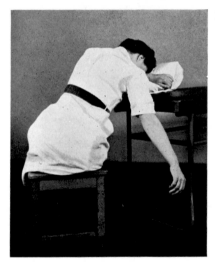

XX. Positions for arm movements

(*a*) Position for backward swing of arm; and position for forward swing of the arm

(*b*) Position for sideways swing of the arm

(*see* p. 319)

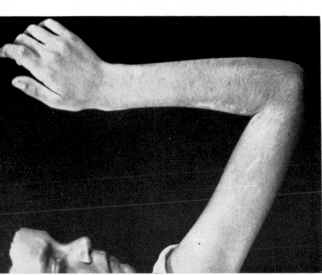

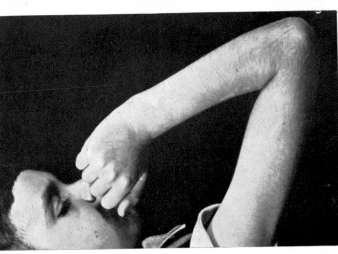

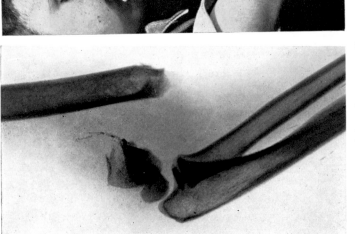

XXII. Supracondylar fracture of the humerus complicated by fibrosis of the capsule

(a) Range of flexion when plaster removed   (b) Range of extension when plaster removed

(5 weeks)

(see p. 346)

XXI. Supracondylar fracture of the lower end of the humerus Progress seen in Plate xxii a, b, c and d (see p. 344)

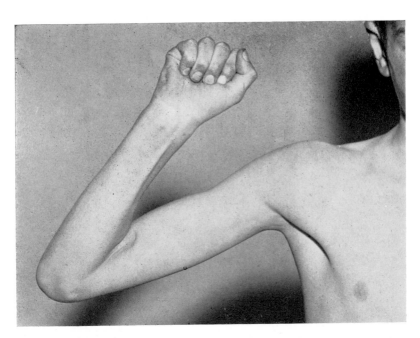

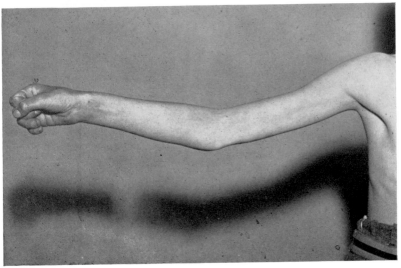

XXII. (c) Range of flexion one year later
(d) Range of extension one year later
(see p. 346)

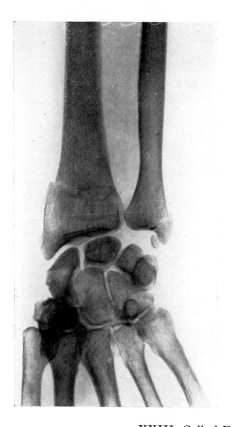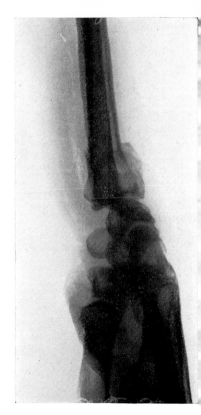

XXIII. Colles' Fracture (*see* p. 371)

(*a*) Showing radial displacement and
fracture of the styloid process of ulna

(*b*) Showing backward displacement
and tilting of the lower fragment

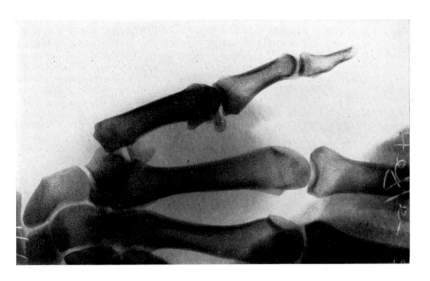

XXIV. Bennett's Fracture Dislocation (*see* p. 374)

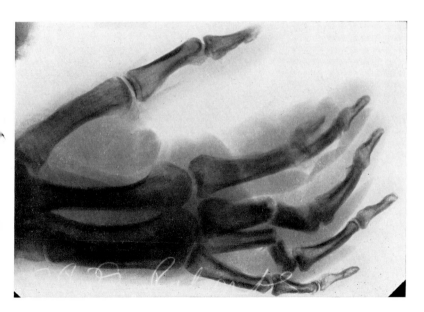

XXV. Fracture of the phalanges (*see* p. 375)

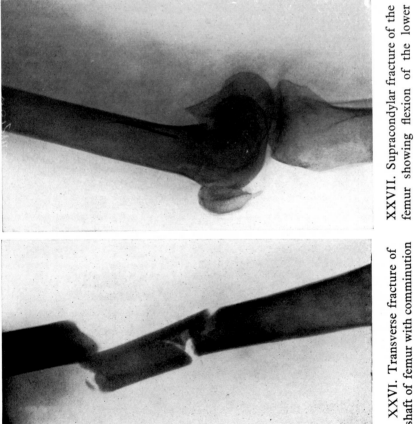

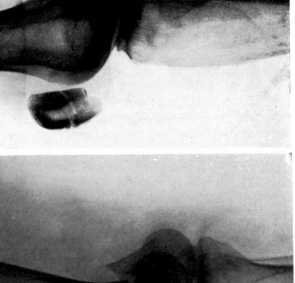

XXVI. Transverse fracture of shaft of femur with comminution and lateral displacement (*see* p. 391)

XXVII. Supracondylar fracture of the femur showing flexion of the lower fragment (*see* p. 391)

XXVIII. Transverse fracture of the patella without displacement (*see* p. 413)

This type of work is used as soon as movements are allowed beginning with manual, self and sling assistance. This can be progressed to pulleys in two to three weeks in the case of fractures and dislocations, but almost at once in rotator cuff lesions.

The purpose of this type of work is to maintain and increase range of movement.

Free exercises are used throughout the treatment and can be combined with apparatus work so that they help both to increase range and strengthen muscles. Supervision is required to eliminate 'cheating'.

At the beginning of treatment pendulum movements and attempted elevation and rotation in the lax stoop position are probably most suitable. Pendular movements in lax stoop sitting and standing are easier and less painful. There is no danger of re-dislocation or dis-impaction, because the tone of the muscles will prevent this. The exceptions are in dislocation of the acromio-clavicular joint and fractures of the clavicle. In the former they are not used until the coraco-clavicular ligament is healed or the suspensory muscles are hypertrophied since the scapula would drop if the arm is allowed to hang by the side. In the latter the weight of the arm would produce movement at the fracture site.

If the lesion is a partial or complete rupture of the rotator cuff, movements begin with lax stoop standing, elevation and rotation (see p. 322), because it is essential to maintain range without producing pain.

Arm circling in the stoop sitting or standing position is given early because it alternately contracts and relaxes all the muscles round the shoulder and, therefore, makes movement easier.

In most shoulder injuries free abduction in side lying can be given at once using a short lever and progression to a long lever, and then to a weight in the hand. Medial and lateral rotation begin at once often in lying or sitting with the elbows straight, but rapidly progressed to the elbow bent to a right angle in order to eliminate rotation of the forearm.

Later, free exercises are given in the form of games and functional activities, because the patient is more likely to forget the arm if he is interested and he is better prepared to return to work if the arm is used for everyday activities. In such lesions as fractures of the surgical neck of the humerus elderly patients should, within a day or two of the accident, be encouraged to dress themselves, wash, try to do the hair, and do simple jobs about the house. Competitive work in the form of class activities is usually introduced about three weeks after the injury if the joint has been moved from the beginning, slightly later if the arm has been immobilized.

Resisted exercises are essential to strengthen the muscles. They also have the value that they work the weak groups while obtaining relaxation of tight antagonists. Movement is often limited by tight adductors and medial rotators, gentle resistance to abduction and lateral rotation as soon as these movements are begun often obtains a better range and avoids the pain which results from attempted movement against tight muscles.

Thus a small amount of manual resistance can be given from the beginning of treatment except in cases of unimpacted fractures of the surgical neck of the humerus and fractures of the clavicle where strain would be felt at the fracture site and might interfere with healing.

If there is muscle spasm the 'contract-relax' and 'hold-relax' techniques can be used provided they do not cause pain. Usually about three weeks after injury stronger resistance can be applied and self-resisted pulleys, poles and balls may be used. Patients who for some reason did not start physiotherapy for some weeks are likely to present with stiff joints and atrophied muscles and for these progressive weight lifting can be used.

LESIONS OF THE ROTATOR CUFF AND
SUBACROMIAL BURSA

Lesions of the rotator cuff and bursa occur most frequently in middle-aged and elderly people. This is explained by the fact that in these years circulation to all tissues is diminished, but particularly to those subjected to the greatest strains and stresses. The cuff and bursa fall into this group since they are repeatedly compressed especially on movements demanding powerful contraction of the deltoid producing an upward thrust of the head of the humerus. They tend, therefore, to show degenerative changes leading to weakening and loss of balance between the cuff and deltoid. Even minor injuries are then likely to lead to slight or severe tears which do not heal easily because the circulation is impaired. Such lesions are particularly liable to occur in manual workers over fifty years who are using the arms for heavy work demanding powerful deltoid action. They are usually the result of a fall on the shoulder or outstretched hand and may also occur while lifting or throwing a heavy weight.

The lesion most often occurs in the tendon of supraspinatus though any part or all the cuff may be involved. It may be a tear of some of the fibres of the supraspinatus tendon or it may be of the whole tendon thickness. If the superficial fibres are torn the floor of the bursa will also be involved and exudate will invade the bursa distending it and giving rise to pain. If there is a complete rupture the joint and bursal cavities will communicate and the bursa will not be distended because fluid will escape into the joint cavity.

Partial or complete ruptures give rise to pain, tenderness and inco-ordination of shoulder movement, except in some cases of incomplete rupture in which there has been progressive degeneration over a long period and the remaining part of the cuff and biceps have been gradually hyper-trophied to take over the work of the supraspinatus.

Pain often comes on some hours after injury particularly if the main changes are related to the bursa, since it will be some time before the bursa becomes distended with fluid. It is felt in the shoulder, but there is also a dull aching pain at the insertion of deltoid. This referred pain probably is due to the fact that the fifth cervical nerve supplies not only supraspinatus, deltoid and the bursa, but also the skin over deltoid. The pain is often worse at night when the arm becomes warm in bed. Pain is experienced not only at rest and at night, but also on movement when unless the bursa is acutely distended there is a painful arc between 60° and 120° (see p. 315). If the tendon of supraspinatus is not completely ruptured pain will be felt on attempted abduction of the arm from the side.

Tenderness will be experienced on palpation over the site of lesion, in the case of supraspinatus just between the anterior part of the lateral border of the acromion and the greater tuberosity.

Inco-ordination of movement arises because of the inhibition of the cuff. If the arm is abducted the bursa and upper part of the cuff are compressed, this causes a painful arc of movement, the supraspinatus is therefore in-hibited and the powerful contraction of deltoid pulls the humerus up instead of out. The arm is consequently abducted by lateral rotation of the scapula and lifted by elevation of the point of the shoulder. Should there be a complete rupture there is still greater weakness of the cuff.

The same painful arc of movement exists when the arm is lowered to the side. There is a painful 'catch' and the arm is either dropped to the side or twisted into lateral rotation so that compression of the soft tissues against the acromion or coraco-acromial ligament is avoided.

Some little time after the rupture *muscle atrophy and limitation of range* may appear. Since movement is difficult and painful the posterior fibres of deltoid, the rotator cuff and the long head of triceps will show atrophy. This will result in undue prominence of the spine of the scapula. At first passive movements are full, but after three to four weeks if treatment is not given these tend to become reduced as a result of adhesions in the bursa and contracture of soft tissues. These are due to failure to put the shoulder through its full range owing to pain.

Treatment

The particular points to note in using physiotherapy in the treatment of these lesions are the ease with which full range is lost and the need to hypertrophy the remaining part of the cuff to compensate for the rupture which is unlikely ever to heal fully.

In the maintenance of the full range it is important not to increase irritation by compression of the damaged tissues; exercises must, therefore, be done without producing pain and the positions chosen will be stoop standing or sitting, side lying and lying (see p. 319). These may be preceded by heat if it proves helpful to relieve pain and obtain relaxation, but if the patient is suffering from night pain, heat may increase discomfort and should be avoided.

Exercises to hypertrophy the remaining part of the cuff should also avoid giving pain. Lateral and medial rotation against manual and auto-resistance are important and resisted work for triceps and the long head of biceps must be included.

Great care should be taken to gain co-ordination of movement (see p. 315). This again involves avoiding painful movements which would bring about inhibition of the cuff. The patient should make a conscious effort to hold the head of the humerus steady in the glenoid cavity while lifting the arm.

FRACTURES OF THE SURGICAL NECK OF THE HUMERUS

These fractures occur most often in elderly people as a result of a fall on the hand, and according to which way the patient falls the shaft may be adducted or abducted in relation to the head (see Plate XVIII). In many cases the bone ends are impacted on one side or the other giving stability, with the result that movement in a small range is possible without excessive pain. If impaction does not occur the fracture is unstable; the bone ends move over one another on movement of the shoulder and movement, even in a small range, is very painful. In the latter case considerable displacement of the fragments may occur at the time of injury.

Treatment depends on the age of the patient and the stability of the fracture

If the patient is elderly immobilization is rarely desirable even if there is no impaction and considerable displacement. This is because there is usually a good deal of bleeding and oedema and the shoulder will rapidly become stiff. A surprisingly good range of movement can be obtained with considerable displacement if adhesions, contractures and atrophy are not allowed to develop. For this reason the usual method is to rest the arm in a large arm sling with an axillary pad. If the fracture is stable exercises for the shoulder begin at once; the sling is taken off for exercises and discarded as soon as the arm is comfortable without it. If the fracture is unstable the sling is worn for three weeks, finger, wrist, forearm and elbow movements are given from the beginning, but the shoulder movements are delayed for ten days to three weeks, by which time sufficient callus will have formed to ensure that the two bone ends move as one.

If the patient is young and the fracture is not impacted then the surgeon may attempt reduction since the shoulder is less likely to become stiff and a perfect result is more important. The arm is then immobilized, with a large axillary pad, in a large arm sling and bandaged to the side for three weeks, and shoulder movements delayed for this time.

Serious complications are not common in this injury, but a stiff shoulder and nerve lesions may occur and in addition the fracture may be accompanied by dislocation of the shoulder and fracture of the greater tuberosity. A stiff shoulder should be avoided if early active movements are carried out, but if for some reason these are not possible, prolonged physiotherapy may be required to restore movement.

Nerve lesions are usually cases of neurapraxia and will be recognized by failure of the muscles to harden on attempted contraction and loss of sensation in the skin supplied by the nerve.

Physiotherapy. This aims at the prevention of a stiff shoulder and restoration of the patient to as near the pre-accident condition as possible. With suitable treatment and co-operation on the part of the patient return to full normal activities should be possible in eight to twelve weeks.

Treatment follows the principles set out at the beginning of this section (see p. 316), but a few special points will be discussed here with special reference to the elderly patient.

Before the exercises are begun infra-red irradiation and gentle massage are used to assist the patient to relax and to disperse the oedema which might otherwise lead to adhesion formation. The best position to choose is probably sitting because the patient is usually elderly and is happier in this position. Very often the patient is frightened and still a little shocked and it is, therefore, particularly important that she should be encouraged, made welcome to the department, and the objects of the treatment carefully explained. Each new exercise should be demonstrated on the uninjured limb so that the patient understands exactly what is required and movements should be taken slowly and gently. The amount of movement depends on the patient and the degree of pain, but usually assisted active medial and lateral rotation with the arm by the side and elbow flexed to a right angle, assisted arm elevation through flexion with slight resistance given at the hand, particularly on the downward phase of the movement, and lax stoop sitting arm swinging forwards and backwards and sideways and arm circling are sufficient shoulder movements for the first day. The movements are within the limit of pain and in the case of rotation the patient should not feel a grinding sensation at the site of fracture. If this occurs the movement must be omitted.

All finger, thumb, wrist, forearm and elbow movements are checked; these aid the circulation and so promote absorption, they also lessen the danger that the patient will cease to use the arm through fear, which might result in serious atrophy and stiff joints. Biceps shortens very rapidly and often the exudate gravitates to the elbow so that the elbow easily loses full extension. This movement should, therefore, be carefully checked. Before the sling is reapplied rhythmic contractions of muscles round the shoulder are taught and the toilet of the axilla and bend of the elbow attended to. With the sling in position it is necessary to see that the arm is relaxed as many patients hold the arm up and to the side and do not take advantage of the support of the sling.

Patients need very careful instructions as to what they may and should do at home. It should be made clear that the sling is not essential and that it should be taken off and the shoulder movements practised several times during the day. The arm may be used for dressing, washing, etc., and the movements of other joints and rhythmic contractions done frequently.

Daily progression is made. Lying and side lying abduction, starting with a short lever, are added the next day, self-assisted elevation, through flexion is taught and elevation encouraged against the resistance of gravity. The patient is encouraged to try to get the hand behind the back and to wash the back of the neck while lateral rotation may be encouraged from the lax stoop sitting position (see p. 318). Gradually more free exercises are introduced including such exercises as standing with back against a wall, rotation of the arm, forearm rotation with a light pole to strengthen biceps, and elbow pressing back to strengthen triceps. The two latter exercises are important to prevent the head of the humerus dropping in the glenoid cavity (see p. 317). Elevation of the arm will be assisted if the patient tries to reach light objects from shelves above the level of the shoulder, dust high objects and possibly tie up tall plants in the garden.

About two weeks after the injury self-assisted pulley work is introduced and in three to four weeks the patient should, if physically fit, join a class and start occupational therapy.

It is not necessary to give much resistance to the muscle work for the first six weeks because the weight of the arm provides sufficient work.

During the treatment a watch should be kept for nerve lesions. Any suspicion that this may have occurred must be reported to the surgeon immediately. Treatment will then be started on the lines discussed in Chapter XIII (see p. 267).

FRACTURES OF THE GREATER TUBEROSITY

Two main types of fracture may be distinguished here. Firstly, there is the contusion fracture, which often accompanies a fracture of the surgical neck of humerus (see Plate XVIII), or a dislocation of the joint. In the latter injury the greater tuberosity impinges against the acromion when forcible abduction is carried out before the humerus can rotate into a position in which the greater tuberosity passes beneath the process. Secondly, there is the avulsion fracture in which forced adduction of the arm while the rotator cuff is actively contracting, results in tearing off a flake of bone at the insertion of the supraspinatus. In the first case the rather large fragment usually slips back into position. In the second case, spasm of supraspinatus may retract the fragment into the space between the head of the humerus and the acromion. The two therefore present rather different problems.

Contusion fractures or those in which the fragment is not displaced are stable fractures and redisplacement is unlikely, fixation is, therefore, unnecessary and the fracture is treated like a soft tissue injury, in a similar way to fractures of the surgical neck of the humerus. The essential difference is in the age of the patient, since these fractures may occur at any age especially where they accompany a dislocated shoulder, and in the fact that they are painful fractures in which the pain tends to persist, often for two months or more until the fracture is consolidated. This pain is usually referred to the insertion of deltoid, although tenderness is felt over the greater tuberosity.

The pain may be due to several factors. Damage to the floor of the subacromial bursa is almost certain to have occurred due to its connection to the greater tuberosity (see p. 313). If the lateral wall of the bicipital groove has been involved in the fracture, the tendon of biceps may be irritated by callus and ease and freedom of movement is reduced. Thus interference with the normal function of the shoulder may develop in these injuries.

For these reasons early active movements are most important and full range in the humero-scapular joint should be obtained within a week. Movements must be gained without increasing pain and should, therefore, be done in side lying and stoop standing (see p. 319). Exercises for biceps are also essential to maintain free movement of the humerus on the tendon.

Avulsion fractures with displacement require reduction or abduction of the arm will be permanently impaired. Open reduction is often undertaken and the fragment is sewn or screwed into position. Post-operative treatment follows the lines of the contusion fracture; a sling until the arm is comfortable without it, and early active movements. If conservative treatment is used the arm is abducted and retained in the position in which the hand lies opposite the mouth until such time as the fragment is firmly united, often a matter of six to nine weeks. It is difficult then to carry out the usual physiotherapy since active movment and certainly active elevation, is liable to displace the fragment. Active contractions of deltoid and movements of other joints must be practised. Care of the patient and the splint is most important because, if an abduction arm-splint is used, it is difficult to retain it in the correct position.

DISLOCATION OF THE SHOULDER JOINT

In most patients this injury is caused by a fall on the outstretched hand, a fall or blow on the back of the shoulder, or violent lateral rotation of the arm. The head of the humerus is driven forward and a sub-coracoid dislocation results. Occasionally as the patient falls he twists towards the side of the outstretched hand, and the head of the humerus driven backwards, comes to rest below the spine of the scapula.

The extent of damage varies. The capsule is always torn in a first dislocation. Most usually it is torn at its attachment to the humerus, but occasionally it is torn from the rim of the glenoid cavity, and in this case part of the glenoid labrum may be detached. In addition there may be tearing of some part of the rotator cuff and stretching and even rupture of muscle fibres. Occasionally as the head of the humerus is driven forward it may strike against the anterior rim of the glenoid cavity and a depressed fracture of the postero-lateral section of the head may result.

If the capsule is torn from its attachment to the neck of the humerus it will heal readily because there is a good blood supply. Provided repeated stretching by full elevation and lateral rotation is not allowed excess fibrous tissue, which would later limit movement, will not be formed. If, on the other hand, the labrum is detached re-attachment to the rim of the glenoid cavity is unlikely to occur since it is an avascular structure. This together with the possible defect in the humeral head probably predisposes towards recurrent dislocation.

Complications, to which this dislocation is particularly liable, are damage to the circumflex nerve, injury of the rotator cuff, fracture of the greater tuberosity and myositis. Care should be taken to detect these complications. It requires some skill to locate a deltoid paresis, for some patients have the power to abduct the arm without using the deltoid. The best way to detect the paralysis is to support the arm in a few degrees of abduction, then while palpating the deltoid with the fingers ask the patient to adduct the arm and then to try to abduct it. The adduction ensures relaxation of the muscle if it is not paralysed, attempted abduction detects clearly any contraction after relaxation.

Treatment

Opinions differ as to how these dislocations should be treated after reduction. Some surgeons believe in a minimum period of immobilization and early active movements while others prefer to keep the shoulder immobilized for three weeks.

Early Movement. Those surgeons who believe in early movement do so on the grounds that they will prevent muscle atrophy and adhesion formation. They claim that recurrent dislocation does not occur because movements have been started at once, but because of the defect in the labrum and that consequently no advantage is gained by keeping the shoulder at rest.

After a dislocation of the shoulder, young people do not usually require set exercises. Once the dislocation has been reduced, they will often move the arm freely through its full range. In this case the only purpose of physical treatment is to check that nerve injury is not present. Consequently, for a few days active movements throughout the arm and particularly the power to contract the deltoid should be tested. It is wise to warn these patients not to stretch the arm above the head for three weeks so that stretching of the healing capsule is prevented. In older people and in some young patients there is considerable synovitis and bruising and the patient may be unwilling to move the arm. In these cases physical treatment is necessary. The patient is equipped with a large arm sling which he wears for a few days. This rests the damaged soft tissues and allows the synovitis to subside.

Physiotherapy is begun about twenty-four hours after the injury. The patient is placed in a comfortable position and heat and massage are given to the shoulder and arm to relieve pain, gain relaxation and promote absorption of traumatic exudate. All active movements of fingers, thumb, wrist and forearm are practised and rhythmic contractions of deltoid, biceps and triceps taught. Within a day or two of the injury active shoulder movements are started. These are most important because they maintain the strength and tone of the muscles which keep the head of humerus in its correct relationship to the glenoid cavity. Medial and lateral rotation exercises are particularly important because they keep the two layers of the subacromial bursa moving over one another and prevent stiffness of the shoulder, while lateral rotation prevents contracture of the medial rotators and anterior part of the capsule. They should, however, be carried out with the arm in adduction so that there is no pressure on the labrum or stretching of the torn structures. Active abduction is equally important and care should be taken to see that there is correct co-ordination between the deltoid and the supraspinatus muscles. Usually abduction is not encouraged beyond shoulder level for fourteen to twenty-one days. Any further abduction necessitates lateral rotation, but this is unwise in abduction for two to three weeks following the injury. Elevation in flexion should be practised, but should be limited to 90° for the first ten to twenty-one days in order to avoid stretching and excess fibrous tissue formation.

Provided they do not cause pain, resisted exercises should be given for those muscles which hold the head of the humerus up in the glenoid cavity, that is for biceps, triceps, coraco-brachialis and deltoid. The object should be to obtain full range in all directions by three weeks after the injury.

Immobilization for three weeks

Exponents of this method prefer immobilization to early movement on the grounds that this will give the labrum and capsule a chance to become firmly healed. The arm may be supported in a large sling and bandaged to the side by several turns of bandage, leaving the hand free, or a collar and cuff beneath the clothes may be worn. If the dislocation is a posterior one the arm is fixed in lateral rotation and about 45° of abduction by means of a plaster spica.

During the period of immobilization it is most important to stimulate the circulation of the limb and reduce muscle atrophy. The fingers, thumb, wrist and forearm muscles must be exercised, and rhythmic contractions of biceps, triceps, deltoid and rotator muscles carried out for five minutes hourly. Shoulder bracing and shrugging should also be practised. If a collar and cuff is worn gravity-assisted shoulder movements may also be given. When the plaster or bandage is removed exercises are directed to regaining the range, strength and co-ordination of movement.

Treatment of Complications

Circumflex nerve lesion will be treated on the lines indicated in Chapter XIII (see p. 271).

Myositis results from damage to the muscles at the time of dislocation. If, after reduction, voluntary movement is particularly painful there is almost certain to be some myositis. In this case active movements must be very gentle, and if they still cause pain, should be omitted for a few days.

Damage of the Rotator Cuff is very common in older patients. It is treated on the lines indicated (see p. 324) limiting the range of abduction and lateral rotation to 90° for the first ten to twenty-one days.

Fracture of the Greater Tuberosity is the result of the impingement of the tuberosity against the acromion and any displacement is usually overcome when the dislocation is reduced. Treatment is then similar to that indicated for these fractures (see p. 327) again limiting the range of abduction and lateral rotation.

Recurrent dislocation of the shoulder is a not uncommon complication, though its cause is as yet uncertain. It appears to occur most often in young people in many of whom the muscles are in excellent condition. It is possible that in some patients there are defects in the rim of the glenoid cavity or in the head of the humerus, or the glenoid labrum and capsule may have failed to re-attach to the rim of the cavity.

With the exception of the first dislocation, the ease with which the dislocation occurs, varies from patient to patient. In some it happens on the simplest movement, in others some abnormal strain is necessary to provoke its occurrence. Subsequent dislocations are almost always intracapsular. They are not, therefore, accompanied by soft tissue damage and there is little, if any, bruising or swelling. Sometimes the patient is able to reduce the dislocation himself, sometimes he requires help. Although it may cause little pain, it does cause a great deal of inconvenience and, for this reason, treatment is eventually sought. The only treatment of any avail is surgical. Several different procedures are used. In Bankart's operation the glenoid labrum is repaired and the bony rim of the glenoid cavity is gouged out. In the Nicola operation, the tendon of the long head of biceps is divided and the proximal end is threaded through the head of the humerus and then sutured to the peripheral part. In the Putti-Platt operation the tendon of subscapularis is divided. Its distal end is fixed in front of the joint over-lapped by the proximal part of the capsule and the proximal end is then sutured near to the greater tuberosity. This shortens the structures at the anterior aspect of the joint and full lateral rotation and abduction of the shoulder are never obtained.

In each case it is usual to bandage the limb to the side for four to six weeks and only then to commence active shoulder movements. During the period of immobilization active exercises of all joints not immobilized are essential and rhythmical contractions of muscle groups of the limb should be practised repeatedly. When the bandage is discarded, every possible step should be taken to regain shoulder movements. The methods which should be employed are those which are used following a fractured surgical neck of humerus. If the Bankart or Putti-Platt operations have been per-formed, no attempt should be made to regain the last few degrees of lateral rotation, since the anterior structures have been deliberately shortened.

DISLOCATION OF THE ACROMIO-CLAVICULAR JOINT

This joint is most often dislocated as a result of a fall on the point of the shoulder. The degree of displacement depends on the ligamentous injury. If the acromio-clavicular ligament only is torn, the scapula and clavicle are still held together by the trapezoid and conoid ligaments and little downward drop of the scapula can occur. This dislocation shows as a slight lump over the acromio-clavicular joint. There is tenderness over the line of the joint and possibly a little swelling.

If the injury is more severe and the trapezoid and conoid ligaments are torn, the scapula, as a result of the weight of the arm, drops downwards and forwards and the acromial end of the clavicle may lie an inch higher than the acromion. In this case the clavicle is no longer stable and can be moved backwards and forwards.

Treatment

If the arm is elevated, the dislocation is reduced. Healing of the liga-ments, however, takes a long time and is difficult to obtain, and during this period every movement of the arm causes re-displacement. There are, therefore, three alternatives in treatment.

The most usual method is to ignore the dislocation and encourage the patient to practise free, active movements and to keep the shoulders well braced back.

The arm is rested in a large arm sling for a few days to allow the inflamatory reaction to subside. Full-range, free, active movements are then started, supporting the outer end of the clavicle for the first few days. Resistance is gradually added to build up strong muscles to support the joint and hold the shoulder up and back.

A second method is lengthy fixation to encourage healing of the ligaments. A pad of felt is applied over the joint and under the point of the flexed elbow and the two pads joined by a strap. To prevent the strap from slipping off the top of the shoulder, a second strap may be taken from the anterior aspect of the first strap round the body to the posterior aspect. This apparatus has to be maintained for a minimum of six weeks. In order to prevent the shoulder and elbow from becoming stiff during this period the patient should be given daily exercise. The joint will not redislocate if two precautions are taken. The patient should be in the lying position for the movements, and the outer end of the clavicle should be held down firmly while the arm is moved.

Operative treatment forms a third alternative. Different procedures are advocated. A long pin or screw may be inserted through the acromion across the joint into the clavicle and active exercises may then be begun at once. Alternatively the conoid and trapezoid ligaments may be replaced by bands of fascia. In this case the arm is immobilized by pads and strapping for three to six weeks and after this time active exercises are begun. The results of these methods of treatment are usually good.

FRACTURES OF THE SHAFT OF THE HUMERUS

These fractures may involve the upper or middle third of the shaft.

UPPER THIRD OF THE SHAFT

If the fracture is in the upper third, the upper fragment tends to be abducted and laterally rotated while the lower is adducted and drawn up so that it lies anterior to the upper. Reduction is, therefore, necessary to obtain compression of the granulation tissue. Once reduced, compression will be maintained by the tonic action of the muscles and fixation will not be required. Usually a large arm sling and axillary pad are used for ten to twenty-one days and active shoulder movements are then started.

MIDDLE THIRD OF THE SHAFT

A fracture in the middle third of the shaft presents different problems and there is a considerable variety of opinion as to how these should be treated. Spiral, oblique and transverse fractures all unite rapidly owing to the fact that vascularity in this region is particularly good. Compression is obtained by the tonic action of biceps and triceps. The main danger is of angulation of the fragments with consequent stretching of granulation tissue if the shoulder is moved and this danger is particularly apparent in transverse fractures. Simple splinting is most often used to prevent this angulation. This is in the form either of a U-shaped plaster (see Fig. 39) or plaster slabs extending from the acromion and axilla to the elbow or a complete plaster extending from the acromion to the wrist. These splints are retained for five to six weeks.

Alternatively no splint is worn, but a small arm sling is applied holding the humerus vertical so that the fractured ends lie opposite each other and compression is obtained by tonic action of biceps and triceps. If a sling only is used and the fracture is a spiral one in which hinging will not occur, the sling is gradually discarded after three to four weeks. The patient first takes the arm out of the sling for simple activities such as dressing and feeding. If, however, the line of fracture is transverse, and particularly if the elbow is stiff, there will be strain at the fracture site if the arm hangs by the side or an attempt is made to move the elbow vigorously. In these cases the sling is retained as a protection for three months, although movements are encouraged as in the previous case.

Another method of treatment is by an intramedullary nail. This usually gives greater stability and quicker union.

Physiotherapy. If a U-shaped plaster or plaster slabs are used, finger, wrist, forearm and small range elbow movements can be given at once and rhythmic contractions of biceps and triceps should also be practised while, if the plaster does not extend beyond the acromion, a small amount of shoulder movement can be obtained if the patient leans forward. When the plaster is removed treatment follows the usual lines.

If a small arm sling only is used, finger, wrist and forearm movements are taught and practised at once. Elbow movements are important because the contraction of the flexors and extensors stimulates compression and therefore callus formation. Although the shoulder is not immobilized, shoulder movements are not commenced for about three weeks since they may produce angulation. At three weeks the patient is encouraged to lean forward and swing the arm forwards and backwards while the physiotherapist supports the arm at the level of the fracture site. Usually at

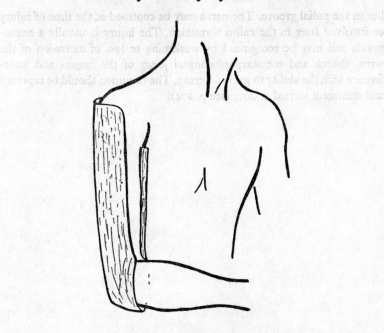

FIG. 39. U-SHAPED PLASTER FOR SPIRAL FRACTURE OF THE
SHAFT OF THE HUMERUS

about the fourth week an abduction swing is started. Progression is made at six to eight weeks by giving assisted active movements in all directions in the lying position. Full movements should be obtained by the eighth week.

Should intramedullary nailing be the method of choice it is usual to start movements of all joints of the arm within forty-eight hours, though rotation of the shoulder may be omitted for seven days. Range in shoulder and elbow should be full in two weeks.

COMPLICATIONS

Although most fractures of the shaft of the humerus unite rapidly, *delayed union and non-union* do occur. These may be the result of extensive comminution with dead bone fragments, of interposition of soft tissue, or of interference with the blood supply of the lower fragment. In such cases the fracture is either fixed by an intramedullary nail or pure splinting fixing both elbow and shoulder is used.

A second possible complication is that of *damage to the radial nerve* as it lies in the radial groove. The nerve may be contused at the time of injury or involved later in the callus formation. The injury is usually a neurapraxia and may be recognized by weakening or loss of extension of the wrist, thumb and metacarpophalangeal joints of the fingers and interference with the ability to grip and grasp. The condition should be reported and treatment started at once (see p. 274).

Chapter XVI

INJURIES OF THE ELBOW RADIUS AND ULNA

INJURIES ROUND THE ELBOW

There is probably no joint of which it is more important to understand the structure and function than the elbow joint. Its structure makes it peculiarly liable to complications when it is damaged and special precautions have to be taken when physiotherapy is used in the treatment of injuries of the joint. Indeed the physiotherapist may well feel she is faced with a series of negatives as far as the treatment of this joint is concerned—do not push movement, do not force, do not use any passive stretching or allow the patient or his relatives to do so, do not use massage. In spite of this some lesions round the elbow do require physical treatment and it is important to know what not to do and why, as well as what to do.

The function of the joint is to assist in prehension (grasp) by permitting objects to be brought nearer to or further from the head and trunk. To fulfil this function the joint must permit flexion and extension, but it must be stable and side-to-side movement should not occur. It is, therefore, a hinge joint in which the shape of the surfaces is such that flexion and extension are possible, but side movement impossible; the capsule is relatively loose in front and behind, but strongly reinforced at the sides by medial and lateral ligaments and the muscles are massed on the anterior and posterior aspects to produce flexion and extension.

While flexion and extension are important for prehension their range need not be full. Few people ever use the full possible range of either movement. Provided the arm is not needed for vigorous games the middle range of movement is adequate. On the other hand the muscles producing the movement should be strong. This particularly applies to the extensors. Considerable weight is put on the elbow as the body is pushed up from lying to sitting or to standing from sitting, the extensors providing the

337

thrust and preventing the elbow buckling under the body weight. The same applies if the arm is used to push a heavy object. The triceps is the powerful extensor and it is attached very strongly to the forearm. Its tendon attaches not only to the superior surface of the olecranon, but it has strong expansions which blend with the deep fascia of the forearm and especially with that covering the anconeus. The anconeus attaches to the upper third of the shaft of the ulna so it will be realized that triceps has an extensive attachment. If the extensors are injured or if they atrophy from disuse there will be weakness of the elbow and this will impair function.

Functionally the joint may be considered to consist of three parts: the humero-radial articulation, the humero-ulnar, and the radio-ulnar. All three are contained within one capsule. While flexion and extension take place at the first two simultaneously, pronation and supination take place at the third. It must, of course, be remembered that the latter movement also occurs throughout the length of the radius and ulna and at the inferior radio-ulnar joint also and these must be intact for the movement to take place. The long axis of the forearm makes an angle of approximately 170° with the long axis of the arm. This is known as the *carrying angle*. It means that when the elbow is flexed the distal end of the ulna remains lateral to the axial line of the humerus, consequently to reach the mouth the shoulder is medially rotated and the forearm pronated. Movement, therefore, occurs in all three components of the elbow joint. The carrying angle disappears in pronation when the forearm may be seen to be in line with the arm. The angle is important since its presence allows the elbow to fit snugly into the side when carrying a heavy weight while the object swings clear of the hip. The fact that in pronation the long axis of the forearm is in a straight line with that of the arm is also important since it means that power can be transmitted directly from the shoulder. It will be noticed that in all powerful actions the forearm is used in the pronated position. Decrease in the angle does not matter provided it is not too great. Increase is, however, important because the ulnar nerve, lying on the posterior aspect of the medial condyle, may be gradually stretched as the angle increases.

Pronation and supination are extremely important movements and they are liable to be limited if the elbow is injured since the superior radio-ulnar joint is within the capsule of the elbow joint.

The synovial membrane of the joint is extensive and has certain reduplications which, together with pads of fat, fill in the unoccupied spaces of the joint. Observation will show that there are non-articular areas at the point where the articular surface of the olecranon joins that of the coronoid to complete the trochlear notch, nor is the head of the radius perfectly congruent with the capitellum of the humerus. Folds of synovial membrane are present in both these areas. In the latter case the folds cover the periphery of the articular surface of the superior aspect of the head of the radius. If, as a result of chronic lesions of the joint, these folds become hypertrophied, or they are displaced as a result of sudden inco-ordinate movements, nipping may occur. This is one possible cause of 'tennis elbow' (see p. 354).

The blood supply of the joint is particularly rich. The joint receives its nutrition from an anastomosis formed by branches from the brachial, radial and ulnar arteries. This may be one of the factors which is responsible for the extensive swelling which usually follows injuries round the joint. It is also of considerable importance if the brachial artery is damaged. The branches from the brachial artery which help to form the anastomosis are given off along the course of the artery, the profunda brachii artery arising just below the axilla. Consequently if the main artery should be involved in injuries around the elbow the circulation in the forearm can be maintained through the anastomosis, provided the other vessels are healthy (see Fig. 40).

The Nerve supply. In close relationship to the joint are three great nerves, median, ulnar and radial. Nerve injury is, therefore, a very possible complication of elbow injuries. The ulnar nerve lies on the back of the medial epicondyle separated only from the elbow joint by the posterior fibres of the medial ligament. It can be readily damaged in fractures of the medial epicondyle or stretched if an abduction force is applied to the forearm or the forearm bones are dislocated. Increase of the carrying angle will also stretch the nerve. The median nerve and brachial artery lie together in front of the humerus and elbow joint, separated from them by the thin medial part of brachialis. Fractures of the lower end of the humerus or dislocation backwards of the elbow may, therefore, cause damage to either or both. The radial nerve and its posterior interosseous branch lie on the lateral side of the anterior aspect of the joint on the capsule and the posterior interosseous branch is also in close relationship with the upper end of the radius as it winds round to the back of the forearm between the superficial and deep fibres of the supinator. These can also be involved in dislocation or fractures.

Injuries of the Elbow, Radius and Ulna

The fascia of the forearm is particularly tense on the flexor aspect of the forearm where there is a special process, the bicipital aponeurosis, given off from the medial side of the tendon of biceps and passing down and medially to blend with the deep fascia on the ulnar side of the forearm. This is of great significance since extensive swelling beneath the fascia cannot expand outwards and must, therefore, press inwards, so being very liable to compress the veins, lymphatics and arteries, thus obstructing the arterial inflow and the drainage from the forearm.

The position of ease of the elbow is one of approximately 90° flexion. This is the position which is commonly used therefore to rest the elbow after injury. If this position is maintained for long there is a tendency for biceps to shorten making it difficult to obtain extension when the splint or sling is removed. Therefore, as soon as is permitted, gentle active movements should be given to prevent this shortening.

Physiotherapy in Elbow Injuries

If the previous points have been considered it will be realized that not very many recent injuries round the elbow reach the physiotherapy department; this especially applies to children in whom the danger of a stiff elbow is very slight. Some patients do, however, require physical treatment and while it is essential to know what to do it is also important to know what not to do.

In most recent injuries there is *some limitation of movement* and attention is given to regaining full range; in elbow injuries this is *not of great importance* since full range is not essential. On the other hand to push movements is probably to produce a stiff elbow and is, therefore, to be avoided. Most elbow injuries result in considerable damage to the soft tissues; muscles may be torn, connective tissue stretched and ruptured, ligaments damaged and periosteum stripped from bone. Healing of these tissues takes place by fibrous tissue formation, but too much movement causes excessive fibrous tissue formation and the result will be a thickened and stiff elbow. The guiding rule is, therefore, to allow movements to recover on their own, giving the patient only simple free elbow flexion and extension and forearm rotation exercises and avoiding any forcing, pushing or passive stretching. The patient and, if he is a child, his parents, should be warned about this.

Myositis ossificans is always a possibility, particularly in the case of children in whom the bone cells are especially active. In most cases the periosteum is stripped up away from the bone as the soft tissues are stretched by the force producing the injury. When the fracture or dislocation is reduced the periosteum is restored to the bone, but if vigorous movements or passive stretching are given it may be elevated again and the sub-periosteal haematoma resulting from bleeding beneath the periosteum will ossify resulting in formation of new and unnecessary bone, which may interfere with movement. This then is another reason why too early and too vigorous movements are to be avoided.

Occasionally myositis ossificans occurs without apparent cause and if exercises are being given these should be stopped, the patient simply using the arm gently without set exercise. The process must, therefore, be recognized. Its signs are usually tenderness over the anterior aspect of the joint, spasm of biceps on attempted movements and very painful and limited movements. Any of these signs should be reported immediately.

All injuries are likely to show muscle atrophy with the need for *exercises to restore the muscles to normal*. This equally applies to elbow injuries. Usually the extensors are most affected as the arm is rested in flexion and this is especially so in fractures of the olecranon with or without damage to the triceps expansion. Exercises are, therefore, given to strengthen the muscle, with extra attention to triceps. The exercises should be carried out in the range available and should be progressive in order to strengthen. Resistance will be delayed for two to three weeks if the triceps has been sutured. If in the later stages weights are used care should be taken to see that the weight cannot throw a strain on the joint.

Partly owing to the extensive damage to the soft tissues and partly due to the rich blood supply, injuries to the elbow are usually characterized by *marked swelling*. This can be dangerous because the tight fascia does not permit the fluid to distend the tissues outwards; it, therefore, presses inward and may constrict the circulation, interfering with the arterial supply and the venous and lymphatic drainage of the forearm. Arterial obstruction may also be the result of damage to the brachial artery and/or its accompanying network of sympathetic nerve fibres. Two particular points, therefore, emerge. The physiotherapist should do all she can to *help to relieve oedema and promote drainage* and in addition she must keep *a careful watch for any signs of circulatory obstruction.*

To relieve swelling the limb may be elevated so that the elbow lies above the level of the heart; the plaster or sling need not be disturbed in order to achieve this. The patient should be taught the easiest way to do this so that it can be done at home. If there is no splint, massage to the arm and lightly over the posterior aspect of the elbow (excluding the site of fracture) will help to promote drainage. Effleurage, and squeezing kneading are the most effective manipulations. Rhythmic muscle contractions and movements of the digits, wrist and shoulder will also help to reduce the swelling.

The signs of circulatory obstruction are usually pain, pallor and pulselessness. *Pain* is felt on attempted movements if there is ischaemia, since the fatigue products fail to be removed from the tissues. It will also be experienced if an attempt is made actively or passively to extend the fingers with the wrist extended. This will stretch the ischaemic and fibrosing tissues. Occasionally pain is not experienced. This will be due to ischaemia of the nerves and is most likely if the sympathetic network is irritated and all the large and small vessels are, therefore, constricted.

Pallor is due to the diminished inflow of arterial blood. If the swelling or vaso-constriction continues, the fingers will become blue as the blood already in the part gives up its oxygen. This will be accompanied by swelling due to damage occurring to the vessel walls as the oxygen tension becomes low. Blisters may then appear on the tips of the fingers.

Pulselessness develops as obstruction increases. If the ischaemia is due to swelling it continues until the swelling subsides. If it is due to thrombosis of a damaged brachial artery the pulse will return, though often only weakly, as the collateral circulation becomes established.

To allow arterial obstruction to develop and continue is to ask for severe damage to the limb; it must, therefore, be detected. If any of the signs are even suspected the patient must be taken at once to the surgeon or the casualty department so that any pressure on the elbow can be immediately released. If for any reason this is not possible, all splints or dressings and bandages should be removed and if the elbow is flexed it should be allowed to extend to an angle at which the pulse is present. Heat to the cold hand should not be given since this will only increase metabolism and swelling will not be relieved.

It has been seen that the major nerves of the arm are very vulnerable and in all elbow injuries a *careful watch should be kept so that any signs of nerve involvement* can be reported immediately. The patient is asked if the hand feels normal and the skin sensation should be tested. A check on the ability to extend the wrist and thumb and fingers at the metacarpophalangeal joints will test the radial nerve. To test the ulnar nerve the patient extends the middle or ring finger and then attempts to move it from side to side. Testing the pincer grip will test the median nerve. A watch must be kept for trick movements. Thus, in attempting the pincer grip, the thumb may be adducted so that the side of the terminal phalanx instead of the palmar surface is approximated to the index finger. Careful palpation of the muscles is necessary as the patient attempts to do the required movements. If a nerve lesion is present physiotherapy will probably be ordered and it will be on the lines indicated in Chapter XIII.

Treatment of most injuries round the elbow, therefore, mainly consists of gentle free exercises for elbow flexion and extension and forearm pronation and supination, progressive strengthening exercises for triceps, elevation and gentle massage if there is much swelling, and a careful lookout for signs of circulatory or nerve involvement. There are of course exceptions; more chronic lesions, such as tennis elbow, may require deep localized massage, electrotherapy or ultra-sound therapy and manipulations (see p. 354).

FRACTURES AROUND THE ELBOW JOINT

A variety of injuries can occur round the elbow, some more common in children, others in adults. The most usual fractures seen in children are the supra-condylar fracture, fractures of the medial epicondyle, fractures of the lateral condyle and fractures of the neck of the radius. Adults more usually sustain a 'T-' or 'Y-' shaped fracture of the lower end of the humerus, fracture of the capitellum, fracture of the head of the radius and fracture of the olecranon.

The main difference between these two groups from the physiotherapist's point of view is that children rarely receive physical treatment except in cases where complications arise, whereas it is usual for adults to require treatment. The explanation of this lies mainly in the fact that children's joints stiffen less readily and regain movements more rapidly. Adhesions are much less prone to form in the young and soft tissues much less readily lose their elasticity and pliability. Again, children are much more likely to forget that a limb has been damaged and will use it more freely in games and school activities without need for any encouragement. In addition, in some elbow injuries, the tendency to excessive callus and bone formation is more noticeable in children than in adults, because all cells are more active. Movement in the early days is apt to encourage this and it is safe to say that it is wiser to fix these fractures in the young for longer than in adults and then to allow movement to recover in its own time and to avoid set exercise or other forms of physical treatment.

Nevertheless children do occasionally attend the physiotherapy department and the main points about their fractures should be known.

FRACTURES IN CHILDREN

SUPRACONDYLAR FRACTURES

These fractures are the result of a fall on the hand. The fracture line is usually transverse as seen on the antero-posterior X-ray and the lower fragment and forearm are most often displaced backwards. Often there is also lateral displacement, angulation and rotation of the lower fragment. Reduction is therefore necessary. Immobilization is not necessary to obtain compression since this will be obtained by the tone of biceps and triceps, but simple splinting is often used to control the lateral position of the fragments. Some surgeons do not consider any splintage necessary. If splinting is used it consists of a posterior plaster slab extending from the axilla to just proximal to the wrist, moulded round the sides of the limb, but not extending on to the front of the elbow. For cases of backward displacement the elbow is flexed, usually to about 60° but rarely more, at least to begin with, to avoid the danger that swelling might cause circulatory obstruction. The rarer forward displacement is treated in extension at about 170° for the first one to two weeks. The splint is maintained for three weeks. If a splint is not used a collar and cuff only is applied (see Plate XXI).

At the end of three weeks the plaster is removed, but protection is needed for a further three weeks until the fracture is consolidated to avoid the child damaging the arm again. But at this stage the child is allowed to take the arm out of the sling for use of the hand in school activities (excluding gym and games), dressing and washing.

This fracture is particularly liable to complications. Ischaemic contracture, nerve injury, myositis ossificans, increase or decrease of the carrying angle and stiff elbow are all possible.

Ischaemic contracture may be due to injury to the brachial artery by the sharp edge of the upper fragment. The artery may be contused (see Fig. 40, p. 345) and this can be followed by thrombosis occluding its lumen or by irritation of the sympathetic nerve fibres around it. Simple thrombosis, though producing a cold pale hand and forearm with absence of the radial pulse for some minutes, will do no permanent harm, because the collateral vessels will dilate within twenty to thirty minutes and the limb will regain its normal temperature and colour though the pulse may remain weakened. But thrombosis may be complicated by spasm of the other vessels following irritation of the sympathetic network, or by obstruction of the vessels resulting from swelling or a haematoma beneath the bicipital aponeurosis (see p. 339). In this case, unless these are relieved, the circulation is not restored in time and a much-reduced blood supply is inadequate for the muscles and nerves. The muscle fibres die and are gradually replaced by fibrous tissue which tends to contract leading to clawing of the fingers and flexion of the wrist. The nerves show degeneration and there will be motor and sensory paralysis. It is essential that diminished circulation should be

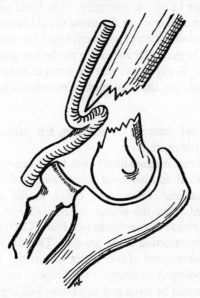

FIG. 40. BACKWARD DISPLACEMENT OF FOREARM AND INVOLVEMENT OF BRACHIAL ARTERY IN SUPRACONDYLAR FRACTURE OF THE LOWER END OF THE HUMERUS

recognized at its onset before harm is done since the surgeon will take immediate steps to deal with it. The first step is to remove all wool, bandage or splints covering the front of the elbow, then if the fracture has not been fully reduced, this is done. Should the circulation not be restored within the next hour the artery is explored, if necessary the fascia is divided, but if this is not successful the artery is freed and painted with an anti-spasmodic. If the artery is punctured or thrombosed a segment may be excised.

The median nerve with the brachial artery passes over the sharp edge of the upper fragment and may be damaged. Should injury occur it is most likely to be a neurapraxia. The radial and ulnar nerves are less likely to be damaged.

Myositis ossificans is not common but it does however occur and should be detected, since its presence will be increased by vigorous movements.

345

When the collar and cuff are removed for use of the hand at the end of three weeks, it will be found that the patient is very unwilling to move the elbow which is very stiff. Attempt to move results in spasm of biceps; there is marked tenderness at the front of the joint and if the elbow is X-rayed a fluffy shadow may be seen in the region of the lower part of the brachialis. If myositis ossificans does occur the elbow should be rested in a sling until spasm of biceps has disappeared, and active exercises omitted. Flexion may be regained later by gradually increasing the flexion position in a collar and cuff and when the X-ray shows that the ectopic bone has a clear outline and mature architecture the mass may be removed if it is interfering with flexion.

A stiff elbow is not common in children, but occasionally the healing process involves the capsule.

The line of fracture is exceedingly close to the capsule which is attached just above the radial and coronoid fossae, and in the process of repair, granulation tissue and callus may easily invade the capsule. This will be recognized when the plaster is removed and movement begun, by a startling limitation of movement (see Plate XXII, (a) and (b)), only a few degrees in any direction being possible. The important point to note here is that encouragement of movement will irritate and increase callus formation and consequently decrease the range of movement. If it is left alone, the capsule will be freed and movement will begin to recover when the time comes for absorption of unnecessary bone (see Plate XXII, (c) and (d)). Hence the physiotherapist should not, in this case, continue active elbow exercises. The child is allowed to use the arm and the position is explained to the parents by the surgeon, but no specific exercises are given.

If a child with a supracondylar fracture is sent to the physiotherapy department treatment will be on the lines set out on page 340. If a collar and cuff or plaster slab is worn, finger and shoulder exercises are taught so that the child can do them at home; it is important that a responsible relative should be shown the exercises. A very careful check should be made to detect any signs of circulatory involvement or nerve lesion. The presence of pain, alteration in sensation, change of temperature or colour, swelling in the hand and inability to extend the fingers with the wrist extended must all be reported at once. Movements of the hand and wrist must be compared with those of the other side and any weakness reported. When the plaster or sling is removed elbow and forearm movements are begun, but they are free and no forcing or stretching is permitted. Any tenderness, spasm or decrease in range of movement again should be noted and reported.

FRACTURE OF THE LATERAL CONDYLE

This fracture occurs in young children in whom the epiphysis has not yet joined the diaphysis. The fracture line includes the lateral epicondyle, capitellum and part of the trochlea (see Fig. 41). If no displacement occurs union will be satisfactory, and it is sufficient to prevent movement of the elbow by the application, for about three weeks, of a collar and cuff with the hand below the chin. In some cases, however, spasm of the extensor tendon rotates the fragment so that it faces laterally and the raw fracture surface does not lie opposite its bed, so that bony union cannot

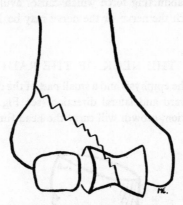

FIG. 41. LINE IN FRACTURE OF LATERAL CONDYLE

occur. If nothing is done, union occurs by fibrous tissue. Then, when the radius thrusts up against the capitellum, the fibrous tissue gradually yields and the lateral epicondyle moves laterally. The forearm therefore takes on an increasing deviation from the axis of the arm, and the increased carrying angle so formed is liable, over a period of years, to cause an ulnar neuritis through gradual stretching of the ulnar nerve, as it lies on the postero-medial aspect of the joint. For this reason, open reduction, sometimes combined with internal fixation, is necessary. Once reduced, protection is gained by a collar and cuff, retained for three to four weeks. Physiotherapy is rarely needed, but if ordered it is carried out on the lines indicated for the supracondylar fracture.

FRACTURE OF THE MEDIAL EPICONDYLE

This injury occurs in the adolescent and is due to an abducting violence applied to the forearm. The medial epicondyle is torn off, and may show only slight displacement, or it may slip into the joint cavity when the medial side is opened by the violence. Without displacement, the only treatment is rest and protection supplied by a collar and cuff, but, if the fragment lies in the joint cavity, reduction is necessary. Under general anaesthesia the fingers and wrist are extended and the elbow abducted. If the fragment is not pulled out of the joint by this manoeuvre a strong faradic stimulation of the flexors may be successful. Some surgeons prefer to excise the fragment of bone since recovery is usually very slow in this fracture and appears to be hastened if the epicondyle is excised.

If physiotherapy is ordered it follows the lines set out for the previous fractures, but the particular complication to be looked for here is ulnar nerve injury. The abducting force which causes avulsion of the epicondyle may also stretch the nerve or the nerve may be later irritated in the roughened groove.

FRACTURE OF THE NECK OF THE RADIUS

In this fracture, the epiphysis and a small part of the diaphysis are usually displaced in a forward and lateral direction (see Fig. 42). If allowed to remain in this position, growth will carry the head further away from the

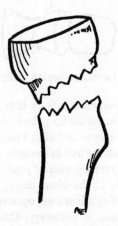

FIG. 42. FRACTURE OF THE NECK OF THE RADIUS

ulna with increasing dislocation of the superior radio-ulnar joint and permanent limitation of pronation and supination. Reduction is, therefore, necessary. This is followed by the application of a collar and cuff for three to four weeks. Physiotherapy is rarely ordered, but, if it is, it will follow the same lines as previously described.

FRACTURES IN ADULTS

'T' or 'Y' shaped fractures of the lower end of the Humerus

These fractures are often the result of a fall on the hand in which the ulna, being forced up, splits the lower end of the humerus. There may be vertical and transverse fracture lines and the fragments may be impacted or separated. Reduction is very difficult and often restoration of a normal articular surface is impossible. Treatment, therefore, depends upon whether such restoration is possible or not. If good alignment can be obtained by reduction, re-displacement is prevented by immobilization in plaster for three to four weeks. The plaster covers about two-thirds of the circumference of the limb in order to avoid the danger of constriction of the circulation, and it extends from below the axilla to just proximal to the wrist. While in plaster active shoulder, finger, thumb and wrist movements should be practised and a careful watch kept for circulatory obstruction or nerve involvement. When the plaster is removed the elbow is likely to be very stiff and recovery will be slow. Full range of movement is seldom regained. Exercises will aim at strengthening the muscles and helping the restoration of some movement.

In those cases in which good alignment of the articular surfaces cannot be obtained, the best way to gain a satisfactory result seems to be by early active elbow movements. These will help to remould the articular surfaces and prevent the intra- and extra-articular adhesions which would other-wise tend to form. Surprisingly good results are obtained in this way. These fractures may, therefore, simply be rested in a large arm sling and elbow movements commenced at once. These are kept within the limit of real pain, but can usually be progressed daily.

FRACTURES OF THE CAPITELLUM

This fracture is usually the result of violence which forces the radius up against the capitellum. A varying-sized fragment is detached and will obstruct flexion of the elbow. Reduction by open operation is necessary and is usually followed by retention of the elbow at 90° by a large arm sling or a collar and cuff for three weeks. Physiotherapy involves the same principles, but the elbow, though not fixed in plaster, should not be moved under three weeks, unless such movements are especially ordered by the surgeon.

FRACTURES OF THE HEAD OF THE RADIUS

These fractures arise as a result of a fall on the hand with the forearm

Injuries of the Elbow, Radius and Ulna

in the abducted position. The head of the radius is 'struck' by the capitellum and, according to the force, a more or less severe injury results. There may simply be a small vertical crack fracture, or fissure, with no displacement (see Fig. 43). Alternatively the lateral part of the head may be fractured and this fragment may be depressed, tilted forward or displaced laterally. Not uncommonly the head is comminuted (see Fig. 44). In all cases there will be damage to the articular cartilage. The fracture is not the only injury since the abducting force may stretch or tear the medial

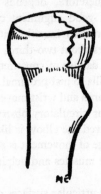

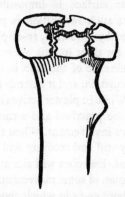

FIG. 43. CRACK FRACTURE OF
THE HEAD OF THE RADIUS

FIG. 44. COMMINUTED FRACTURE
OF THE HEAD OF THE RADIUS

ligament of the elbow joint and other soft tissues on the medial side of the joint. There will therefore be considerable traumatic exudate.

If the ligament is irritated by excessive movement it will never heal properly, fibrous tissue will be formed, it will become adherent, and a stiff elbow with limited extension will result. London points out that extension may also be limited because the head of the radius tends to slip sideways before it breaks and as it does so it damages the extensors at their attachment to the humerus. Scarring results and restricts their normal movement over the epicondyle during flexion and extension of the elbow. There are therefore two main injuries: the fracture and the damage to the extensors and the rupture of the medial ligament and, according to which the surgeon considers the more important, so different methods of treatment may be used.

If the ligamentous damage is considered to be the more important, the elbow is immobilized in plaster for three to four weeks. During this time the usual physiotherapy routine may be carried out. When the plaster is removed active movements are encouraged, but they should not be pressed to the point at which they elicit pain and muscle spasm.

If the fracture, extensor injury and cartilage damage are thought to be more important, early movements without immobilization, or excision of fragments are the methods chosen. In the case of a *fissure fracture* displacement does not occur though the cartilage will be damaged. Fixation is not required and the fracture is treated like a soft tissue injury. Rest for the traumatized soft tissues and cartilage is gained by the use of a sling for ten to fourteen days. Physiotherapy usually begins at once. It follows the usual lines, namely encouragement of free active pronation, supination, flexion and extension, but though gentle persuasion to greater effort is often needed, no forcing or passive movement is permitted. Full rotation of the forearm is usually obtained in a few weeks, but full flexion and extension of the elbow are often delayed and may never be obtained. This is due to the inevitable damage of the hyaline cartilage covering both articular surfaces.

In the case of the *marginal fracture*, if the fragment is slightly depressed or impacted no fixation is needed and the fracture is treated in the same way as the fissure type. If the fragment is displaced, unless something is done, it will unite by fibrous tissue in a tilted position, giving rise to an enlarged and irregular articular surface which will later show osteo-arthritic changes. Open reduction is sometimes necessary and many surgeons prefer to excise the whole head, because in doing so the damaged articular cartilage is removed and osteo-arthritis prevented. Pronation and supination will not be affected if the neck of the radius is left intact within the annular ligament. The radius cannot ride up because it is firmly connected to the ulna. The medial and downward direction of the fibres of the interosseous membrane would also resist the tendency.

Following the operation the patient is liable to hold the arm still, through fear of pain and as a result of muscle spasm. This will naturally result in the formation of scar tissue and in limitation of movement. A few days after the operation the patient is therefore sent to the physiotherapy department for supervision of movements. As a rule he is wearing a sterile dressing and sling or collar and cuff with the forearm supinated and the elbow in a position of flexion between 90° and 45°.

Again movement should not be forced, but much practice and encouragement should be given to the movements of the elbow and forearm, particularly supination. This latter movement is often difficult to obtain and, as it is a most important movement in everyday activities, a careful watch must be kept that its range steadily increases. All the other principles of physiotherapy in the treatment of fractures not immobilized must be followed.

In the third type of fracture of the head of the radius, the *comminuted fracture*, reduction would obviously be impossible. Small bone fragments are often widely scattered. Excision is, therefore, necessary and the after-treatment follows the lines of the previous fracture.

Two complications may occur in these fractures. Occasionally, following operation, calcium is deposited in the capsule of the elbow joint and movement becomes very limited. If movement does not gradually increase this should be suspected and reported since active exercises will only increase the deposit. Movements are then omitted for some days and only resumed with great caution. The second complication is that of injury to the ulnar nerve occurring as a result of the abducting force. Tests for ulnar nerve involvement should, therefore, be carried out (see p. 342).

FRACTURES OF THE OLECRANON

Fractures of the olecranon are the result either of direct violence, such as a fall on the elbow, or of muscular action, the elbow being forcibly flexed when the triceps is actively contracting. The type of fracture produced is either comminuted or transverse. What really matters, however, is not the type, but whether or not there is a separation of the fragments. This can only take place if the expansion of triceps is torn. If the triceps is torn, the patient will not be able to extend his elbow voluntarily, while, if the triceps is intact, there will be the ability to contract the muscle although it may be uncomfortable to do so.

If the triceps is not torn, the fracture may be ignored and the lesion is treated as a soft tissue injury. There will be much bruising and swelling, very often an olecranon bursitis and movement will be painful, and so rest is essential. This can be adequately obtained with a pressure bandage for the joint and a large arm sling. Rest will be continued until the inflammation subsides (often about a fortnight) but, during this time, the venous and lymphatic circulation may be stimulated, to aid absorption, by means of heat applied proximally to the injury and exercises to all joints except the elbow. Organization may be prevented by rhythmic contractions of the flexors and extensors of the elbow. Towards the end of this period, gentle, active assisted elbow movements may be started. Triceps is the important muscle in any fracture of the olecranon and special attention must be paid to it.

When triceps is torn, a different problem is presented. Then the spasm which results retracts the upper fragment, tilting it so that it often becomes locked in the olecranon fossa. The gap between the fragments and in triceps is rapidly filled with blood, and, if nothing is done, the blood will clot, organize and become turned into fibrous tissue. Later, with constant movement of the elbow, the fibrous tissue will stretch and triceps will be lengthened and its power reduced, so that it will finish its contraction before full extension is obtained.

In older people the small fragment is usually excised and the triceps expansion firmly sutured to the upper end of the ulna. In younger people the fragment may be replaced and secured by means of a screw. Some surgeons prefer to suture both the bone and triceps.

The after-treatment depends on the type of operation. In the first two methods the condition is treated as a soft tissue lesion. The arm is rested by means of a large arm sling with the elbow at a right angle for a few days and movements are commenced at once.

If the bone is sutured immobilization is necessary until union is sound. A plaster extending from axilla to wrist, with the elbow flexed to a right angle, is applied. This is retained for approximately five weeks.

The main object of physiotherapy is to maintain the tone and power of triceps. Loss of tone and power will rapidly occur as a result of inhibition from pain. It is also the result of lack of use, especially when the elbow has been immobilized for five weeks. Rhythmic contractions should be carried out many times a day and active extension started as soon as the surgeon permits. At first the exercises should be free using slings or a smooth surface to support the arm and eliminate friction and the force of gravity, but as soon as possible resistance should be added. This not only increases the work for triceps, but also produces relaxations of biceps. If the triceps is repaired, resistance may be added about three weeks after the repair; if the arm is immobilized it may be added as soon as the plaster is removed.

DISLOCATION OF THE ELBOW

This injury is liable to occur at any age. In a large percentage of patients the forearm bones are driven backwards, but in addition they may be displaced medially or laterally. The injury is usually recognized by the fact that there is an abnormal contour in the elbow region, the olecranon is out of its normal relationship with the epicondyles of the humerus and there is immobility at the elbow, the joint being held rigidly at about one hundred and thirty degrees of extension.

As in most dislocations a great deal of soft tissue damage must be produced. The capsule of the joint will have been torn and brachialis will either be torn or it will have stripped up the periosteum from the anterior aspect of the coronoid process. According to the direction of the dislocation the medial or lateral ligaments will have been stretched or ruptured and sometimes the common flexor tendon will avulse the medial epicondyle. Fractures often accompany the dislocation particularly fracture of the head of the radius or of the capitellum or coronoid. Any of the nerves may be damaged and the brachial artery may also be involved.

The first essential is that the *dislocation should be reduced* so that stretching of vessels, nerves and soft tissues is relieved. This must be followed by *rest* for the soft tissues so that healing with the minimum amount of fibrous tissue can take place as rapidly as possible. The reduction allows any elevated periosteum to fall back into place so that sub-periosteal haematomata do not form or are only very small. If a fracture of the head of the radius has occurred it is excised later when the swelling has subsided. Rest is obtained by a sling, collar and cuff or posterior plaster slab depending on the stability of the elbow after reduction. The presence of fractures may reduce the stability. Rest should continue until the tissues have healed, usually about three weeks, but during this time hand and shoulder exercises should be practised frequently. Forearm rotation is also important, but elbow movements, particularly in the case of children, are usually postponed for two to three weeks. If allowed before this time they should be free active movements very gently carried out. A careful watch should be kept for signs of nerve involvement or circulatory obstruction. When the sling or plaster is removed elbow movements continue in a wider range.

TENNIS ELBOW

Tennis elbow is a condition characterized by pain on the lateral side of the elbow, often radiating into the forearm and hand. Much discussion has arisen as to the cause of the condition and it is now widely accepted that there is a variety of possible lesions responsible.

The name 'tennis elbow' arises from the fact that the condition was first described as a tennis player's injury, but the symptoms occur in many other sports and occupations, particularly those which involve tight gripping and rotational movements of the forearm or repeated extension of the wrist.

Wiles has classified the causes into intra-articular and extra-articular lesions. In the first group he suggests that the lesion is a nipping of a synovial fringe displaced by sudden movement of the elbow. If a tag of synovial membrane is caught, it will swell and may become ulcerated. Thus every time the same movement is repeated, pain will result.

Many different conditions can be gathered together in the extra-articular group. Some cases may be the result of direct trauma to the lateral epicondyle setting up a periostitis; others may be due to a chronic inflammation of a bursa between the common extensor tendon and the lateral aspect of the radio-humeral joint. Yet others may be strain of the lateral ligament of the elbow or of the muscle fibres of the extensor group. One of the most widely accepted theories as to the causation of tennis elbow is that there is a partial tear at the junction of the tendon of the extensor carpi radialis brevis with the periosteum of the lateral epicondyle. As the tear begins to heal, it is again broken down by movement. The constant unequal pull on the periosteum and the repeated breaking down of healing tissue results in a type of 'fibrositis' at the teno-periosteal junction. This may quite likely be aggravated by the deposit of toxic substances. Some authorities firmly believe in a toxic element in this condition and state that there have been many cases in which toxaemia has been present.

The main signs and symptoms are those of pain, tenderness and inability to use the hand and forearm effectively. *Pain* varies in its onset. If the condition is intra-articular, pain usually comes on suddenly following movement, passes off with rest, but re-occurs with resumption of the same activity. If the lesion is extra-articular, pain comes on gradually, the patient noticing its presence after some activity. There is also aching and discomfort on the lateral side of the elbow which gradually becomes worse until it is impossible to continue with the particular movement. In both groups pain tends to radiate down the centre or lateral side of the posterior aspect of the forearm into the dorsum of the hand and the middle finger. In the intra-articular group, pain is increased by pronation and supination of the forearm and by extension of the elbow, even if the extensors of the wrist and fingers are relaxed. In the extra-articular group, pain is not felt on pronation or supination and only on extension if the extensors are stretched by flexion of the wrist and fingers.

Tenderness is a good guide to the actual lesion, since its site will depend on the tissue affected. If the lesion is a nipping of a synovial fringe, tenderness will be acute on the postero-lateral aspect of the forearm over the radio-humeral joint. Should the lesion be a strain of the muscles, tenderness will be palpated if the muscle belly is lifted and squeezed between the finger and thumb. If the lesion is a periostitis or a partial tear of the extensor carpi radialis brevis attachment, tenderness will occur over the anterior aspect of the lateral epicondyle, thickening may then also be felt. Should the extensor carpi radialis longus attachment be at fault, the tender spot will be over the lower part of the lateral supracondylar ridge. If the trouble is confined to the lateral ligament, tenderness will be felt just below the lateral epicondyle. Sometimes there is general diffuse tenderness over the whole extensor group. This is most likely to be present when the condition is acute.

Limited movement will be present in the intra-articular lesions both in pronation and supination and in extension. There is no limitation of movement in the extra-articular lesions except of full extension if the extensor muscles are at the same time stretched by full flexion of the wrist and fingers, but there will often be weakness of grip; the housewife, for example, complaining of being unable to lift the teapot to pour out the tea.

TREATMENT

Treatment clearly depends upon the type of lesion and a careful examination is always made first to isolate the structure affected.

Lesions of the synovial membrane. In early cases a single manipulation is often entirely successful and physiotherapy is unnecessary. In later cases, where the synovial membrane is oedematous and shows a raw, unhealed patch, rest is necessary to gain healing. This may be obtained by strapping until all pain and tenderness have subsided. The physiotherapist may then be called in to supervise the gradual resumption of activity.

Lesions of the muscle belly. Strain or rupture of a few fibres of one or other of the extensor muscles will be treated like any other strained or 'pulled' muscle. Exudate will be removed by heat and massage, organization prevented by active contractions and relaxations, and over-use prevented by cessation from the activity which is causing the trouble until pain and tenderness have completely disappeared.

Periostitis. This can only be cured by complete rest, obtained by preventing the common tendon of origin of the extensor muscles from pulling on the epicondyle. These cases are usually treated by means of a cock-up splint or plaster, holding the wrist in extension until extension of the wrist against the plaster ceases to cause pain. Again physiotherapy is rarely required.

Tear at teno-periosteal junction. This type is most commonly treated by hydrocortisone injections. Following the injection the area may be very painful for a few hours but pain quickly subsides leaving the elbow free from pain. Discomfort may recur at about seven to ten days and a second injection may be necessary. For some patients physiotherapy may help. Since a partial tear is causing continual unequal pull on the periosteum and traumatic 'fibrositis', the principle here is to prevent this pull and obtain firm healing of the tendon and firm re-attachment to the epicondyle. This may be obtained in several different ways. *If movement is prevented*, then the lesion will heal firmly. This may be the method of choice and is carried out either by strapping the arm, from mid-forearm to mid-arm, with the elbow slightly flexed, or, more effectively, by splinting the wrist in extension, using a large arm sling and abstaining from any activities which would move the tendons. Four to six weeks immobilization will result in an apparent cure. Cyriax points out, however, that healing will occur in the short position of the tendon and resumption of activity may well cause future rupture and re-occurrence of symptoms. An alternative method is to irritate the site *so that much fibrous tissue is formed ensuring firm attachment of tendon to bone*. This may be done by really deep massage at the site. It is, however, open to the same objections as in the previous case.

Probably the most satisfactory way is *to rupture the tendon completely* so that it will heal by fibrous tissue and lengthening will result. Breakdown may be obtained by manipulation when no further treatment should be required, or by repeated stretching preceded by measures to soften the area. This is where the physiotherapist can be of most use. The blood supply in the region of the lateral epicondyle may be first increased by the use of deep-heating or the constant current. The tendon and fibrous tissue may then be stretched and softened by deep frictions, given transversely across the anterior aspect of the lateral epicondyle. Alternately the micro-massage effect of ultra-sound can be used. The attachment is then completely ruptured by sudden adduction of the forearm on the arm with the elbow extended. A more effective manipulation is (*a*) flex wrist and fingers and pronate forearm, then (*b*) sudden full extension of elbow, while holding position (*a*). Three or four treatments should be sufficient to effect a cure.

If none of these measures is successful surgical measures can be tried. Either the extensors are detached from the lateral epicondyle and supracondylar ridge, or the extensor carpi radialis brevis tendon is lengthened by an oblique or Z cut near the wrist.

Bursitis. A chronic bursitis may be dealt with by deep heating and massage as in other cases of this condition.

Sometimes in the last two lesions the methods advocated prove unsuccessful and the condition persists. *Surgical treatment* may then be necessary to fulfil the same principles. Excision of the bursa for example will effectively relieve the condition. Excision of the attachment of the extensor carpi radialis brevis or division of the tendon will result in healing by fibrous tissue in a lengthened position. This produces the same effect as manipulation. Such operations will be followed by active exercise to maintain range.

FRACTURES OF THE RADIUS AND ULNA

Fractures of the shaft of radius and/or ulna arise as a result either of angular or twisting strains, or of direct violence. If the radius is fractured, displacement depends on the level of fracture. If this takes place above the level of the insertion of pronator radii teres, then the supinators are attached to the upper fragment and the pronators to the lower, and so the upper end of the radius will be supinated, the lower end pronated, and an obvious deformity of the forearm will be seen. Should the fracture line be below the pronator insertion, then the upper fragment will be in mid-position, since both supinator and pronator teres are attached to it, while the lower fragment will be pronated by pronator quadratus. If the ulna alone is fractured, the upper fragment is flexed by brachialis. If the radius is fractured and the ulna intact, the fragments will be rotated as before and the lower fragment tends to be displaced upwards and towards the ulna, since the long tendons of the thumb, passing from the medial side of the forearm, wrap round the lower end of the radius and consequently on contraction displace it medially, while any extension of the wrist pushes the lower fragment upwards.

Reduction is essential since any shortening of one bone will lead to sub-luxation of the inferior radio-ulnar joint and interference with pronation and supination. Angulation will also impair these movements. Reduction is difficult and sometimes open reduction is necessary, when the bones are usually immobilized by plates and screws or in the case of the ulna by an intramedullary nail.

To obtain bony union *immobilization* is necessary because rotation of the radius would otherwise occur, the granulation tissue would be stretched and there would be non-union. Thus if open reduction and plating has not been necessary pure splinting is required. A plaster of paris splint is usually applied. This extends from the metacarpal heads to the upper third of the arm. The elbow is flexed to a right angle and the wrist dorsiflexed. The forearm is in mid-position if the fracture is distal to the insertion of pronator teres and in full supination in the event of a fracture proximal to the pronator teres insertion.

Union is usually slow because the shafts of the bones are not very vascular and, if only one bone is broken, impingement of fragments is difficult to maintain. Six weeks are needed in children and twelve or more in adults, before union is sufficiently firm to withstand rotational strains especially if the elbow or wrist are stiff.

If the bones are immobilized by a nail or plate a similar external splint may be required, but some surgeons allow the limb to be free, except for a large arm sling, until the joints of the elbow, forearm and wrist are moving in a full range, usually about ten to fourteen days after the operation. The limb is then encased in a plaster splint similar to that used in the conservative treatment.

In those cases in which there is a lengthy period of immobilization, physiotherapy is particularly valuable especially for the first few weeks of immobilization and when the plaster is removed. It follows the same principles as the other fractures treated by plaster splinting, but certain special points should be noted.

The stimulus to union may be assisted if vigorous contractions of the long flexor and extensor tendons of the fingers and wrist are practised frequently. This will draw the bone ends together impinging them on one another.

Since the plaster extends to the metacarpal heads, care must be taken to see that it does not impede full range movements of the metacarpophalangeal joints of the fingers and thumb, and strict attention must be paid to obtaining normal range and power in all joints of the digits.

The plaster is an extensive and heavy one, and full movement of the shoulder and shoulder girdle is difficult and there is a natural tendency to cease to perform these movements. The result will be atrophied and weakened muscles and limited range of movements in the joints. Full range active movements of these joints must be insisted on. At first they may be given in lying, but should soon be carried out in sitting and standing.

It is easy to forget the limb when so many muscles and joints are fixed. To prevent this the patient must be encouraged to use the arm as normally as possible.

There is one serious and special complication to be watched for—a severe ischaemia can arise if the plaster presses a little too tightly on the muscles of the forearm. These, being superficial, may rapidly be rendered ischaemic while the radial pulse remains intact. The muscles will quickly become necrotic and replacement by fibrous tissue will result. If the condition is not detected, the fibrosed muscles will contract, and the long extensors and flexors will draw the fingers into the clawed position and the wrist into flexion. Nerves may also be involved and a paralysis of the small muscles of the hand will contribute towards an unsightly deformity.

Within a matter of six to twelve hours irreparable damage will be done for which no treatment is of any avail. It is, therefore, essential that the physiotherapist should be on the watch for the onset of this ischaemic condition. As in vascular damage at the elbow, the outstanding evidence will be pain, swelling, drop in temperature and change in colour of the fingers.

Chapter XVII

INJURIES ROUND THE WRIST
AND HAND

Injuries of the wrist and hand are very common and in a great many cases physiotherapy will help in their rehabilitation. An understanding of the anatomy of this region is, therefore, necessary.

The functions of the hand are prehensile and non-prehensile, but to fulfil these it must in each case also act as a tactile agent. Without this its ability to move and grasp are of little value.

PREHENSILE FUNCTION

Prehension is the act of grasping and holding an object and man's hand is well equipped for this. Wynn Parry divides grasp into two types, grip and pinch. It might be said that the first is a power and the second a precision grasp.

In grip the fingers are flexed towards the palm and surround the object which is grasped in the hollow of the hand formed by the carpal and metacarpal arches. In strong grips both the thenar and hypothenar eminences are contracted to reinforce the grip. The thumb may be used across the fingers to reinforce the power of the fingers and to lock them in flexion. Such a grip is used in wringing out a cloth. More often the grip is used to hold a tool and manipulate it. In this case the little and ring fingers grasp the handle of the tool and press it against the stabilizing thenar or hypothenar eminence, according to which direction the tool points, while the thumb and index finger lightly grip and guide the tool. The middle finger often helps in both actions.

For grip of this type the wrist is nearly always held in the neutral or slightly dorsiflexed position and with a varying degree of ulnar deviation according to the size of the object gripped.

In the pinch grasp the object is lightly held between the tips of the thumb and fingers and in this position may be finely and precisely manipulated.

361

If the object is large like a tennis ball the digits are spread out and slightly flexed; if small, it is held between the ring finger and thumb or the thumb and index, while the remaining fingers are used for support and stability. In many very fine delicate movements, such as picking up small beads with a pair of forceps, the forceps are grasped by the thumb and index supported by the middle finger and steadied by the ring and little fingers, which are flexed at the metacarpo-phalangeal joints and extended at the inter-phalangeal joints. In activities such as writing the object is grasped and moved by the thumb and index, and the hand is supported, to give stability, on the ulnar border of the little finger and palm while the middle finger helps to support and move the pen.

In all forms of the pinch grasp the wrist is held in extension and lateral movements of radial and ulnar deviation usually form part of the movement.

In most of these positions there is slight ulnar deviation and medial rotation at the metacarpo-phalangeal joints.

For good grasp certain requirements are essential

In every case except the hook grasp, in which an object like the handle of a suitcase is gripped by the flexed fingers only, *abduction, flexion, medial rotation and adduction of the thumb are all required.*

The thumb is carried away from the palm of the hand; this allows the thumb to surround the object and at the same time gives the opponens pollicis a better pull. Then flexion of the thumb tautens the posterior oblique ligament of the carpo-metacarpal joint so fixing the ulnar side of the metacarpal which, as it continues to flex therefore rotates medially swinging the padded surface of the thumb towards the fingers. To a varying extent the thumb is then moved towards the fingers and held against the object by the adductor pollicis. In the precision (pinch) grasp this adduction is only weak, but in the grip (power) grasp the adduction demands a strong adductor pollicis. Usually in prehension the tip of the thumb is flexed and a strong flexor pollicis longus is required, otherwise in the pinch the thumb tends to slide down the object.

In all prehension the fingers are flexed. In *grip* the ring and little fingers are almost fully flexed bringing in not only the metacarpo-phalangeal and inter-phalangeal joints, but also the carpo-metacarpal joints. These latter, unlike the gliding carpo-metacarpal joints of the index and ring digits, are hinge joints so that there is a greater range of movement in these joints. The middle and index fingers are much less fully flexed, the amount of flexion depending on whether these fingers are used for power or to guide and direct the tool. Less flexion is required of all the fingers in '*pinch*'.

The important point here is that whereas full flexion is required of the joints of the ring and little fingers if the hand is to be fully useful, much less is required of the middle and index fingers.

Ulnar deviation and rotation of the metacarpo-phalangeal joints are important and care must be taken to maintain these movements.

The power of grip is provided by the long flexors, the flexor digitorum profundis having the greatest power since it has an extensive fleshy origin.

When the *ulnar side of the hand is used for support and as a balancing agent,* while fine precision movements are undertaken by the thumb and index finger, a powerful *hypothenar eminence and flexor carpi ulnaris* are required. This is often forgotten when re-education of the hand is being carried out.

Very important for grasp are the *carpal and metacarpal arches* in order to allow the object to be held in the hollow of the hand. For this reason the bones are firmly held together partly by their method of articulation and partly by ligamentous and muscular ties. The various articulations do not form a straight line; each joint lies on a slightly different plane from its neighbour. The base of the second metacarpal is set well back, wedged between the trapezium and capitate, because the trapezoid does not extend so far distally as either of the other two bones. In this way sideways gliding and splaying out of the metacarpals is prevented.

The carpal bones form a hollow on the palmar aspect partly due to their shape and partly because they are firmly held together on this aspect by the flexor retinaculum. The metacarpals are held together at their bases by the interosseous ligaments and at their heads by the superficial and deep transverse ligaments of the palm. In addition the intrinsic muscles and long flexor tendons will help to hold the bones together.

NON-PREHENSILE FUNCTIONS

The hand is used in many other ways than that of grasp. It is for example a means of expression on its own, not only through the tools it can grasp and manipulate. When talking, acting, singing, the hands are in constant use. They are also used as a very valuable pushing means and as a clamp. The brushing or pushing action mainly requires extension of the wrist and fingers. As a clamp there is usually strong ulnar deviation of the wrist and abduction of the little finger and the muscles of the hypothenar eminence and flexor carpi ulnaris are again important.

Often the fingers are needed for tapping movements. In these movements the interossei are particularly important because they allow flexion of the metacarpo-phalangeal joints without flexion of the inter-phalangeal joints. This action is seen in typing, playing the piano and many wind instruments.

TACTILE FUNCTION

The ability to recognize sizes and shapes of unseen objects, textures and consistencies, variations in temperature, is essential if the hand is to be of any use. It is of little use having the power of grip if the hand is not able to distinguish the type of object which is to be gripped. The safety of the hand depends on its ability to detect heat, cold and painful stimuli.

Sensibility is more essential in some areas than others. Thus it is essential on the palmar aspect of the thumb, the lateral side of the index and ring fingers, where they oppose the thumb, and the ulnar side of the little finger and hand. If the hand is badly damaged and much skin lost, skin transfers taking with them the nerve and blood supply, may be necessary and when a severely damaged hand is reconstructed the surgeon bears in mind this point.

JOINTS AND MUSCLES

The wrist, like the elbow, has within its capsule a second joint, in this case the *inferior radio-ulnar joint*. Thus damage in the region of the wrist is liable to affect rotation of the forearm as well as the movements of the wrist. This seriously affects the use of the hand since the movements of pronation and supination determine the position in which the hand can be used.

The wrist joint itself is a condyloid joint permitting some 80° of flexion, 90° of extension, 35° of ulnar deviation and rather less, about 25°, of radial deviation. These movements do not take place solely at the wrist joint but are considerably augmented by movement at the intercarpal joints particularly during flexion and ulnar deviation. It is not possible by observation to determine the exact range occurring at the wrist or intercarpal joints. It should, however, be realized that loss of movement at the wrist can often be compensated for by increase of the movement in the carpus and also that apparent decrease of movement may in fact be due to trouble in the carpus rather than in the wrist.

Radial and ulnar deviation are important movements. The former is usually combined with extension and the latter with flexion. It is important therefore, that these movements should not be forgotten in the rehabilitation of the injured hand.

The metacarpo-phalangeal joints of the digits are also condyloid joints.

Those of the fingers lie on the arc of a circle, hence as the fingers are extended they diverge from one another and they converge as they flex. In addition as the fingers flex, they do so in the direction of the thenar eminence so that the little finger flexes to the greatest extent. In re-educating finger movement these points are important. The metacarpo-phalangeal joint of the thumb, although similar in type differs, somewhat in shape, being compressed palmar-dorsally; thus flexion and extension is often of smaller range at this joint in the thumb than in the fingers.

It will be noticed that when the metacarpo-phalangeal joints are in the flexed position, abduction and adduction of the fingers are not possible. This is due to the fact that the articular surfaces of the metacarpal heads are flat on their flexor surfaces and the collateral ligaments are taut. These ligaments extend from the pits and tubercles on the dorsal part of the side of the heads forward and downward to the sides of the bases of the phalanges; they are therefore relaxed in slight flexion and taut in full flexion and extension.

Both extrinsic and intrinsic muscles of the hand are vitally important. The extrinsic muscles mainly provide the power and range of movement, the intrinsic stabilize and produce fine movement. As has already been seen certain muscles have particular importance in the different types of prehension.

Movement of individual fingers alone is difficult

This is at least partly due to the fact that the four tendons of extensor digitorum are joined on the dorsum of the hand by three oblique bands just proximal to the metacarpal heads. It is difficult, therefore, to flex one finger while keeping the others extended and vice versa. This is one reason why an injured finger is seldom immobilized in extension since this is liable to limit the movement of the undamaged fingers and is certainly why it is so important to train the patient to exercise all the undamaged fingers.

NERVE SUPPLY OF THE HAND

The muscles of the thenar eminence and the first and second lumbricales are supplied by the *median nerve*. This nerve also supplies the lateral half of flexor profundus digitorum, the flexor sublimis and flexor longus pollicis. For this reason if the nerve is injured above the elbow both pinch and grip are impaired. 'Pinch' is most seriously affected since for it the thenar muscles are essential. Grip will, of course, be impaired by loss of the reinforcing and stabilizing action of the thumb and by the loss of the flexors of the index and middle finger, but it is less affected because flexion of the little and ring fingers is still strong, since flexor profundus digitorum and the lumbricales to these fingers are intact. Both grips will be affected by the loss of ability to recognize textures, etc., due to the loss of cutaneous sensation on the lateral side of the palm and essential areas on thumb, index and middle fingers.

The Ulnar Nerve supplies the remaining intrinsic muscles, the medial half of profundus and the flexor carpi ulnaris together with the important skin area on the ulnar side of the little finger and hand. There is serious impairment of grip since there is marked loss of power in the two medial fingers. Pinch is less seriously impaired. In the precision grasp of objects involving a fairly firm pinch, weakness will result from loss of the adductor, but in the delicate pinch this will be less noticeable. Weakness will also result from instability of the index and middle fingers due to paralysis of the first and second dorsal interossei allowing the fingers to fall away from the object. The stabilizing effect of the ring and little fingers and ulnar side of the hand will be diminished due to sensory loss and paralysis of the hypothenar muscles, medial two lumbricales, interossei and flexor carpi ulnaris.

The radial nerve supplies all the extensors of the wrist and metacarpophalangeal joint but the interphalangeal extension is carried out by intrinsic muscles. Loss of the ability to extend the metacarpo-phalangeal joints makes release of an object difficult. The less important skin area on the lateral side of the dorsum of the hand and adjacent three and a half digits are the areas of sensory distribution. Paralysis of extensor carpi radialis and ulnaris prevents extension of the wrist, a movement essential to give the flexors of the fingers the strongest pull, therefore interfering with both pinch and grip. The loss of abductor pollicis longus weakens pinch if the object to be grasped is large and necessitates wide abduction of the thumb.

THE TENDON SHEATHS

Both flexor and extensor tendons pass through osseo-aponeurotic tunnels as they cross the wrist and carpus; they are, therefore, equipped with synovial sheaths. The extent of each sheath depends on the degree of excursion of the tendon. The flexor tendons of the digits also run through similar canals in the fingers. In the case of the thumb and little finger, the shortest and most mobile of the digits, the sheaths at the wrist and fingers will be long and consequently they will be continuous with each other. For the less mobile ring, middle and index fingers the sheaths are shorter, consequently the sheath at the carpus terminates round the tendons for the finger about the middle of the metacarpus and a separate sheath is present in the fingers. There is thus an area in the palm of the hand in which the tendons for these fingers have no sheaths, but are simply surrounded by loose areolar tissue.

The Palmar Aponeurosis. Palmar Compartments and Spaces

The palmar aponeurosis is the direct continuation of the palmaris longus, extending forwards from the flexor retinaculum and dividing into four slips for the fingers, each of which divides into superficial and deep layers over the proximal end of the flexor sheath. The superficial layers are joined to the skin while the deep blend with the fibrous sheaths of the tendons and the deep transverse ligament of the palm. The aponeurosis is firmly connected to the skin and so by anchoring the skin improves the grip. It also serves to protect the underlying tendons, nerves and vessels. From the medial border of the palmar aponeurosis two septa are given off. One covers the hypothenar eminence, the other is lateral to the hypothenar muscles reaching the fifth metacarpal, thus enclosing the hypothenar space. From the lateral border of palmar aponeurosis two septa are given off. One is on the surface of the adductor pollicis reaching the third metacarpal and, with the septum from the medial border encloses the middle palmar space and flexor tendons. The other septum from the lateral border of the palmar aponeurosis is a thin layer over the thenar eminence enclosing the thenar space. The deep palmar space lies between the adductor pollicis and the first dorsal interosseous. These spaces are important because the septa of firm fibrous tissues are tough and resistant to infection and, therefore, tend to prevent the spread of any form of infection from one part of the hand to another.

PHYSIOTHERAPY IN WRIST AND HAND INJURIES

Physiotherapy is of importance in the rehabilitation of these injuries.

Encouraging the patient to use the thumb and fingers at once

Injury to the wrist, carpus, metacarpus or one or more fingers almost always results in difficulty in moving the undamaged digits. If the wrist or carpus is painful the fingers are not willingly moved, because good movement of the digits involves movement of these joints (see p. 361). If one finger is damaged and has to be immobilized it is not easy to move the neighbouring finger (see p. 365). If the fingers are not used they rapidly become stiff.

Damage to the wrist and hand nearly always entails considerable injury of the soft tissues with the result that these injuries are *painful*. Unless the hand is supported, movement is therefore avoided by the patient and quickly organization occurs with scarring and adhesion formation. This may be a cause of the stiff and painful hand met in Sudeck's atrophy.

Extensive *oedema* usually follows injuries in this region and quickly tends to gravitate into the dorsum of the hand and the fingers. This again hampers movement and if not rapidly relieved leads to a stiff hand.

To prevent stiffness which may incapacitate the hand for long periods, two rules should be followed: oedema should be prevented or relieved as soon as possible, and all joints not immobilized should be actively exercised immediately or at least as soon as any plaster has dried. The exception to this early movement arises if skin grafting has been necessary when movements have to be postponed until the graft has taken.

Oedema can usually be relieved by elevation of the arm and it is important that the patient is taught how best to do this and warned not to allow the hand to hang down for any length of time. If oedema persists and tends to become chronic it may be dealt with by the use of wax with the arm in elevation and the hand in a heat cradle, followed by deep massage and active movements. Faradism under pressure is also useful.

There is no doubt that the best method is to get rid of any swelling at once by vigorous active movements. If the injury is of soft tissue only, support as far as the metacarpal heads leaving the fingers free, will make movements less painful and the patient will be more willing to carry them out many times a day. If the bones are fractured, immobilization may be necessary, but the digits are most likely to be left free.

Active exercises of all joints not immobilized require to be taught and the patient's co-operation is essential. It is necessary therefore to explain why they are so important. A careful watch must be kept to see that all joints are moved through their full range in every direction of which they are capable.

Regaining functional use is a second equally important object

It depends not only on retaining a mobile hand with strong muscles and good sensation, but also on the ability and willingness of the patient to use the hand as normally as possible from the time of injury. Thus as soon as the injury has been dealt with by the surgeon, if any immobilization or dressings allow, the patient should begin to use the hand for ordinary activities, dressing, feeding, jobs about the house, and, if a workshop is available, for activities as nearly resembling his normal occupation as possible. Ideally the best means of treatment is return to his work, if possible.

Strengthening Muscles

Strengthening is usually necessary since some reduction in function has almost certainly occurred. Active exercises started at once will help to lessen atrophy, but use of manual resistance and apparatus should be quickly added for the muscles of the wrist and intrinsic and extrinsic muscles of the hand. If there is nerve involvement the particular muscles affected will receive special attention (see p. 271).

Complications

These must be carefully watched for and three points require especial care. Any hand injury, but particularly those involving the soft tissues only, may be followed by *Sudeck's atrophy*. If the injury does not appear to be progressing as it should and if, six to eight weeks after injury, there is pain, swelling, hyperaemia, obliteration of skin creases, changes in skin temperature and colour, with marked loss of movement, a report should be made at once since the use of hot wax, elevation and exercise will usually relieve the symptoms and prevent months of incapacity.

Many wrist and hand injuries are due to a fall on the hand and in some of the cases the shoulder has been jarred at the time of accident and the subacromial bursa and rotator cuff damaged. This injury has not necessarily been detected because of the more severe injury and greater pain at the hand. If not detected and dealt with, the subsidiary injury may lead to *prolonged disability from a stiff and painful shoulder*. From the very commencement of physiotherapy therefore, a careful check should be made on the movements of the shoulder and shoulder girdle and any pain or tenderness reported at once so that treatment can be given.

A third complication of hand injuries is that of *sepsis*. This is a very likely trouble since many of these injuries are works accidents in which the skin is broken, pieces of metal or dirt enter and crushing lessens the vitality of the tissues since blood vessels may be thrombosed and ruptured, and swelling may impede the circulation. This is a problem for the surgeon which he usually tackles by wide incision with excision of devitalized tissues, but the physiotherapist may be asked to help with the use of ultraviolet therapy. Ultra-violet may be used for its sterilizing and healing properties. If the skin is broken the physiotherapist requires to take antiseptic precautions in whatever treatment she is giving.

Points in using Exercise Therapy

With few exceptions exercise must be active and no forcing or passive movements should be given at any stage. Forcing stiff joints simply increases sero-fibrinous exudate from tight capsules and ligaments and is likely to increase the adhesion formation. Passive movements which produce pain are resisted by muscle spasm and if pushed, will result in tearing of soft tissues with increase of inflammatory exudate. Thus more harm is done by this type of movement. An exception to this rule is the use of the accessory movements as described by the late Dr. Mennell. These movements serve to loosen the capsule from the bone, gently stretching it, so making active movements easier.

Very careful examination should be carried out before the exercises are started so that an assessment can be made, noting the range in the different joints, the strength of the muscles and the strength of the various types of grasps. A plan can then be made bearing in mind the ranges required and the particular muscles needed if the hand is to be of functional value (see p. 362). Any sensory change requires particular notice and if present the patient must be warned to take care to avoid damage from heat or sharp objects and to look out for signs of slight skin injury.

Use of Splints

If splints are being used, in addition to the usual care of fit and comfort, a check should be made to see that they are not impeding the necessary movements. Thus following immobilization for a Colles' fracture, for example, the plaster should not prevent full range of flexion in the metacarpo-phalangeal joints, and full abduction and opposition of the thumb. The splint should never hold the metacarpo-phalangeal joints hyperextended or the palmar ligaments and lumbricales will be stretched and flexion essential for grasp will be very difficult to regain. Splints should not lessen the carpal and metacarpal arches or grasp will again be seriously interfered with. As far as possible inter-phalangeal joints should be immobilized in at least a few degrees of flexion. This is the position of ease in which the collateral ligaments are relaxed. Occasionally errors do arise and it is the physiotherapist's duty to be aware of these points and to report at once if anything appears unsatisfactory. On the whole it may be said that whereas fractures of the wrist and carpus usually require immobilization, fractures and soft tissue injuries to the metacarpals (excluding the first) and phalanges, palm and fingers are often not immobilized, or where splinting is necessary it is kept to the minimum possible or used for a short time only for the relief of pain.

COLLES' FRACTURE

This fracture, involving the lower end of the radius, was first described by Abraham Colles. The exact injury consists of a fracture of the lower end of the radius one inch above the wrist joint, with dorsal and radial displacement. It is often associated with a fracture of the styloid process of the ulna, a tearing of the medial ligament of the wrist, or a subluxation of the inferior radio-ulnar joint with tearing of the triangular fibro-cartilage (see Plate XXIII, (a), (b)).

The most usual age group is the middle-aged or elderly and the fracture occurs most commonly in women, particularly in the domestic worker, who is liable to fall off a chair, steps or stool while dusting or cleaning, and who automatically puts out her hand to save herself. As a result, the injury occurs with the wrist in dorsiflexion and radial deviation, so that the lower fragment of the radius, which is driven up and impacted into the upper fragment, is also displaced backwards and to the radial side and tilted backwards (see Plate XXIII, (a), (b)). The alteration in position of the lower fragment may cause an unsightly deformity, in which the hand appears radially displaced, leaving the head of the ulna to stand out as a definite prominence. The lower fragment forms a 'lump' at the back of the wrist with a hollow above and below, while the hollow normally present on the front of the lower end of the forearm is lost as the fragment tilts back. The typical appearance resembles the shape of a fork and is often known as the 'dinner-fork' deformity.

The severity of the displacement and therefore of the deformity depends on the violence and the exact position of the hand at the time of accident.

Reduction is necessary if there is displacement or an unsightly deformity persists.

Immobilization must follow reduction. Union will occur without lengthy fixation, but when the spicules of dead bone at the fracture site are removed by the phagocytic cells, the fragment tends to slip; a deformity will then develop and subluxation at the inferior radio-ulnar joint will result in permanent limitation of pronation and supination. Fixation is therefore usually retained for a period of from four to six weeks. If the patient is old and arthritic, the minimum time is used. Immobility may be obtained by light metal splints or by plaster of Paris. If plaster is used it may be complete or it may be a dorsal slab moulded well round the borders of the forearm. The advantage of the slab is that it allows for swelling, but as the swelling subsides it will tend to become loose and will need re-bandaging. The essential point is that the wrist must be fixed, but not the joints of the fingers, although some surgeons prefer to include the elbow to maintain pronation of the forearm. Splints usually extend from just distal to the elbow to the heads of the metacarpals of the four fingers on the posterior aspect, and to the scaphoid and pisiform on the anterior aspect. Some surgeons prefer to carry the plaster or anterior splint into the palm of the hand, but all leave the thumb quite free, so that its full range of movements can be performed, and all are careful to avoid fixing the metacarpophalangeal joints of the fingers. The wrist is usually immobilized in the neutral position though there is some variation in this. It may be found in slight dorsiflexion or alternatively in slight flexion and ulnar deviation.

Physiotherapy

This is usually ordered both during the period of immobilization and when the plaster is removed.

During immobilization physiotherapy is usually required only for the first one or two weeks until the patient understands what he has to do. The particular points to note in this period are active movements of the thumb and fingers, the comfort of the splint and the development of complications.

Movement of the digits is important because this fracture is often accompanied by considerable swelling, which tends to gravitate into the dorsum of the hand and into the digits. This makes movement difficult and unless care is taken full range may not be obtained and the undamaged thumb and fingers may become stiff. In addition movement of the digits may at first cause discomfort at the wrist. The patient must, therefore, be taught active finger and thumb exercises including such exercises as trying to press the tips of the fingers into the palm of the hand or against the plaster, full flexion of the metacarpal-phalangeal joints with the fingers straight, parting and closing the fingers, full abduction and opposition of the thumb. After a day or two, normal use of the arm and hand should be added, excluding heavy lifting. The plaster should be protected by suitable gloves when doing jobs which would result in it getting wet or dirty. The reason for the exercises must be explained and the patient should continue to attend for treatment until the arm is being used normally and there is full range at all the joints of the digits.

The Splint must be checked because with excessive swelling it may easily become too tight. Later if a dorsal slab is used it may, as swelling goes down, become loose and re-bandaging is necessary. The splint should not impede full movement of the thumb and fingers and if the elbow is free, that joint too should enjoy a full range.

Complications which may develop during the period of immobilization are a stiff shoulder, spontaneous rupture of extensor pollicis longus tendon and a median nerve paresis.

A stiff and painful shoulder due either to injury at the time of accident or to lack of use of the arm may gradually become apparent. If the shoulder is exercised in its full range from the first day of treatment this rarely occurs. Should there be any pain or tenderness it must be reported at once.

Spontaneous rupture of the tendon of extensor pollicis longus occasionally occurs three to six weeks after the accident. It may be the result of the gradual fraying of the tendon as it moves in a roughened groove and will be recognized by inability to extend the terminal joint of the thumb which tends to remain in the flexed position. It should be reported as suture of the distal part of the tendon to the short extensor may be carried out by the surgeon.

Nerve injury is not very common, but occasionally the median nerve may be contused and a complaint of numbness, paraesthesia and weakness of grasp should be noted and reported. It is wise to test the function of the intrinsic muscles daily.

When the plaster is removed some stiffness is usually found in the wrist and inferior radio-ulnar joints with weakness of the muscles of the wrist and hand. Exercises will be needed to deal with this. These are often more comfortable if preceded by wax or hot-water baths.

Complications which should now be looked for are non-union and Sudeck's atrophy.

Non-union of the styloid process of the ulna frequently occurs, though the radius always unites. It leads to tenderness over the site of the fibrous tissue union making movements of the wrist, involving extension and radial deviation painful. In the course of time this disappears, but it can often be lessened by counter-irritation at the site of tenderness.

FRACTURES OF THE SCAPHOID

The scaphoid of all the carpal bones is the most often fractured. This is probably partly due to the fact that it extends into both rows of the carpus, hyperextension of the wrist therefore may readily result in fracture. This usually occurs at the thinnest point, the waist of the bone. Another characteristic of the scaphoid is that it has no muscular attachments except that of the short abductor of the thumb to the tubercle. Consequently the fracture does not result in displacement but, on the other hand, there is little natural stability. Since the bone is nearly entirely articular there is very little periosteum, consequently the vascular supply is poor. Such blood vessels as there are mainly enter towards the distal end of the bone. The smaller the proximal fragment, the poorer its circulation and the slower will be the union.

Reduction is not usually necessary but owing to the lack of muscle attachments and consequently absence of compression, immobilization until consolidation has occurred is required. The splint must therefore be a PURE splint. It extends from the upper third of the forearm to the metacarpal heads on the dorsal aspect of the hand and to the proximal crease on the palm. The thumb is included as far as the interphalangeal joint. To avoid any shearing stress on the callus the wrist is dorsiflexed and the thumb abducted. Immobilization is continued for eight to twelve weeks.

The only likely complication is that of non-union, either due to failure to immobilize adequately or for sufficient length of time, or because avascular necrosis of the proximal fragment occurs.

Physiotherapy will be similar to that needed for a Colles' fracture. Treatment is required for the first few days of immobilization and when the plaster is removed. Its purpose is to ensure full use of the digits, elbow and shoulder followed by normal use of the arm, and later to restore full range and strength.

FRACTURES OF THE METACARPALS AND PHALANGES

Bennett's Fracture

A fracture-dislocation of the base of the first metacarpal (see Plate XXIV) is sometimes seen in the physiotherapy department. It is usually the result of a force driving the thumb across the palm. The line of fracture runs from the flexor side of the shaft up proximally to the articular surface. Spasm of the long flexor and extensor tendons of the thumb causes the main fragment to slide proximally leaving the tiny fragment only articulating with the trapezium. A plaster alone is insufficient to immobilize the fracture, since, as the swelling subsides and some atrophy occurs, the plaster becomes slightly loose and the fragment is again retracted. The usual method is to apply a plaster of Paris splint with the wrist in slight extension and the thumb in the 'grasp' position. The plaster extends as far as the metacarpo-phalangeal joint of the thumb leaving the terminal joint free so that it can be repeatedly exercised. Incorporated in the plaster is a loop of wire to which the thumb may be attached by means of adhesive tape and lamp wick so that traction is applied. Because the wrist is in extension, the plaster is not drawn towards the fingers, but will remain in position.

This is maintained for four to six weeks, but union is not consolidated in less than three months, and heavy work is not allowed under this time.

During the period of immobilization active exercises for the fingers, terminal joint of the thumb, elbow and shoulder are necessary and when the plaster is removed physiotherapy will be directed towards regaining full range of movement in the carpo-metacarpal and metacarpo-phalangeal joints of the thumb.

Fractures of the other Metacarpals

These usually result from a blow on the knuckles or on the dorsum of the hand. The fracture line may be through the base, shaft or neck of the metacarpal. If the force is direct the fracture line will be transverse; if the forearm is rotating at the time of a blow on the knuckles the fracture may be spiral.

Treatment depends upon the presence or absence of displacement. If there is no displacement reduction and immobilization are not necessary and the fingers may be moved at once. Usually, however, there is considerable pain and the patient will be more comfortable and movements easier if the hand is strapped or a posterior plaster slab is applied for two to three weeks. The metacarpo-phalangeal joints should be left free and finger exercises and use of the hand carried out from the beginning.

Should there be much displacement reduction and immobilization are required; if this is difficult, internal fixation by means of an intra-medullary wire may be necessary.

A transverse fracture of the neck of the fifth metacarpal is a fairly common injury. In this case the head of the metacarpal is nearly always tilted towards the palm. This necessitates reduction followed by immobilization by means of a strip of plaster extending from the wrist to the tip of the finger on the dorsal aspect. The metacarpo-phalangeal and proximal inter-phalangeal joints are flexed to a right angle. This splint is retained for two to three weeks.

Fractures of the Phalanges

These fractures are the result of direct violence and, especially in the case of the terminal phalanx, are often accompanied by soft tissue injury (see Plate XXV). To avoid deformity and stiffness, they are usually treated by a short plaster the length of the digit, applied with the inter-phalangeal joints flexed to a right angle. The exception to this is in the condition of mallet finger, when a tiny flake of bone is torn off and retracted by the long extensor tendon. This injury occurs if the tip of a finger is forcibly flexed when the extensor is actively contracting. To bring the fragment near to its bed, the tip must be hyperextended, but the proximal inter-phalangeal joint is flexed. The fixation period for fractures of the phalanges is usually three weeks.

An outstanding feature of hand and finger injuries is oedema. This is most noticeable in fractures of the metacarpals. The fluid tends to distend the lax tissue on the dorsum of the hand, and gravitate into the fingers. It hampers movement, organizes and much fibrous tissue is formed. Limitation of movement in the metacarpo-phalangeal joints is particularly serious. If flexion of these joints is limited, a good grip is impossible and the use of the hand is much impaired. The physiotherapist must be especially careful to encourage active movements of these joints if they are free, laying particular emphasis on flexion and on getting the fingers right down into the palm of the hand. She should also give the patient advice not to allow the arm to hang down while swelling is present and from time to time to support it in elevation. When the dorsal slab is removed attention should be paid to any thickening on the dorsum of the hand. Measures, such as inductothermy, ionization with potassium iodide, or with heparin or renotin, deep massage and almost continuous active exercise should be used to soften and stretch.

Another very important point where one finger is injured is to remember that fixation of one tends to limit free movement of the others. This is why the finger is almost always fixed in flexion. If it were fixed in extension, not only would it be difficult to regain flexion, but flexion of the other fingers would be impossible. For this reason it is most important that the patient should be encouraged to carry out full movements of all joints of the uninjured fingers and thumb, making sure that full range is obtained. Co-ordination of the hand is also a very important point.

TENDON INJURIES

Injury of tendons at the wrist or in the hand are fairly common and they demand not only skilful surgery, but also careful physiotherapy.

Flexor Tendons

These are most commonly severed in the fingers, but may also be damaged in the palm or at the wrist. The injury may be caused by such accidents as pushing the hand through a window, a fall on glass or metal, sharp tools, crushing, or blast, often from fireworks. Sometimes the injury is a severance of one tendon only, but often, especially at the wrist, several tendons, nerves and arteries are all involved. In crush and blast injuries bones and joints may also be damaged.

A single tendon at the wrist is treated by suture. This will be done at once if the hand is seen within six hours of the accident and there is no crushing of soft tissues or soiling of the wound. Suture is always delayed if other tissues are involved or there is obvious infection. Following suture the hand is immobilized in slight flexion either by bandage or plaster for three weeks. At the end of three weeks exercises may be started. It is unusual to begin exercises before this time because a sutured tendon will not withstand strain for three weeks and too early movement appears to produce more adhesions rather than less. Exercises aim at regaining movement of the tendon and full range at the wrist. At first no movement occurs and it is necessary to demonstrate the movement on the unaffected wrist. Sometimes extension is limited due to flexor contracture; resisted extension will help to relax the flexors and obtain extension. Five to six weeks following the suture, more vigorous exercises can be given and resistance added to flexion exercises.

Multiple tendon injury at the wrist is nearly always followed by considerable scarring and flexor sublimis digitorum tends to become adherent to the skin with the result that the proximal inter-phalangeal joint cannot be passively extended if the metacarpo-phalangeal joint is extended at the same time. It is essential that the scar tissue should be loosened and stretched. This can be done by massage with oil, active exercises, including resisted work for the extensors of the wrist and fingers, and splinting in between treatments in the best position that can be obtained. Treatment should be given twice daily and the splint adjusted as the position improves.

Tendon rupture in the palm is often the result of falling with the hand outstretched on to glass or sharp metal. Suture is usually satisfactory, because the surrounding tissues are elastic and the suture line can be buried in the lumbricale muscle, so reducing the tendency to adhesions. Treatment is similar to that of divided tendons at the wrist.

Division of tendons in the fingers presents a different problem because at this position the tendons pass through fibrous sheaths and if an attempt is made to suture one or both, adhesions are almost bound to form, severely limiting movement of the tendons and upsetting function. For this reason, a tendon graft is usually done. The tendon of palmaris longus, plantaris or one of the extensor tendons of the toes may be used. The graft is sutured to the tendon in the palm of the hand where adhesions will be less serious and is threaded through the flexor sheath and sutured to the base of the terminal phalanx, the distal end of the severed tendons being removed. The hand is then immobilized with the fingers flexed slightly more than the normal resting position for a period of three weeks. When the splint is removed there is rarely any active movement at the interphalangeal joints of the affected fingers and all the fingers are inclined to be stiff.

Physiotherapy

If the operation has had to be delayed there may be stiffness of the joints and scarring, and the surgeon will not do a graft while these are present. Pre-operative physiotherapy will be directed towards loosening scar tissue and regaining movement at the joints. Massage with oil and passive movements are, therefore, necessary.

When the joints are free the operation is carried out. There is some difference of opinion as to when movements should be started postoperatively, but usually they are not begun for three weeks since early movement does not seem to hasten recovery. When physiotherapy is ordered the splint, if still worn, is removed and if the wound is healed wax baths are given; if not, hot saline baths can be used. The patient is encouraged to move the fingers in the baths. Massage with oil may then be given to the palmar scar if it is healed and adherent. Active exercises begin with encouraging the patient to move the unaffected fingers; free and resisted movements of each joint should be given as these restore range and make it easier for the patient to move the affected finger, since normally the fingers work together. The patient is then encouraged to try to move the affected finger, each joint separately and all the joints together. This needs to be tried on the same finger of the sound hand first. Easy occupational therapy with the finger in a double finger stall with its neighbour, will encourage natural use.

About the sixth week resistance may be added and stronger occupational therapy in the form of carpentry, modelling and pottery undertaken. If the joints are stiff passive movements can be given to each joint separately with the other joints flexed. At this time it is also safe to use Faradism to help to get the tendon moving. No heavy strain should be taken on the tendon for eight weeks or the graft may break. At this time (eight weeks) passive stretching may be used if there is a flexion deformity. General use of the hand must be stressed throughout and if the occupation is suitable or the firm for which the patient works has a remedial workshop the patient should return to work early; he is much more likely to make a speedy recovery this way.

Tenosynovitis

Extensor Tendons

The extensor tendons are most often damaged on the dorsum of the hand or over the phalanges, occasionally an extensor tendon is avulsed from the base of the distal phalanx producing a condition known as mallet finger. In fractures of the shaft of the metacarpals the tendons may become involved in callus formation. Normally the tendons heal well, but since they are surrounded by little soft tissue and are so close to the bone and joints these structures also may be damaged at the time of injury.

Rupture of extensor tendons is dealt with on the same lines as the flexor tendons, but, as they do not pass through fibrous sheaths in the fingers, grafting is not normally necessary. Immobilization is usual for ten to twenty-one days and is then followed by active exercises; by the fourth week gentle resistance is added and this is progressed daily. Work for the intrinsic muscles is important because the interrossei and lumbricales insert into the extensor expansion. Occupational therapy and normal use of the hand are both important. Stretch should not be applied to the tendon for six to eight weeks and exercises and occupational therapy should for the first one to two weeks of treatment be carried out in inner range.

Mallet finger, so called because following avulsion of the extensor tendon the tip of the finger drops into flexion, shows loss of power to extend the terminal phalanx actively though passive extension is possible.

If this condition remains untreated, it becomes a great nuisance to the patient and the finger gets in the way of movements of the hand. Usually it can be completely cured by immobilizing the finger in such a way as to bring the tendon against the bone from which it has been torn. The finger is therefore fixed for four to six weeks in plaster with the tip hyperextended and the proximal interphalangeal joint flexed. It is to be expected that, when the plaster is removed, the joints will be stiff and full range will not be immediately restored. Treatment by physiotherapy is, therefore, required to strengthen the power of the lumbrical and to regain full movement of the inter-phalangeal joints. Since fibrous tissue formation and shrinkage of the capsule will result in a certain amount of limitation of movement, wax and deep massage may prove helpful, but persistent active exercise will be the most effective treatment. No forcing should be allowed, but the patient is encouraged to perform normal activities about the house and garden, and to resume his normal occupation, provided that it is suitable.

TENOSYNOVITIS

Inflammation of the tendon sheaths may occur on either aspect of the wrist and may be acute or chronic.

Injuries round the Wrist and Hand

Acute Tenosynovitis

This is usually the result of a blow or wrench, but it may occur from unaccustomed use or prolonged strain.

Usually the sheath becomes distended with fluid and sometimes fibrin is deposited so that roughening of the normally smooth opposing surfaces develops and adhesions may form.

The condition usually clears satisfactorily with rest, but in the case of athletes the treatment is modified because, as Featherstone points out, adhesions would be a serious disability. In these cases treatment consists of strapping and rest for twenty-four to thirty-six hours. It is then followed by the use of short-wave diathermy, deep transverse frictions and exercises.

Chronic Tenosynovitis

This is probably the result of over-use of the affected tendon in a new occupation or in one which is resumed after a period of rest. Thus, for example, it is seen in cleaners in the extensor and abductor tendons of the thumb.

Thickening of the sheath gradually develops. Often tiny fibrous nodules are formed, either attached to the lining of the sheath or free within it. These are sometimes known as melon-seed bodies.

The condition is characterized by aching and pain on the performance of any movement which causes the tendon to be moved within its sheath. Thus, if the extensor tendons of the wrist are affected, gripping is painful and the patient tends to become incapable of continuing his work. Thickening of the sheath can be seen and felt and crepitation is often present.

Since the condition of the sheath is preventing the tendon from moving easily and painlessly within it, the main principle of treatment is to restore the ability to move freely. There are two ways of doing this, the choice lies with the surgeon in charge of the case. In the first place, if the condition is due to over-use, rest may restore the condition of the sheath. This will be achieved by fixing the hand in such a position that the tendon cannot possibly be used. For example, if the extensor tendons of the wrist are affected, the hand must be fixed in flexion, so that when gripping, the synergic action of these tendons is avoided. If this method is to be successful, prolonged immobilization is required; often six weeks or more are needed to produce the required effects. If the splint is removable, physiotherapy will be of value to stimulate the circulation and promote softening and absorption of the thickened tissue. Various measures can be used, including direct heating by short-wave diathermy, stimulation of circulation by constant current applications, and relieving congestion by counter-irritant measures. One method, useful to promote hyperaemia and smooth the lining of the sheath, is deep friction as advocated by Cyriax. Immobilization has the disadvantage of requiring a long period of time to ensure success, and it often prevents the patient from continuing his work.

A second method advocated by Cyriax is the use of deep frictions alone. He claims that the method ensures quick and satisfactory results, and avoids the use of splintage. During the period in which the manipulation is being used, the patient should avoid the movements which cause pain.

Stenosing Tenosynovitis (De Quervain's Tenovaginitis)

This condition affects the sheath of the abductor and short extensor of the thumb as they lie in the groove on the lateral side of the styloid process of the radius beneath the extensor retinaculum. The condition is a localized thickening of the sheath occurring most commonly in people whose occupation involves continual gripping movements.

The thickening can be palpated and is often visible. Active abduction of the thumb is painful as also are passive movements which stretch the tendon sheath, such as opposition and flexion of the thumb with ulnar deviation of the wrist.

The most successful method of treatment is to incise the sheath and so diminish friction. Occasionally a section of the sheath may require excision. Splints are not usually applied and, according to the surgeon's wishes, physiotherapy in the form of active movements may begin the day after the operation or when the sutures are removed.

Trigger Finger (Digital Tenovaginitis Stenosans)

This is a very similar condition, but it occurs in the flexor tendon sheaths of the thumb or fingers. There is a constriction of unknown origin at the mouth of the fibrous sheath and the tendon is swollen proximal to this constriction. It is difficult therefore for this part of the tendon to enter the sheath. There is tenderness at the base of the finger and sometimes a nodule can be felt. The finger tends to become locked in flexion and can only be extended passively or by a great active effort. At the moment of release a snap can be heard. The treatment is usually to incise the sheath and active movements should follow.

Chapter XVIII

INJURIES ROUND THE HIP

The hip joint is one of the most important joints of the body. It transmits the weight of the body, plays an important part in the regulation of posture, and is necessary for normal locomotion and such activities as sitting down and climbing stairs. It is therefore constructed in such a way as to be stable and yet permit a wide range of movement. This is unusual, joints normally being built either for stability, when mobility is sacrificed, or for mobility when stability is reduced. The dovetailing of the two features is achieved by the bony structure. The joint is stable because the socket is deep and the depth is increased by the acetabular labrum. It is also mobile because the articular surface of the head of the femur is more extensive than that of the acetabulum. In addition the neck is much narrower than the head and therefore does not impinge on the rim of the acetabulum during the wide range of movement of the joint.

Stability is also gained by the presence of the very strong capsule and ligaments and by powerful muscles. In standing the line of gravity passes behind the centre of the joint, consequently the trunk tends to rotate back on the femoral heads. To counteract this the capsule is thickened on the front and is reinforced by the ilio-femoral and pubo-femoral ligaments. Between the upper attachments of these two ligaments is a gap, but this is filled in by the tendon of Psoas and Iliacus.

When standing on one leg the pelvis would tend to drop towards the unsupported side giving an unsteady joint. This is prevented by powerful abductor muscles which work from the femur on the weight-bearing side, on to the pelvis checking the drop and even raising the pelvis on the unsupported side. Weakness of this muscle group would lead to instability.

If the hip joint is moving, stability is gained by contraction of the short muscles holding the head of the femur in the acetabulum. These are the lateral rotators of the hip which lie across the posterior aspect of the capsule. They are assisted by the gluteus medius and minimus.

The position of least stability of the hip is that of flexion and adduction. In this position the greater part of the head of the femur is no longer in the acetabulum, but rests against the posterior part of the capsule. If then a force is applied in the long axis of the femur dislocation can readily occur.

Deformity at the hip. The characteristic position of a painful hip is one of flexion, adduction and lateral rotation. This is due to several factors. All three extra-capsular ligaments are placed so that their fibres run spirally around the neck of the femur and become taut on medial rotation and extension. If there is inflammation or effusion in the joint the ligaments will be relaxed by adopting the opposite position of lateral rotation and flexion—this is, therefore, said to be the position of ease of the joint.

The most powerful muscles are the flexors and adductors though as man gradually becomes more adapted to the erect posture the extensors are becoming stronger. Pain in the hip causes spasm to prevent movement and the hip is therefore held in flexion and adduction, often reflex inhibition being present in the extensors and abductors.

Blood supply. While most joints are very richly supplied with blood from an extensive anastomosis around the joint, the hip joint is not so well supplied. The capsule and synovial membrane receive an extensive blood supply from the various vessels around the joint, but the head of the femur gets its nutrition from two main sources only. Vessels run in the longitudinal folds in the synovial membrane at the postero-superior and postero-inferior aspects of the neck of the femur and enter the neck just proximal to the articular surface of the head from whence they turn towards the centre of the head and anastomose with branches of the nutrient artery of the shaft. A single twig from the obturator artery runs in the synovial sheath of the ligament of the head and supplies the small area of bone around the fovea capitis. This usually anastomoses with the other arteries, but in some people this is a relatively poor anastomosis. Fractures of the neck of the femur may seriously damage the vessels entering the head from the synovial membrane and, since the supply from the single vessel of the ligamentum teres is insufficient to maintain the life of the head, avascular necrosis will result.

Nerve supply. The hip joint is supplied by three great nerves: the femoral through its branch to rectus femoris; the great sciatic through the branch to quadratus femoris, and directly from the obturator nerve. There may be branches from the superior gluteal nerve, but these have a small distribution. It would appear, therefore, that irritation of the nerve endings will provoke spasm of the flexors, lateral rotators and adductors supplied by these nerves and will be one of the reasons for the characteristic deformity of the joint.

PHYSIOTHERAPY IN HIP INJURIES

Injuries around the hip may be treated by internal fixation, traction, plaster, or simple recumbency, but whatever methods are used certain points must be noted if the foregoing facts are understood. The characteristic *deformity* which tends to develop must be prevented if possible because muscles and ligaments quickly shorten and in addition a deformed hip will lead to compensatory deformities of the lumbar spine and knee. In older people particularly, the hip joint, just like other joints, rapidly becomes *stiff* due to contractures, spasm, and adhesions. Both deformity and stiffness are serious since they interfere with the normal function of the joint.

In addition pain in the hip is always made worse by weight-bearing, consequently the patient, if he is allowed to bear weight, will tend to *limp*. A limp may also be the later result of weak muscles and limitation of joint range.

Four main objects of treatment by physiotherapy, therefore, emerge. Attention to the posture of the hip; strengthening of all the muscles, but particularly the extensors and abductors; maintenance of the joint range; and re-education of functional activities, particularly walking.

Position of the hip. Patients who are confined to bed, with or without traction, are usually in a position of modified half lying for the greater part of the time. This position encourages flexion deformity, therefore several times a day the patient should lie completely flat if possible for periods of half to one hour. If the surgeon permits, often after several weeks, she should also lie in prone lying for twenty to thirty minutes daily. Treatment should, as far as possible, be given in the lying position and the co-operation of the nursing staff must be gained to see that this position is taken up during the day. When the patient is allowed up, long periods tend to be spent in the sitting position. Care must, therefore, be taken to train the patient in the importance of getting up and lying down frequently so that hip flexor contracture does not occur. A second difficulty both in lying and half lying, unless traction is being used, is the tendency for the leg to roll out, increasing the danger of lateral rotation deformity. Some surgeons like a wooden bar to be fitted to the slipper which should be worn in bed; this effectively prevents rotation. Here again careful instruction is given to the patient to try to keep the leg so that the knee cap is facing up and not in or out. If medial rotation as an exercise is permitted this should be taught and practised regularly, but in some hip injuries rotation exercises are not allowed. When the patient is allowed to start weight-bearing great care must be taken to see that she does not walk with the leg laterally rotated and the hip flexed.

Strengthening of the Muscles. This can usually be begun as soon as the traction has been applied or the internal fixation completed. The abductors are exercised in lying, and if movement is permitted abduction can be started by taking the weight of the limb in slings or by hand. If movement is not permitted rhythmic contractions should be taught first on the un-injured limb and then on the affected side. It is easy for the patient to trick abduction by elevating the side of the pelvis; this must be watched for. Another satisfactory way of exercising the abductors is to press the foot down against a board so simulating their action as muscles which control the pelvis (see p. 382). As soon as the surgeon permits progression is made by turning the patient on to the unaffected side so that the abductors can be exercised against gravity. In doing so it is usually wise to support the leg so that it does not fall into adduction or lateral rotation.

Extension exercises are also important. These can be begun with rhythmic contractions of gluteus maximus and the hamstrings. Thigh pressing against the mattress will also help. The leg can be lifted and pressed down against slight resistance. If side lying is allowed extension can be done in this position, the weight of the limb being taken manually or by slings. Later, when prone lying is possible, extension against gravity is added. Tricking by tilting the pelvis on the opposite hip should be checked.

Exercises for the hip flexors and other muscles of the leg should also be given.

Maintenance of joint range. If the hip injury has been treated by internal fixation it is usual to allow hip movements to be started almost at once. these may be begun with the weight of the limb taken and a short lever should be used first where possible. One of the first movements will be assisted hip and knee flexion and extension and this should only be later progressed to flexion of the hip with a straight knee. If the hip should be stiff prior to a fracture, straight leg lifting should not be attempted since it will strain the fracture site. If the injury is being treated by traction, hip movements can still be done, flexion and extension being gained either by sitting up and lying down or by assisted hip and knee flexion if the method of traction allows. Abduction can also be performed in traction. If the hip is immobilized in plaster, rhythmic contractions of the hip muscles and exercise of all joints not immobilized will help to stimulate the circulation and prevent adhesion formation.

Re-education of Functional Activities. In all injuries of the lower extremity the patient tends to walk badly when he is first allowed to take some weight on the damaged leg. This may be due to pain, muscle weakness, fear and limitation in joint range. This has been fully dealt with later (see p. 421), but the special points to note in hip injuries are the development of a lunging gait due to weakness of the abductors and a tendency to walk with the leg laterally rotated and with a forward lean of the trunk. These should be prevented by exercising the muscles and checking posture before weight-bearing is allowed, but in spite of this they do develop if the patient is not watched. To avoid a lunging gait great care is taken to teach the patient to control the pelvis before he is allowed to walk. To do this he should stand between the parallel bars taking most of his weight on his hands. He then lifts the uninjured leg so that only the toes are touching the ground while consciously contracting the abductors of the injured hip and preventing the pelvis dropping to the unaffected side. When he can do this he can start taking slow steps checking this point at every step.

The use of a mirror will correct the tendency to flexion of the trunk at the hip and lateral rotation of the leg.

There is a great tendency to hurry off the leg on to the uninjured one and the patient must be trained to bring each foot an equal distance through so that the same time is spent on each foot. Crutches should be used until full weight-bearing is allowed and the pattern of walking is correct.

FRACTURE OF THE NECK OF THE FEMUR

A fracture of the neck of the femur is a particularly common injury in elderly people. It can occur near the head, or anywhere between this point and the junction of the neck with the shaft. Thus such names as sub-capital, transverse cervical and intertrochanteric are often heard. If the fractures are high in the neck, they will be intra-capsular. The exact site of the fracture has a direct bearing on the bony displacement, the speed of union, and upon the subsequent fixation. If the fracture is within the capsule, then the attachment of the strong capsule to the lower fragment will lessen the amount of lateral rotation of the leg which would otherwise take place when the break occurs. The blood supply to the upper fragment is more likely to be impaired in an intra-capsular fracture causing union to be slow.

Fracture of the Neck of the Femur

Many fractures of the neck of the femur are not displaced, while others show some displacement but are impacted. These are often treated by rest in bed without immobilization for six weeks.

In elderly patients in whom there may be considerable osteoporosis there is usually separation of the fragments. The limb will then rotate laterally and the fractured surface of the lower fragment usually faces forward and lies in front of the femoral head. If this displacement is not reduced union cannot occur. Immobilization is essential since without it both rotational and angulatory stresses will occur and will lead to non-union. The usual method of preventing these stresses is by means of internal fixation with a three-flanged nail. This has the advantage that no plaster fixation is needed. The patient can get up the first day and the dangers of prolonged bed rest are avoided. The operation is not a very lengthy one neither is it accompanied by much shock since the hip joint is not opened. An incision is made on the lateral aspect of the thigh centred just below the lower margin of the great trochanter. When the correct position has been made certain by use of a guide wire and radiography, the nail is driven in from just below the great trochanter through the neck into the centre of the head. It just enters, but does not pass through, the compact shell of bone covering the head. No form of external fixation is necessary, but some surgeons like the patient, when in bed, to wear a shoe with a cross bar. This bar rests on the bed and prevents rotation of the leg. Should the fracture be a low one, particularly if trochanteric, a McLaughlin nail-plate is used.

The patient is usually lifted out of bed to sit in a chair the first day and begins to walk as soon as she can do so without pain, often about forty-eight hours after the operation. Elderly patients do not manage crutches or sticks easily and a walking aid is most commonly supplied. As much weight is taken on the injured leg as the patient feels she can manage.

If the home circumstances are suitable the patient is discharged as soon as she is able to manage with the aid.

Physiotherapy

Physiotherapy is entirely active and aims at restoring the pre-accident condition or even at an improvement of this. To this end the range of movements in the hip and knee must be maintained, muscles must be kept as powerful as possible and the ability to sit down and stand up, walk and manage stairs must be restored. In quite a few instances elderly patients who have not previously been getting out at all can be taught and encouraged to do so following the accident.

Range of Movement. If active movements are not begun at once there is a tendency, particularly in old people, for the hip and knee to become increasingly stiff. Hip and knee flexion and extension are therefore begun on the first or second day and a day or two later abduction is added. For the first few days the weight of the limb should be taken by slings or by the physiotherapist so that assistance is given to the movements.

Exercises should be done in lying and side lying. In the latter case care should be taken as the patient is turned to see that the injured leg does not fall into adduction or lateral rotation.

When the patient is sitting out of bed on the first day the knee should be bent to a right-angle though for some of the time the leg should be supported to prevent oedema. Hip and knee movements should be full range by the seventh day.

Strength of Muscles. As far as possible the muscle condition, which is likely to be impaired by disuse, should not only be maintained, but should be improved in many of the patients so that the strength is greater than before the accident. Particular attention must be given to the flexors, abductors and extensors of the hip, the quadriceps and calf muscles and the intrinsic muscles of the feet. Rhythmic contractions of these groups and concentric work can begin on the first day. Progression is made by adding in assisted and then free exercises. Active hip flexion, knee extension, ankle and foot movements can be done in sitting so bringing in the resistance of gravity. Manual or weight resistance to hip exercises is not usually given before the sixth week and then it is begun using a short lever, progressing to a long lever about the eighth week.

Straight leg lifting should not be given; with so long a lever there is too much strain on the site of fracture and the exercise is too strong for very elderly patients.

It is hardly necessary to say that exercise once daily is not enough. The co-operation of the patient is essential so that exercises are practised at regular intervals throughout the day. To ensure this a written list of home exercises, properly taught, is essential.

Walking. The patient is taught to walk using the aid and when she can manage this, progression is made, if possible, to two sticks. Some very elderly patients never progress to this stage: others may eventually become able to walk without aid or sticks.

In all cases training is given in sitting down and standing up and managing stairs. If possible the patient should be encouraged to go out. If she is fit enough to do this but afraid to do so she should be taken out the first time by the physiotherapist and subsequently by a reliable friend or relative.

General Routine. For the first day or two and as long as necessary, after the accident, breathing exercises are given because elderly people are particularly liable to chest complications. General light exercises for the head and trunk are valuable to stimulate the circulation and improve posture and work should include strengthening arm exercises.

When the patient is able to get about easily using a walking aid, is doing the exercises properly and will obviously be able to manage at home, she is usually discharged, but told to return six weeks after the accident. Resisted exercises are then started.

Sometimes, especially if there is comminution, the head and neck of the femur are excised and an Austin-Moore prosthesis is substituted.

Fracture of the neck of the femur is not common in young people but when it does occur it is usually treated in traction.

DISLOCATION OF THE HIP

The most common type of dislocation is that in which force is applied along the long axis of the femur when the hip is flexed and adducted. The head of the femur is then resting against the capsule and the force pushes it through. It lies at first behind the acetabulum, but gradually glides up on to the dorsum of the ilium. This is a common occurrence in road accidents. The passenger in the front seat, sitting with one leg crossed over the other, is flung forward and the knee strikes the dashboard. The injury involves tearing of the capsule and sometimes of the ligament of the head often damaging the blood vessels entering the head. Occasionally the posterior rim of the acetabulum is fractured as the head is forced back and there may be damage of the great sciatic nerve lying immediately behind.

An anterior dislocation is less common but may occur if force is applied when the hip is abducted. This is not often accompanied by fracture.

A central dislocation will be produced by a fall or blow over the great trochanter driving the head of the femur through the floor of the acetabulum. The capsule is not torn, but the acetabulum floor is fractured and often comminuted.

Treatment

Early reduction of the dislocation is necessary to relieve the strain on the blood vessels and other soft tissues. It is usually followed by traction for three to six weeks. This rests the hip, relieves spasm and pain and allows time for healing of the tissues. In some cases after reduction skin traction is used for forty-eight hours. When the patient can lift the leg and rotate it with comfort he is allowed out of bed and begins partial weight bearing, progressing to full weight bearing as soon as he can do so without pain. Some surgeons prefer to immobilize the hip in a plaster spica especially if there is a central dislocation and it is thought wiser to omit reduction and accept a limited joint range.

If traction is used hip movements within the limit of pain are usually begun early, in one to two weeks in order to prevent scarring of the soft tissues and reduced range of movement. Flexion and extension, abduction and adduction can be practised together with rhythmic contractions of the quadriceps and all muscles round the hip. A careful watch should be kept for increasing pain or decreasing range which would indicate the onset of a myositis ossificans. Toe and foot movements, exercises for the other leg, trunk and arm exercises are also given.

The patient is usually allowed up between the fourth and sixth week and begins partial weight-bearing increasing the distance walked and the amount of weight taken according to the freedom from discomfort and pain.

There are *complications* common to all these types of dislocations. Avascular necrosis of the head of the femur may develop as a result of damage to the blood vessels. Myositis ossificans is not uncommon because there is much tearing of muscles and ligaments in both posterior and anterior dislocations, particularly if the patient was tense at the time of the accident. Osteoarthritis, developing a few years later, is very likely as a result of roughening of the articular surface of the acetabulum. Damage to the sciatic nerve is not common, but does occasionally occur in posterior dislocations, particularly if complicated by fracture of the acetabulum.

The physiotherapist should keep a careful watch for any signs of nerve lesion, complaints of paraesthesia or loss of sensation, weakness of leg muscles or the hamstrings. These must be reported at once and the usual treatment is then started (see p. 275).

early he will be non-weight-bearing with crutches for four to six weeks, and probably in either case he will be allowed to begin taking full weight at eight weeks and may be discharged and back at work in nine or ten weeks after the accident.

A further advantage of this method is that hip and knee movements can be begun almost immediately provided the method of traction will allow. This is due to the fact that a stable fracture is present once the nail is fitted. Stiffness of the knee is, therefore, much less of a problem.

It may be wondered why this method is not always used, but it has to be realized that it does involve surgery and however well carried out any operation carries the very small risk of fatal embolism or infection. Not all patients, even if the fracture is suitable for surgical treatment, will be willing to be treated this way.

PHYSIOTHERAPY IF TRACTION IS USED

There are four phases in the treatment by physiotherapy: the first, a lengthy period while fixation is by traction, often lasting twelve weeks; the second period before the patient is allowed up, but when all splintage is removed; the third, when the patient is ambulant but using crutches or a weight-relieving caliper; and the fourth, when full weight may be taken.

PHASE ONE

Recumbency with traction continues for a long period and therefore the patient requires physical treatment.

Owing to the fact that the knee is often kept extended (though it should not be hyperextended) for all or part of the time the *quadriceps muscle is likely to be affected*. It may become adherent to the shaft of the femur, especially if there has been injury to the deep surface of the muscle by sharp fragments of bone at the time of accident. It may lose its ability to lengthen if the knee is never carried through its full range, and full-range movement is impossible even if a splint which allows knee movement is used. Certainly, if unexercised, the quadriceps will atrophy and trouble will then arise when the patients begin to walk. These things can be prevented or at least lessened if contractions and relaxations of the muscles are practised regularly and often; five minutes out of every hour is a useful guide to give the patient. The time at which contractions are commenced varies with the wishes of the individual surgeon, but it is usually within the first two weeks of immobilization. At first grating at the fracture site will be heard. This should cease by the fifth week indicating that callus has formed. If it is still present it should be reported. After a few weeks contractions may be given against the resistance of the hand placed just above the upper border of the patella. Full relaxation must be stressed if full elasticity is to be retained. Relaxation can also be gained by resisted work for the hamstring muscles, when this is possible.

For many reasons *the knee on the affected side is liable to become stiff*. This may be due to adherence or loss of elasticity of the quadriceps muscle. It may be the result of gradual shrinkage of the capsule, or it may be due to congestion in the blood vessels, as a result of diminished movement, producing excessive exudate of tissue fluid with consequent fibrous tissue formation. It may be the result of a sero-fibrinous exudate from the damaged soft tissues if the fracture line is low, or from the synovial pouch caused by the skeletal traction pin if it has been inserted through the femoral condyles. Continual slight movement of the pin, owing to incorrect alignment or unequal pull, will result in tissue reaction and adhesion formation particularly if the pin is near the synovial membrane. If the pinholes are continually being opened, it is difficult to avoid sepsis. A further cause of knee stiffness is fixation of the patella to the patellar surface of the femur. This may result from lack of quadriceps exercises or may be due to damage to the knee at the time of the accident.

One of the disadvantages of a stiff knee is the strain which results when the patient walks or attempts to gain movement in the joint. This strain may be felt at the fracture site, which may yield more readily than the joint. For this reason it is important to limit the stiffness and to regain as wide a movement as possible before the patient becomes ambulant. It is impossible to prevent some stiffness, but it may be considerably lessened by contractions and relaxations of the quadriceps and hamstrings groups, by passive movements of the patella, by vigorous movements of the toes and foot, and exercises of the body as a whole, which all serve to maintain a brisk circulation of blood and lymph. Contractions of the extensors and abductors of the hip will also help to prevent adhesion formation, through their pull on the ilio-tibial tract. Small-range knee movements may be begun between the second and eighth week, according to the wishes of the surgeon, if the method of fixation allows. This will help to lessen the danger of joint stiffness.

The posture of the foot is another serious consideration. If it is supported by a rigid foot-piece, absence of toe movements is liable to result in weakening of the intrinsic foot muscles and contracture of the long flexor and extensor tendons, so that clawing of the toes occurs, and this will seriously affect gait and comfort. If no support is used and the foot is not exercised, the continual force of gravity is liable to cause dropping of the foot and stretching of the dorsiflexors with adaptive shortening of the plantar flexors. These deformities can definitely be prevented by exercise. Vigorous and oft-repeated dorsiflexion followed by relaxation will ensure strong muscles and prevent drop foot. A flat board may be placed against the sole of the foot, and, against this, toe-parting and closing, toe-flattening and lumbrical action may be practised. This will also have the effect of maintaining normal pressure and cutaneous sensations and of maintaining the good condition of the plantar fascia which would otherwise soften. It will be remembered that this fascia is vitally important for the support and protection of the shape and structures of the sole of the foot. In addition these exercises, together with inversion and eversion and plantarflexion movements, will maintain the strength of all the extrinsic and intrinsic muscles of the foot, so that when walking is recommenced, the foot is used correctly and pain and flat foot do not develop.

As usual, when a patient is confined to bed for any length of time, *general musculature is weakened, circulation slowed* and respiration becomes shallow. Breathing and general exercises are therefore necessary. These are best given in a class for the whole ward, so that games can be used and interest and competitive spirit roused.

It is reasonable if a patient is confined to bed for a long time, for him to become *mentally and physically lazy*. His co-operation then is difficult to obtain for the essential part of the work, especially when, as soon as the traction is removed, much effort is needed. For this reason he must work throughout the whole period of recumbency. General exercise in groups can be arranged and diversional occupational therapy is most important.

In the case of older patients, if crutches are to be used, special attention is paid to the *hypertrophy of arm and shoulder girdle muscles* so that correct use of crutches is assured.

If a limp is to be avoided when walking is resumed, it is important to maintain *co-ordination between the two legs*. This can be gained by performing all the exercises alternatively with the two legs, though naturally more is done for the affected leg. Thus toe and foot movements may be done first on the affected side, and then both together, trying to gain equal range and speed. Many of the movements may then be performed reciprocally in the natural sequence of use as in walking.

PHASE TWO

Usually, when the traction apparatus is removed, the patient is allowed to lie free in bed for a week or more before he gets up and starts to walk. This may be to allow time for measurement and fitting of caliper or crutches, or it may be to allow time to gain a greater range of movement in the knee joint, and greater strength in hip and knee muscles. Though the previous work will be continued, more can now be added. Since limitation of knee movement will be present every possible step should be taken *to increase the active range* without straining the site of fracture. Thickenings may be softened by the use of the constant current, or by deep heating, using short-wave diathermy. Stretching of the thickened tissue may be obtained by deep massage. Strengthening exercises for the hamstring muscles will help to regain flexion, and, for the quadriceps group, will help to gain full control of the last few degrees of extension. If range is limited by loss of elasticity of the quadriceps, its circulation may be aided by the use of the inductothermy and it may be taught to relax by means of resisted exercise of the knee flexors.

Since the legs have been in the horizontal or elevated position for many weeks and the circulation has not been subject to normal control, *faintness and giddiness* may be present when the patient stands for the first time, with blood tending to collect in the lower extremities. This can be prevented, during this stage of treatment, by sitting the patient up on the edge of the bed, swinging the legs and carrying out foot and knee exercises for increasing lengths of time.

The normal movements of walking, which may have been forgotten, can now be re-learnt without weight and, if the patient is to wear a caliper, hip updrawing can be taught so that the correct 'caliper' gait can be easily acquired.

If the patient is to use crutches, *crutch exercises may be started*. The patient lies flat and holds the crutches in the usual way. The physiotherapist gives slight resistance against the end of the crutch while the patient presses firmly down on the hand-piece. The crutches may also be lifted and lowered alternately against slight resistance.

PHASE THREE

Work still continues as before, but should be progressed because stronger exercises may be given now that the patient can attend the gymnasium and a greater range can be obtained in hip and knee. Manual resistance is added to muscular exercises, and self-assisted pulley work is used for increase of range. Resistance by weights or springs should not be started until the surgeon gives permission (probably not for another two months), because the callus is not yet firm enough to withstand the strain, especially if the range of movement in the knee is limited.

Walking has now to be taught and, once learnt, progression is made to climbing stairs.

If a patient is wearing a weight-relieving caliper, he must be *taught how to apply it* and how to take care of it, and the physiotherapist must see that it remains a perfect fit. As muscles develop, the ring may become too small and rub the skin or be unable to be pushed right up to the ischial tuberosity, so that it is no longer fully weight-relieving. Occasionally, as the patient bears weight, the ring is seen to be too large and passes proximal to the bony points; this also is unsatisfactory. Instructions are also usually needed about the care of the pressure points, as the skin is apt to become sore and this makes the wearing of the splint impossible.

PHASE FOUR

In this stage it is safe for weight to be taken and the patient has to learn to do this gradually. He may have some difficulty in using the correct pattern of walking, even though he has been practising it during the period of non-weight-bearing. Therefore much attention is paid to *re-education of walking*, taking care to prevent a limp and to correct wrong patterns (see p. 421). Over a period of weeks, progression is made including going up and down stairs, jumping and running.

PHYSIOTHERAPY IF INTERNAL FIXATION IS USED

The physiotherapy which can be given depends upon the method used. If the leg is left free, active movements begin about the third or fourth day and are progressed in a similar way to those used in the treatment of a fractured neck of femur (see p. 388), except that the progress is a little slower. Usually assisted knee movements are not started until the fourth day. Training of walking with crutches begins as soon as ambulation is permitted. Similar treatment to that used for the fracture treated by traction is given if the insertion of the nail is followed by traction.

INJURIES OF THE QUADRICEPS MUSCLE

A severe contusion of the Quadriceps Muscle

This can result from a kick on the thigh in football or when horseriding. The muscle is compressed against the shaft of the femur and considerable bleeding occurs in vastus intermedius as well as in surrounding tissue. Within a few hours the thigh is hot, tense and swollen and later there will be considerable bruising. Knee movements are painful and limited by the intense swelling. Special care has to be taken with this injury because there is a possibility of bone formation within the muscle. The cause of this is uncertain, but passive movements and deep massage will increase the danger. The usual treatment is rest for a few days with firm strapping or an elastic or crepe bandage. The patient is encouraged to contract the quadriceps regularly so that a pumping effect is exerted on the blood vessels and absorption is aided. After a few days exercises are begun and weight-bearing is resumed. The strapping or bandage is removed when the swelling has subsided. Any residual thickening may be dealt with after three weeks when danger of ossification is passed, by ultra-sonic therapy and deep massage.

Rupture of the muscle. This occurs most commonly in rectus femoris. It may be a minor injury resulting in a rupture of a few fibres with pain on contracting the muscle and a small area of deep tenderness, or it may be a more severe injury, occurring in middle-aged or elderly patients, in which the muscle gives way at the lower musculo-tendinous junction. In the latter case the muscle will retract and a gap will be formed which is rapidly filled with blood. Minor injuries are usually treated by strapping and immediate exercise omitting competitive sport.

Unlike most complete ruptures, rupture of rectus femoris is rarely treated surgically since the muscle is not usually in good condition and suture is difficult. Complete rupture is therefore dealt with by rest, with strapping, for a few days, followed by progressive exercises to strengthen the muscle. The muscle will heal by fibrous tissue and will, therefore, tend to be lengthened, but any weakening is masked by increased strength of the other parts of the quadriceps and by the remaining hip flexors.

Avulsion of the tendon. Occasionally the tendon is avulsed from the upper border of the patella. Provided the vastus medialis, lateralis and intermedius are intact, protection by a back splint is all that is required. The patient walks in the splint for two weeks and knee exercises are begun after a few days. If the rectus and intermedius tendon is avulsed then suture is necessary and weight-bearing is delayed for three or four weeks, but knee exercises without weight may be begun in ten to fourteen days, although some surgeons prefer to maintain the limb in a plaster cylinder for some weeks.

For a complete rupture surgical intervention is essential, since the patient will otherwise have great difficulty in straightening the joint while weight-bearing, and will therefore experience considerable disability on stairs.

Chapter XX

INJURIES ROUND THE KNEE

Injuries around the knee joint are exceedingly common and at some point in their treatment usually require physiotherapy. The most frequent conditions to reach the department are traumatic synovitis, sprains of the medial ligament, injury of the menisci, damage to the extensor mechanism, and fractures of the condyles of the femur or tibial plateaux. These will, therefore, be briefly discussed here. To understand the treatment of these conditions some knowledge of the special features of the anatomy of the joint is essential.

During *extension* of the knee the femoral condyles roll forward on the tibia until movement is checked on the lateral side of the joint by the anterior cruciate ligament and by compression of the anterior end of the lateral meniscus. As movement continues on the medial side the femur rotates medially. Finally all movement is checked by compression of the anterior extremity of the medial meniscus and by the medial, lateral and posterior ligaments. The joint is now said to be 'locked' and in the 'close-packed' position. During the first part of extension all parts of the quadriceps muscle are working together, but the end of the movement involving rotation is the work of the vastus medialis since it is attached by the medial expansion to the medial condyle of the tibia. Knowledge of this is important because if for some reason the last few degrees of extension cannot be obtained vastus medialis will atrophy and the support and protection it gives to the medial side of the joint will be lost.

The Synovial Membrane of the knee joint is most extensive. It has been estimated that stretched out, it would cover forty-three square inches of ground. It has in fact many folds and fringes, some filled with fat. Damage of the membrane will be followed by considerable effusion into the joint. This effusion, if extensive, will distend the capsule and so irritate its nerve endings, causing discomfort and diminished use of the joint. This will mean atrophy and loss of power of the quadriceps and hamstring muscles. If an injury becomes chronic, hypertrophy of the membrane and its folds develops. Nipping of these enlarged folds may produce acute exacerbations of synovitis.

The medial and lateral ligaments are strong ligaments at the sides of the joint extending downwards and slightly backwards from the epicondyles of the femur to the tibia and fibula. Both ligaments are separated from the upper end of the tibia before they reach their lower attachment by blood vessels, fibrous tissue and bursae with the result that the tibia normally moves beneath them during flexion and extension of the joint. Should these ligam nts be damaged, organization of sero-fibrinous exudate may bind them to the tibia so that its freedom of movement is impaired and knee movements become painful and limited. If these ligaments are weakened by injury lateral instability of the joint results. Since the lateral side of the joint is the more vulnerable, the knee is likely to be forced medially and the medial ligament is the more often injured. If weight is taken while the ligament is torn or weak a marked valgus deformity will rapidly develop.

The cruciate ligaments are of great importance to the stability of the joint since their chief function is to prevent the femur slipping forwards and backwards on the tibia when the knee is semi-flexed. These can be damaged in severe injury to the joint and, like all ligaments, they do not heal readily.

The menisci are C-shaped fibro-cartilaginous structures lying on the periphery of the articular surfaces of the tibia. They serve to increase the stability of the knee joint by deepening the articular surfaces; they protect the surfaces by acting as shock absorbers and they help to spread a thin film of synovial fluid over the articular surfaces during movement. Both menisci are firmly connected to the intercondylar area of the tibia by fibrous horns. Those of the lateral are attached close to the intercondylar eminence; it is, therefore, nearly circular in shape. The horns of the medial meniscus are further apart being attached in front and behind the horns of the lateral structure. The convex edge of each meniscus is loosely connected to the tibia by the capsule, these fibres forming the coronary ligament. The medial meniscus is less mobile than the lateral. This is because it is strongly connected to the femur by short fibres which extend from the medial epicondyle of the femur to the medial convexity of the meniscus. In spite of this it is more prone to rupture because when the femur rotates during movements of the joint there is torsion in the meniscus since the medial convexity is attached to the femur and the horns to the tibia. The more mobile lateral meniscus is less readily damaged because its mobility is controlled. The posterior part of the convexity of the lateral meniscus is attached to the medial femoral condyle by two bundles of fibres, the ligaments of Humphrey and Wrisberg. Thus when the femur rotates laterally during flexion the meniscus would be drawn centrally, but this is prevented because the tendon of popliteus gives a slip to the meniscus and this, as the muscle contracts in flexion, draws the meniscus backward out of harm's way.

In spite of the functions of the menisci removal does not damage the joint because within a few weeks of a meniscectomy, a new meniscus is formed by the growth of fibrous tissue inwards from the synovial membrane. The regenerated meniscus is very similar in shape to the original structure differing only in that it is narrower and thinner and in being more firmly connected to the capsule. For this reason it is less mobile and less readily damaged.

The patella is a sesamoid bone developed in the tendon of quadriceps. Its function is to give the quadriceps muscle a better leverage by throwing its tendon an increased distance in front of the axis of movement of the joint. It also protects the tendon from friction against the lower end of the femur. For this reason the greater part of its posterior surface escapes from the fibres of the tendon and shows a smooth surface to articulate with the patellar surface of the femur.

During movements of the knee the patella glides on the femur so facilitating knee movement. If the patella becomes adherent to the lower end of the femur, movements of the joint will be greatly impaired and forced flexion can easily fracture the bone. Adherence can occur both in injuries around the joint and in fractures of the shaft of the femur.

The position of ease of the knee joint is one of semi-flexion. This is explained by the fact that all the true ligaments of the joint lie nearer the posterior than the anterior aspect of the joint; they are therefore relaxed in flexion, taut in extension. If there is pain or effusion within the joint the patient will hold the knee semi-flexed so reducing tension and lessening pain. To hold this position the hamstrings will be in a state of increased tone while the quadriceps will be inhibited. Both groups will, therefore, atrophy since neither is contracting and relaxing normally. The quadriceps will show the greatest loss of bulk and power, since as a result of inhibition its metabolism is the more reduced.

The stability of the knee joint is dependent on its ligaments and muscles, not on its bony configuration. In standing with the knees straight the centre of gravity lies in front of the axis of movement. The weight of the body tends, therefore, to hyperextend the joint. This is prevented by tension in the hamstrings and by the ligaments which all lie towards the posterior aspect of the joint. When the knees are flexed the centre of gravity lies behind the axis and the body-weight tends to increase the flexion. This cannot be prevented by ligaments since none lies towards the front of the joint. Powerful muscles are, therefore, needed on the anterior aspect of the joint. These are provided by the quadriceps group which pass over the front of the joint and attach to the tubercle of the tibia and the lower margins of the tibial condyles. Since, in most of our daily activities, the weight of the body passes through semi-flexed knees the condition of the quadriceps is vitally important to the stability of the joint.

Lateral stability of the knee joints is gained by the strong medial and lateral ligaments, while antero-posterior glide of the femur on the tibial plateaux is prevented by the cruciate ligaments.

Due to the fact that the stability of the knee joint depends so much on its ligaments, damage to these ligaments is serious. Ligaments formed as they are of white fibrous tissue do not heal readily and so if injury occurs this damage must be compensated for by hypertrophy of the extensors and flexors of the joint, particularly the extensors which need to be stronger than normal if the joint is to be protected.

PRINCIPLES OF PHYSIOTHERAPY IN KNEE INJURIES

Strengthening Quadriceps

In all knee injuries some temporary decrease in the normal function of the quadriceps must occur. Even in an uncomplicated synovitis of the knee, in which the patient may walk at once, full normal activity is reduced. In some lesions there is considerable effusion and if knee movements have to be postponed, quadriceps can only be used isometrically and atrophy occurs. Inhibition of quadriceps is present in many knee injuries, though its cause is uncertain, and unless rapidly overcome, loss of bulk soon develops. The loss of power and endurance which accompany atrophy are serious since the quadriceps is essential to the stability of the knee joint. If the muscle is weakened a vicious circle is set up; weak quadriceps means an unstable knee, the unstable joint is subject to repeated strains, chronic synovitis develops with diminished use and further muscular atrophy. If the injury involves ligamentous damage quadriceps atrophy is even more serious because ligaments do not heal readily and the muscle must be stronger than normal to compensate for the joint weakness.

Injuries round the Knee

In all knee injuries, whether immobilized or not, whether operated on or not, whether weight-bearing or not, exercises for quadriceps must be started at once. The only exceptions to this rule are in acute pyogenic infections of the joint or where there is a haemarthrosis. The former requires complete rest until infection is controlled by antibiotics and in the latter case exercise is postponed for three to four days until the danger of further bleeding is passed. Blood in the joint, if not rapidly absorbed, will clot, act as an irritant, and become organized with consequent formation of adhesions.

The type of quadriceps exercise depends on whether the knee may be moved or whether it must be kept straight. If it is immobilized in a plaster cylinder no knee movements are possible. If knee movements are not possible the quadriceps can be exercised either by means of rhythmical contraction and relaxation or isometrically, holding the knee straight as the hip is moved, or in case of rectus femoris concentrically in hip flexion exercises. Such exercises as straight leg-raising, leg abduction and leg extension are suitable. The points to watch for when quadriceps is exercised in these ways are, first is the patient really using the muscle and second is he using it often and hard enough. To ensure the first, the exercise must be taught on the uninjured limb insisting that the patient both sees, feels and palpates the contracting muscle. He may then try the exercise on the injured leg. If inhibition is difficult to overcome, Faradism can be used to teach the patient to do the movement. When hip exercises are being done the patient is taught to contract the quadriceps and so brace the knee first and it must be insisted that he does this.

To make sure the patient works hard enough, he must first understand why hard work is necessary. It must be made clear that if the muscle does not work as hard as usual it will lose size and become weaker and then the joint will be weakened. When he understands this point then he is told how often each exercise should be done, how many times a day they should be practised and how they should be progressed. Written instructions are essential and it is valuable to provide a card on which the patient can keep his own record of the progression of the exercises.

When knee movements are permitted then quadriceps can be exercised from knee flexion. According to the degree of stiffness of the knee movements may be commenced in side lying, prone lying, or high sitting. The important point here is that the exercise should be as hard as the muscle can take in the range that is available. Care must be taken to ensure that there is no 'lag'. Thus it is necessary to watch that the patient does complete the full range of extension each time he straightens the knee from flexion. If he cannot do so an easier position or a smaller range should be chosen, as for example knee extension in half lying with the knee supported on a hard sandbag.

To make the work as hard as possible daily progression is essential. As soon as the patient can extend the knee against gravity and hold it straight, resistance, first manual and then by weights or springs, should be added. The method of progression for the weight lifted varies in different physiotherapy departments, but what is of importance is that the work should be progressive and hard enough.

To restore the quadriceps muscle to its pre-accident state or in certain cases to build it up beyond this, requires not only progressive weight-lifting, but also vigorous general activity. Walking, running, jumping, games are all added when the knee injury is sufficiently recovered to permit them. Weight-bearing with an unsupported knee should not be permitted until the quadriceps is strong enough to extend and hold the knee straight against gravity. In addition, effusion should have subsided before these activities are started.

Strengthening other muscles acting on the joint

Though the quadriceps muscle is the most important contributor to the stability of the joint, the ilio-tibial tract and the hamstrings are also necessary to stability and movement. In addition to being powerful flexors of the knee the hamstrings also act to prevent hyperextension, while the ilio-tibial tract stabilizes the lateral side of the joint and can assist in extension of the joint, since it is attached to the tibia in front of the axis of movement of the joint. These muscles therefore require attention. The gluteus maximus and tensor fascia lata acting on the ilio-tibial tract can be exercised whether the knee is immobilized or free. From the time the plaster is dry or the bandage applied, free and then resisted hip abduction and extension can be practised regularly and an increasing number of times in side lying and prone lying. As soon as possible resistance in the form of weights or sandbags can be added. As soon as the patient is allowed to take full weight on the leg, standing on that leg and moving the other gives excellent exercise for the abductors while walking and climbing stairs brings in the extensors, particularly if the knee is immobilized.

If the knee is immobilized the hamstrings must be exercised by rhythmic contraction and relaxation and by using them as hip extensors. When knee flexion is allowed they can be built up by resisted knee flexion exercises against resistance within the range available. A word of warning must be inserted here. If the knee injury is a fracture of the lower end of the femur and the knee is stiff, resisted exercises should not be given until the range is good and the surgeon is satisfied that the union is strong enough, otherwise the fracture site will be strained rather than the knee moved.

Range of Movement

In uncomplicated synovitis of the knee and in most cases of meniscectomy movements are not necessary to maintain or increase range. In neither case does the knee tend to become stiff because synovial fluid does not clot and it is only when there is bleeding into the joint that adhesions tend to form. The knee is flexed when the effusion has subsided in order to permit full-range quadriceps exercises and strengthening exercises for the knee flexors. There are, however, many injuries in which stiffness of the knee does occur, particularly when immobilization for fractures and ligamentous tears has been necessary. This stiffness cannot be prevented, but it can be lessened by rhythmic contractions of the surrounding muscles and vigorous use of all the other joints of the limb which are not immobilized and, where permitted, functional use of the limb in walking and stair climbing.

As soon as the surgeon allows knee movements to begin, a careful examination of the joint should be carried out to ascertain the range of flexion, extension and rotation and to decide the cause of any limitation of movement. Movement may be limited by such factors as adhesions within the joint, actual adherence of the patella to the lower end of the femur or the medial ligament to the upper end of the tibia, thickening around the joint, shortening of the hamstrings and loss of extensibility of the quadriceps.

The persistent practice of knee movements will gradually stretch adhesions and loosen thickening. Extra-capsular adhesions and thickenings can be effectively softened prior to movements by the use of deep kneadings, ultra-sonics, short-wave or constant-current applications. An adherent patella must be freed before mobilizing exercises are started; this can be attempted by passive movements and rhythmic quadriceps contractions. Adherence of the medial ligament is dealt with by carefully localized transverse frictions. Tight hamstrings can often be relaxed by using the 'hold-relax' technique. Loss of the ability of the quadriceps to lengthen adequately has already been discussed (see p. 394).

All these measures are preliminary or additional to the main means—active exercises. Repeated active exercises are absolutely essential and this has to be explained so that the patient will co-operate. However slow the recovery, forcing is not permitted unless expressly ordered by the surgeon. A minimal amount of apparatus should be used—preferably only that which the patient can use at home. Auto-assisted pulleys are of great value and these can usually be rigged up at home; a pool is most helpful and, when the surgeon permits, the patient is encouraged to go swimming if he is accustomed to doing so. If there has been a fracture, while the range is small, care has to be taken not to strain the fracture site and non-weight-bearing games and exercises, assisted and free, are best. Later more vigorous work using body weight can be added.

Re-education of Gait

In most knee injuries attention to walking, climbing stairs, jumping and running is needed at some stage in the treatment. If the knee is immobilized in a non-weight-bearing plaster the patient will require training in the correct use of crutches, in crutch walking and how to use the crutches in sitting down and in climbing steps. If the patient is allowed to bear weight on the limb, but is wearing a back splint or plaster cylinder, he will need to be trained to use the hip-updrawing gait and to avoid swinging the leg into abduction. When the plaster or splint is removed he has to be trained to use a normal gait and avoid a limp (see p. 421).

Re-education of gait is not complete until the patient can run, jump, go easily up and down stairs, in fact until he has perfect confidence in his knee.

TRAUMATIC SYNOVITIS OF THE KNEE JOINT

Acute synovitis is a characteristic of all injuries of the knee. In mild injuries it may be the only obvious effect; in more severe injuries it will be accompanied by partial or complete tearing of ligaments, damage of the cartilages, fractures or dislocation.

A twist or strain of the knee will set up inflammatory changes in the synovial membrane and as a result, effusion into the joint. The effusion gradually develops and is apparent about six hours after the injury. It is easy to recognize because it fills up the hollows around the joint and distends the suprapatellar pouch so that a horseshoe-shaped swelling can be seen. It can be detected by palpation, one hand should be placed on the front of the thigh just above the pouch, the fingers of the other hand lie on either side of the patella and ligamentum patellae. If gentle pressure is given with the hand in a direction towards the foot, fluid will be felt to move against the fingers.

In severe effusions the capsule becomes so distended that its nerve endings are stimulated and reflex inhibition of quadriceps results. The knee is held in the position of ease, that is in semi-flexion since in this position the ligaments are relaxed and there is more room for the fluid.

The hamstring muscles are tense. It is essential that this should not continue for long because loss of power of quadriceps will rapidly develop and the knee will then be inadequately protected and subject to repeated strains (see p. 402). The main object of treatment therefore is to *relieve the effusion* as rapidly as possible. To do this rest and protection from further strain are necessary. A pressure bandage is applied and if the effusion is excessive a back splint is also used. In severe cases weight-bearing is avoided for 24 to 48 hours. The back splint and pressure bandage are removed when the effusion has subsided and the quadriceps is working normally, rarely later than ten days after injury.

The second object is *to prevent loss of quadriceps power*. For this reason physiotherapy is usually ordered. Any inhibition must be overcome, thus quadriceps exercises are started at once. As long as there is marked effusion these should be in the form of rhythmic contractions and straight leg exercises, but manual resistance may be used with the latter. As soon as the effusion begins to decrease the splint and pressure bandage are removed for non-weight-bearing knee exercises.

When unsupported weight-bearing is allowed weight-bearing exercises can be added. Strong resisted exercises are not normally required if adequate treatment is carried out immediately, since atrophy will not then occur and recovery is complete in seven to ten days.

Instruction may be needed in the use of crutches in the first 24–48 hours and in walking with hip updrawing in a back splint.

There is no need to worry about knee flexion since adhesions do not form in a straightforward synovitis and full flexion will be present within a day or two of the removal of the splint.

Sprain and rupture of the medial ligament of the Knee joint

A force, such as a blow on the lateral side of the knee, which abducts the tibia on the femur will strain the medial ligament of the joint. According to the degree of violence the ligament may be stretched and a few fibres ruptured; many fibres may be torn or the ligament may be completely ruptured.

SIGNS AND SYMPTOMS

These vary with the severity of the injury. *If the ligament is stretched or only partly torn* there will be pain on the medial side of the joint and tenderness over the site of damage, most often at the femoral attachment to the medial epicondyle and sometimes over the line of the joint. There is also swelling and bruising over the ligament and a varying degree of effusion. Movement will be painful as the tibia moves beneath the ligament and there will be limitation of the last few degrees of extension, because this puts a stretch on the damaged structure. Valgus strain on the joint will be painful, but there will be no instability.

In the case of complete rupture all the features will be more marked and there will be bleeding into the joint. In addition, if the patient is anaesthetized, the medial side of the joint can be opened up. This is not possible while the patient is conscious because of the pain. When pain and swelling have subsided, if treatment has been inadequate, there will be instability of the joint and weight-bearing will result in a marked knock-knee deformity.

Treatment depends on the type of lesion. If the lesion *is one of stretching only*, the treatment is directed towards protecting the ligament, preventing its adherence to the underlying bone and maintaining the strength of the quadriceps. Thus the knee is usually bandaged with a crepe, or firm-pressure bandage, depending upon whether there is effusion into the joint or not. The shoe may be raised on the inner side of the heel and sole to relieve the strain on the medial side of the knee; the patient is instructed in quadriceps exercises. Massage, including transverse friction, may be given to the ligament.

The essential part of the treatment is the quadriceps drill. This includes rhythmic contractions, straight knee exercises and knee straightening from the flexed position. The knee is not likely to become stiff unless the medial ligament becomes adherent; this is prevented by the knee movements used in maintaining the strength of quadriceps, by using the knee normally, within the limits of the bandage, in walking and activities, and by massage.

If the injury is a partial rupture of the fibres it may be necessary to aspirate the joint and apply a pressure bandage for a few days followed by a plaster cylinder for two to four weeks. This usually extends from the groin to just proximal to the ankle. In this the patient walks and quadriceps drill is carried out regularly. When the cylinder is removed knee exercises are started with particular emphasis on quadriceps work.

Complete rupture is serious because ligaments, not having a good blood supply, do not heal readily, and if the ligament does not unite firmly the stability of the joint is impaired. The injury may be treated conservatively or by surgical repair of the ligament, but in either case the knee is immobilized in a long plaster cylinder for six to eight weeks. It is particularly important that quadriceps exercises should be practised throughout the period of immobilization so that atrophy of the muscle is minimized, since if the ligament is weak a stronger than normal muscle is necessary to compensate for the weakness. When the knee is freed, there will be some atrophy of the muscles round the joint and some limitation of joint movement. Massage to the medial ligament, exercises to build up the muscles, particularly vastus medialis, and exercises to increase the range of the joint will all be needed.

INJURIES OF THE SEMILUNAR CARTILAGES OF THE KNEE

Injuries to the menisci are common particularly amongst young men. The medial meniscus is the more often damaged probably because it is the less mobile of the two. Due to the fact that it is attached to the medial ligament, it has a relatively fixed posterior segment and a mobile anterior part; it cannot, therefore, move as one piece in the way the lateral cartilage does. Many explanations have been put forward as to how the cartilages are damaged, but all are agreed that the main factor is a rotational strain of a flexed knee when it is bearing weight. If, for example, the femur is medially rotated on the tibia the medial cartilage is forced into the posterocentral part of the joint. If weight is then taken the cartilage may be trapped against the top of the tibia and may be split. This fact may explain why the injury is commonest in various occupations and games. If the footballer makes a sudden turn to the opposite side the set of circumstances necessary for a medial cartilage injury is reproduced, because the foot is fixed to the ground by the studs in the boot, then as the femur rotates medially the cartilage may be displaced.

Various types of tears occur: some are longitudinal splits, others transverse tears or tears of the horns. Those which occur at the periphery may heal because they are in direct continuity with the synovial membrane from which granulation tissue may grow. Longitudinal tears cannot heal as cartilage has little reparative properties. Redisplacement of unhealed fragments is likely and locking of the joint may be a more or less frequent occurrence.

SIGNS AND SYMPTOMS

At the moment of injury *acute pain* is experienced and there is often a tearing sensation. The patient usually falls and then finds he cannot fully extend the knee. A few hours later the joint is hot, swollen and tender. If the cartilage is reduced, with adequate treatment the joint rapidly returns to normal, but unless the tear heals subsequent displacement is likely. The second injury may occur on a twist without weight bearing. The reaction is unlikely to be so great even though *locking* may occur. There will be some *effusion and localized tenderness*. If the medial cartilage is damaged this will be over the line of the knee joint just anterior to the medial ligament, but as damage of the ligament often accompanies the cartilage injury there may also be tenderness over the ligament at the joint line or at its attachment to the medial epicondyle of the femur.

The chief feature is the *atrophy of quadriceps* which, after several incidents, may be considerable. Each time effusion and pain occur, reflex inhibition of the muscle results and the atrophied muscle may not be completely restored to normal. Atrophy leads to quadriceps insufficiency, with instability of the knee and greater likelihood of further damage and a chronic synovitis. Thus confidence in the joint is increasingly lost.

Diagnosis of cartilage injury is not easy because the signs and symptoms of the first injury may equally well be those of an acute traumatic synovitis following injury to one of the ligaments. Wiles points out that locking is not a diagnostic sign; it means that the last degrees of extension cannot be obtained. While this may be due to a fragment of the torn cartilage being nipped between the tibia and femur on extension of the joint, it may also be due to extreme distension of the joint or to damage of the medial ligament. Unlocking gives a more certain diagnosis since if, on manipulation, full movement is restored it is likely that some structure has been acting as a block. Often in this case a 'click' may be heard.

TREATMENT

Conservative, provocative, or surgical treatment may all be used.

Conservative treatment is nearly always the method of choice following the first injury. This is partly because the diagnosis may be uncertain, partly because there is a chance of natural healing if the tear should be a peripheral one, and partly because operative interference would not be undertaken while there is acute inflammation of the joint.

If the joint is locked it is manipulated. This may be done in one of several ways. Cyriax, for example, flexes the knee and then applies an abduction strain to open up the medial side of the joint if the medial ligament is damaged. The leg is then rotated to and fro on the femur as the knee is extended.

Following manipulation, strapping or a pressure bandage will be applied to limit effusion, and a back splint may also be used. The leg will be rested for a few days, but non-weight-bearing quadriceps exercises must be started at once to overcome inhibition and prevent atrophy. Rhythmic quadriceps contractions, straight leg lifting, leg extension and abduction, vigorous foot movements should all be practised for five minutes out of every hour. After a few days effusion should have subsided and knee movements are allowed. Weight bearing is also started, but the support of strapping or bandage is retained until effusion has completely subsided.

Treatment must be continued until the quadriceps is back to normal or is stronger than before the injury.

Provocative treatment. In some cases the diagnosis is uncertain. The patient may give a history of a joint which gives way and sometimes locks. There may be slight effusion and there will probably be muscle atrophy. These may, however, be due to other local conditions of the joint such as chronic arthritis in which a hypertrophied synovial fringe may act as an obstruction to full extension.

The patient is, therefore, sent to the physiotherapy department for vigorous quadriceps exercises, general activities and games, including movements which will produce rotation at the knee joint. If there is an unhealed cartilage injury there is almost certain to be a displacement with this treatment and when this occurs the surgeon must be immediately notified.

Surgical treatment. This is usually undertaken either following redisplacement, when the diagnosis of a torn cartilage is certain, or, when the traumatic effusion has subsided, after a primary injury with definite evidence of a cartilage tear. The whole of the cartilage is removed and a pressure bandage is then applied. Many surgeons also use a back splint in addition to the pressure bandage. Physiotherapy is practically always ordered both for the pre- and post-operative stages.

Pre-operative work aims at *bringing the quadriceps to the maximum possible tone and strength,* since the length of recovery depends very largely on the condition of the muscle and joint prior to the operation. It is also essential to get the *understanding and co-operation of the patient* because quadriceps work immediately after the operation is difficult since pain leads to inhibition of the muscle. Much stress is, therefore, laid on the importance of beginning rhythmic contractions as soon as consciousness is regained.

Post-operative routine varies with the individual surgeon, but all agree that quadriceps drill is essential and should begin as soon as the patient returns to the ward. In many patients reflex inhibition is present and this must be overcome or rapid atrophy with loss of joint stability will result and recovery will be delayed. The patient should not be left until he is able to do a good contraction and he must be visited several times during the day to ensure that he is carrying on with the exercise. Once he can do the contractions straight leg-raising is added. The following day manual resistance is begun and by the third or fourth day weight-lifting should be started.

During this time the other muscles round the knee require exercise and gluteal contractions, leg abduction and extension in side lying should be taught and practised.

Some patients show a tendency to oedema in the lower leg and foot possibly because the firm pressure bandage renders venous return more difficult. Foot exercises will help to prevent this and elevation of the leg may be advised for the first ten days. Routine post-operative breathing should also be given for the first few days.

The time at which knee flexion exercises and weight-bearing are allowed vary very much, each surgeon having his own routine. Since the knee rarely becomes stiff flexion need not be a problem. Some surgeons allow knee flexion within the bandage at the fourth post-operative day; many delay it for ten or fourteen days. But when it is begun its purpose is primarily to allow concentric work for quadriceps.

Weight-bearing may be commenced with the pressure bandage on between the first and fourth day or it may be delayed till the tenth day or even longer. It is the opinion of some surgeons that it is better to delay weight-bearing until the quadriceps can extend and hold the knee straight against gravity and there is little or no effusion.

The patient usually attends the gymnasium between the sixth and tenth day where he continues quadriceps drill and non-weight-bearing knee exercises. At ten days he is discharged from the ward and attends as an out-patient unless he is being treated in a residential rehabilitation centre. It is preferable that he should attend for as much of the day as possible having periods of class and individual exercises, and occupational therapy, particularly in a workshop if this is available.

Up to approximately three weeks the exercises are mainly non-weight-bearing and free, mat work, high sitting knee extension, long sitting ball games are all included. The patient usually walks and climbs stairs and these activities should be checked. During weight-bearing an elastic knee bandage is worn if there is any effusion. Most patients are ready for progressive resistance exercises to build up the quadriceps at about three weeks, though some surgeons expect this to start at ten days. The progressive resistance may be given in any one of the accepted methods, provided the method chosen is adhered to. When the patient is doing weight-lifting he is also ready for more vigorous weight-bearing activities. Should the physiotherapist have to make the decision as to when these exercises should begin, judgement can be based on how much the patient is able to do in the way of ordinary activities such as walking and stairs without producing or increasing effusion, and on the strength of quadriceps and the presence or absence of effusion.

The time at which the patient is discharged depends upon his progress and the job to which he is to return. It may be as early as three weeks or as late as twelve. It is probably safe to say that no patient should return to heavy work under four weeks from the date of the operation.

DAMAGE TO THE EXTENSOR MECHANISM
OF THE KNEE (see Plate XXVIII)

Fracture of the patella may be caused by a direct blow or fall on the knee. A transverse or stellate fragment with damage to the articular cartilage results from the squashing of the patella against the femur. The quadriceps tendon is not likely to be ruptured and, depending on the degree of violence, the fragments may or may not be displaced.

Indirect violence is also a common cause of fracture. In this case the usual history is of a middle-aged person stumbling. While his knee is being passively flexed by body-weight he violently contracts his quadriceps to save himself from falling; the result is likely to be a transverse fracture of the patella with rupture of the quadriceps expansion. Quadriceps will go into spasm retracting the upper fragment of bone and muscle. The gap so produced rapidly fills with blood and inflammatory exudate. If nothing is done this clots; the clot will organize and repair will take place by fibrous tissue formation. This will give good union, but with continuous movement of the knee it tends to stretch and the quadriceps will be correspondingly lengthened. When this has happened, the quadriceps will complete its contraction before the knee is fully extended; an unstable knee therefore results.

Treatment

This depends on the type of fracture. If the injury is a *simple fracture without displacement* the blood is aspirated and either a pressure bandage and posterior plaster slab are applied or a plaster cylinder extending from the groin to just proximal to the malleoli. These are worn for two, three or four weeks according to the surgeon. In each case the patient walks in the plaster and after a few days starts quadriceps exercises. If the splint is a back slab only, it can be removed for active non-weight-bearing knee exercises.

If there is *separation of the fragments with rupture of the quadriceps* suture is essential to prevent lengthening of the muscle. The smaller fragment is usually excised. A plaster cylinder is worn for six weeks, the patient practising quadriceps exercises and walking as soon as the plaster is dry.

In the event of the injury resulting in *comminution and displacement of the fragments* there is considerable difference of opinion as to how it should be treated. The fragments may be excised and post-operative treatment is then as for the previous case. Some surgeons do not approve of excision; early movement is then the method of choice so that moulding of the articular surface results. The patient starts knee movements almost at once, but is kept in bed until the quadriceps can extend the knee and hold it straight; he is then allowed up.

POINTS TO BE CONSIDERED IN THE USE OF PHYSIOTHERAPY

Quadriceps Exercises

These will be given whatever method of treatment the surgeon is using In every case they will start with straight leg work and rhythmic quadriceps contractions. Some difficulty may be experienced because reflex inhibition is often present, but it must be overcome if power is not to be seriously impaired (see p. 403). As soon as the surgeon allows a back splint to be removed or a plaster cylinder is taken off, knee extension exercises are begun. These are free or assisted at first done in half lying with the thigh supported so that the knee is slightly flexed and later in sitting on the side of the bed or in high sitting with a firm support beneath the thigh. When the muscle can extend the knee from the position of maximum possible flexion and hold it extended, manual resistance is added. Progressive weight-lifting is next begun. If there is only thirty or forty degrees of flexion, weight lifting is best started with the patient in half lying and the thigh supported on firm sandbags. The amount of weight to be lifted is usually judged by noting the ease or difficulty with which the patient performs the movement, probably three or four pounds will be a reasonable weight. Weight-lifting will be progressed daily by one of the many systems available for muscle strengthening. It is important to adhere to the rules of the particular system chosen so that detailed progress is made and the muscle is worked to its maximum capacity.

In all systems three main points emerge: the weight must be measureable and accurate, it must be increased systematically, and there must be a systematic increase in the number of repetitions. Most authorities also feel that the muscle should be 'warmed up' before weight-lifting is commenced.

Exercises to restore full range

Stiffness of the knee can be a troublesome feature especially if the leg has been immobilized in a plaster cylinder for four to eight weeks. Active exercises of the toes, foot, ankle and hip will stimulate the circulation in the limb and therefore lessen unnecessary fibrous tissue formation. Whatever the method of treatment these should be done many times daily.

Rhythmic contractions of the knee flexors and extensors within the plaster will prevent the sticky exudate from organizing and lessen the danger of periarticular adhesions; they will also check the danger that the quadriceps may lose its ability to lengthen.

As soon as the surgeon permits or when the plaster is removed, knee flexion exercises will be begun. If they are begun early they should be assisted active movements in lying and side lying, the weight of the limb being taken either manually or by slings. Great care must be taken to see that the knee can be fully extended after flexion. Flexion must never be gained at the expense of extension. If these exercises are begun later, more vigorous work can be done. Care should be taken to see that the patella is not adherent and active exercises may be preceded by deep localized massage if there is much thickening around the knee. In cases in which the knee is already very stiff when knee exercises are begun, self-assisted pulley work, slow reversal of antagonists and the 'hold-relax' techniques may all be useful.

Training in Walking

If the patient is weight-bearing in a posterior plaster slab or cylinder there will be difficulty in clearing the ground and the patient tends to swing the affected leg into abduction as he brings it forward. To avoid this, before walking is commenced, the patient is taught hip updrawing first in lying and then in standing, then in slow walking. No sticks or crutches should be needed except for the first few days after the injury. When the plaster is removed the patient, partly from habit and partly because there may be only a few degrees of flexion, will continue to walk with the hip-updrawing gait. This has to be overcome. Once there is sixty degrees of flexion the patient can clear the ground normally. It may be necessary to break up the movements of walking and teach the patient to flex the knee and hip unduly high and then extend it as he swings the leg through.

FRACTURES OF THE LOWER END OF THE FEMUR AND UPPER END OF THE TIBIA

Fractures of the lateral femoral condyle and tibial plateau are the result of violence applied to the lateral side of the knee joint. The lateral condyle of the femur is impacted against the lateral plateau of the tibia occasionally fracturing the femoral condyle, but more often involving the tibia.

The lateral tibial plateau may be depressed and its articular surface comminuted or sometimes a large fragment is depressed, but the articular surface remains intact. The neck of the fibula is often fractured and the medial ligament is torn. Occasionally, the cruciate ligaments and medial meniscus are also damaged.

A fall on the bent knee produces a less common injury, a T-shaped fracture of the femoral condyles in which the transverse line is a few inches above the knee joint and the vertical line runs into the joint.

In each case there is alteration in the alignment of the articular surfaces, bleeding into the joint and damage to the ligaments. There is danger of roughening of the articular surfaces, intra-articular adhesions and weakening of the joint. As a result, though there are many different methods of treatment, all aim at *good union* with early active movements of the joint to smooth out irregularities and prevent adhesions, and *immediate exercises* for the muscles to ensure a strong joint. The knee may be supported in a posterior plaster slab or traction may be applied for six to eight weeks. In the first case the splint is removed daily for knee flexion and extension exercises. If traction is used either the Thomas' splint is fitted with a Pearson's flexed knee attachment or the mattress is in two halves so that the lower section can be removed for knee exercises. Thus for six to eight weeks the patient is in bed, but doing hourly quadriceps drill, toe, foot, ankle and hip movements, and at least once a day knee movements.

Usually at the end of this period the traction or splint is removed and the patient starts assisted weight bearing progressing from crutches to sticks and then taking full weight. Exercises to strengthen the knee muscles and increase range continue and in about three months from the time of injury the patient should be ready for discharge.

Some surgeons prefer at the end of six to eight weeks to fit a hinged plaster. This consists of a below-knee plaster and thigh corset joined by hinges. The advantage of this method is that it affords some protection to the knee while at the same time encouraging knee movement.

Chapter XXI

FRACTURES OF THE SHAFTS
OF THE TIBIA AND FIBULA

ither the tibia or the fibula may be fractured alone, or alternatively both bones can be involved. If only one bone is broken, the essential difference lies in the fact that the fibula does not transmit the weight of the body to the ground while the tibia does so. Thus fractures of the fibula, which are usually the result of direct violence, do not require immobilization. They are most commonly treated like soft tissue lesions, though, if the patient persists in a limp, a short plaster splint from the toes to the tubercle of the tibia may be worn for a few weeks. Fractures of the tibia, on the other hand, require reduction and immobilization and may be considered as requiring treatment similar to that used for fractures of the shaft of both bones.

Fractures of both bones

These may be the result of direct violence, when the fracture is usually transverse and both bones are broken at the same level; or they may be due to a twisting force causing oblique or spiral fractures with each bone yielding at its weakest point, the tibia at its lower end, the fibula at its upper end. In either case overlapping and rotational displacement are likely to occur, and there will also be angulation if both bones are fractured at the same level. Angular and rotatory displacement, if allowed to remain, would produce serious results, as they would cause an alteration in the axis of the ankle joint and mal-use of the foot. Reduction and immobilization are, therefore, necessary. Surgeons vary in their choice of the method and duration of immobilization, but one main factor always taken into consideration is the stability of the fracture. Stability depends on the line of the fracture, muscle pull and the integrity of the ligaments. In these fractures it is the line of fracture which has to be considered. If the fracture line is transverse and the jagged edges of the bone interlock, the fracture is not likely to be re-displaced by muscle pull, but if the line is spiral or oblique the distal fragment may be pulled up by muscle spasm.

Stable fractures are almost always immobilized in a toe-to-groin plaster with the knee slightly flexed and the foot at a right angle. Some surgeons keep the patient in bed for three weeks if there is any uncertainty as to the stability of the fracture. The plaster is retained until there is clinical and radiological evidence of firm union, usually three to four months. Weight-bearing is allowed after six weeks. Sometimes between the second and eighth week a hinged splint is substituted for the plaster. This consists of a below-knee plaster and a thigh corset, the two being joined by hinges. The advantage of this splint is that knee movements are encouraged and it is easier for the patient to get about especially in bus or train. If the long plaster is retained a boot with a convex sole is worn two to three weeks after the injury and the patient is allowed to begin weight-bearing.

If the fracture is unstable the same methods may be used, but weight-bearing is delayed for six to eight weeks and if a hinged plaster is worn it is not applied for eight to ten weeks. In these fractures traction is sometimes used for four to six weeks or internal fixation by intramedullary nail, screws or plate may be preferred. Usually a weight-bearing plaster is then worn for six weeks or longer.

Another method is to put the leg in plaster for two to three weeks and at the end of the period to re-X-ray. If the fragments have not retained their position the tibia is then plated. Some surgeons then like the knee and ankle movements to begin at once and when these are full, usually in about two weeks, a toe-to-groin plaster is applied until union is firm. The patient walks in this plaster. This has one great advantage, if there is full range of movement before the plaster is applied the inflammatory exudate and blood will have been absorbed and stiff joints will not develop so that the period of rehabilitation after the plaster has been removed will be much shorter.

PHYSIOTHERAPY

While the limb is immobilized

Owing to the long period of immobilization, complications with which we are already familiar are liable to arise. As a result of inability to carry out full normal function, *atrophy of muscles will occur*. This will particularly apply to the quadriceps, the calf muscles, the long flexors of the toes and the intrinsic muscles of the foot. The quadriceps will waste if the knee is slightly flexed and vastus medialis cannot fulfil its normal duty of producing the last few degrees of extension. The calf muscles are affected because plantarflexion cannot be obtained either during the period of non-weight-bearing, or during the period of ambulation in the plaster. These muscles are used to strong exercise, as they are responsible for lifting the weight of the body every time a step is taken, and they will therefore atrophy rapidly during a period of disuse. The long flexors of the toes work to convert the segmented lever into a rigid arched lever and in addition the Flexor Hallucis Longus provides the final thrust-off. Thus these muscles will also atrophy. The intrinsic muscles of the foot follow suit because the toe muscles are not being used to fix the toes against the ground, to steady the borders of the foot or to support the arches.

Hence, while all muscles of the leg should be exercised, these four groups must receive particular attention. The *quadriceps* may be exercised by strong attempts to extend the knee in the plaster and by rhythmical contractions, as well as by exercises for the hip muscles such as straight leg raising free and progressively resisted, leg abduction, adduction, extension and rotation. These will have value only if the patient contracts the quadriceps and tries to extend the knee in the plaster while performing the hip movement. When a hinged splint is worn the quadriceps muscle can be exercised from flexion, but manual or weight resistance should not be applied until union is firm.

The *calf muscles* may be exercised by vigorous attempted plantarflexion in the plaster and rhythmical contractions. These exercises must be performed for a period of five minutes out of every hour throughout the day.

Toe-pressing against the plaster platform which usually supports the toes, toe-parting and closing, and attempted lumbrical action will all help to prevent excessive atrophy of the *intrinsic muscles*. The patient should try to hold the correct position of the foot and to shorten and lengthen the sole so that loss of elasticity and adaptive shortening of plantar structures do not occur.

If the tibia is plated and hip and knee movements are given before the plaster is applied, joints should not become stiff, but if other methods of treatment are used *the joints of the foot and ankle, and possibly the knee, may become stiff*. Although the stiffness cannot be prevented, it can be lessened, through the use of vigorous movements of all joints not included in the plaster and contractions of muscles acting on immobilized joints. This stimulates the flow of blood and lymph and prevents exudate from organizing and sticking tissues together.

The patient may also tend to *lose the co-ordination between the two legs,* and the brain may tend to discard the limb which is not performing its accustomed work. This may be prevented by exercising both legs alternately and together.

The fact that the patient does not bear weight on the affected leg does not mean that he is a recumbent. If the boot on the uninjured side is raised, he can get about using crutches from the beginning, with the plaster swinging clear of the ground.

This *method of ambulation needs teaching* in the first place and a careful watch should be kept to see that it is being carried out correctly. If the crutches are a little too long or if the patient uses them incorrectly there may be undue pressure in the axilla and the radial nerve, as it winds backwards beneath the long head of triceps may be damaged. The patient is taught to take the weight on the hands and to press the crutches against the sides of the chest, not into the axilla. In order to do this, it may sometimes be necessary to hypertrophy the adductors of the shoulders, depressors of the shoulder girdle, and extensors of the elbow.

When the patient is equipped with a boot, *training in walking will be essential*. Certain faults are likely to be committed. These will predispose the patient to limp and cause later trouble. Since the knee is straight or only slightly flexed, the patient will tend to clear the ground by abducting the leg as it is carried forward. This gives an abnormal and conspicuous gait and can be prevented by teaching the patient to draw the hip up as he carries his leg straight through. Again there is a great tendency for the patient to rotate the whole leg laterally as it takes the weight, bringing the foot into the everted position. This not only strains the foot, knee and hip joints, but leads to a similar type of gait when the plaster is finally removed.

During the ambulant stage, crutches are used at first, but are rapidly changed to sticks. The physiotherapist should not allow the patient to use one stick only because if he does so, he will use it on the sound side and lean his weight over it, and thus acquire a faulty posture.

It is obviously not essential to continue this treatment throughout the whole period of immobilization. Once he has learnt the exercises and has proved to be co-operative and trustworthy, he can continue at home, coming from time to time for a check and for the addition of new or stronger exercises.

When the splint is removed certain complications may occur if adequate attention is not given to prevent them. The most likely of these is the development of a limp. This is so serious a complication that special thought should be given to it.

Fractures of the Shafts of the Tibia and Fibula

LIMP

A patient may develop a limp for many reasons, some of which certainly should have been prevented. The limp may be the result of *bad habits* acquired while the limb was in plaster. If proper re-education is carried out, this cause would be obviated.

The patient may limp because it is *painful* to take full weight on the leg for the length of time necessary to bring the other leg forward. The pain will not be at the site of fracture, but will most often be in the sole of the foot, owing to changes which have taken place while the limb was in plaster. Softening of the plantar fascia may have occurred, some atrophy of intrinsic muscles will have taken place, and ligaments and fascia may have shortened and have lost their ability to lengthen. Adhesions around joints and in soft tissues may have formed and, with atrophy of intrinsic muscles, unbalanced action of the long flexor and extensor tendons will have led to clawing of the toes. Pain is, therefore, extremely likely when the rigid support is removed and movement begins to occur. Much of this, though not all, could have been prevented by adequate exercise during the period of immobilization. Pain may also be the result of the weakening and loss of function of the long flexors of the toes so that they fail to support adequately the medial longitudinal arch of the foot (see p. 419).

Limp may also be due to *weakness of the calf muscles* which are not now strong enough to lift the body weight forward in the normal heel-toe gait. Without adequately strong plantar flexors, a normal gait is impossible. With exercise in the plaster, it should be possible to maintain a reasonable power in these muscles.

There may be *insufficient range of movement* in the foot and ankle to allow the normal use of the foot and the patient will walk with a stiff foot. As has been previously seen, this may be lessened by suitable exercise during the immobilization period. Stiffness of the talo-calcaneal joints particularly affect gait. These joints are sometimes known as the 'joints of balance'. Loss of movement here means loss of balance when standing on the affected limb and therefore the patient hurries off this foot as quickly as possible in walking.

Weakness of muscles and ligaments may lead to the use of the foot in the position of weakness, that is the abducted position. This not only throws strain on the medial side of the foot, but puts the flexor hallucis longus at a grave disadvantage, since it no longer acts at right angles over the joints of the big toe and the final thrust-off is in a lateral rather than a forward direction.

Since some general muscular weakness of the leg, as compared with its fellow, must inevitably be present, its reactions are not as rapid. Consequently the two do not work in unison and *co-ordination is defective*.

Lastly there is *fear*. If a rigid support has been worn for many months, its sudden removal gives the feeling of insecurity and fear that something will give way, and it takes considerable encouragement and gradual trial before the patient feels that he can trust the limb. He will, therefore, keep his weight on it for as brief a time as is possible.

Common characteristics of a Limp

Limps vary but there are three features common to most limps. The patient *leans over to the sound side* so that his weight is taken off the affected leg, and he brings the fractured leg through, often without flexing the knee, and puts the foot as one solid piece on the ground, frequently in the abducted position. He then *rapidly brings the good leg forward* as far as, but not beyond, the affected leg, to lessen the time taken on the bad leg. *No attempt is made to transfer the weight forward by raising the heel of the affected side* or thrusting off from the toes. The result is a stiff, ugly gait with unequal length of step, unequal timing, bent spine, loss of correct leverage and strain on muscles and joints. Such a gait is harmful to muscles and joints, is fatiguing, and effectively bars the patient from walking any distance or from taking part in any vigorous activities. Once this limp becomes established, it rapidly becomes a habit and like all habits, it will be extremely difficult to break.

The whole object therefore when the plaster is removed, is to prevent the limp from ever occurring. It can be prevented much more easily than it can be cured. Obviously much is done during the period of immobilization and any steps taken to lessen atrophy, diminish stiffness of joints, maintain co-ordination, and obtain the correct gait allowed by the plaster, will lessen the tendency to limp.

As soon as the plaster is removed, a careful examination is made to estimate the possibility of a good gait. It should be ascertained that the calf muscles are strong enough to lift the weight of the body, that there is a right angle of dorsiflexion and sufficient mobility in the talo-calcaneal joint and all other joints of the foot, and that all extrinsic and intrinsic foot muscles are reasonably strong and the legs used to working in reciprocation. If these points are not satisfactory it should be seriously considered if it would not be better to spend some days building up the muscles and mobilizing the joints and teaching the correct pattern of walking without weight, before walking without support is allowed.

Particular attention to the joints of the foot is always necessary. Not only should exercises to improve range be given in half lying and sitting but to improve balance and mobility, as soon as the patient can take his weight, he should practise standing on the injured leg while moving the other and later should do exercises standing on the narrow side of a form.

As soon as it is considered wise to begin walking, re-education should begin in order to prevent a limp. A patient simply must not be allowed to limp and no step forward should be taken until he can stand on the affected leg and flex and abduct the sound hip. Then, with two sticks, he should walk forward towards a mirror so that he can watch his posture. Equal length and timing of steps can be obtained by marking foot lengths on the floor and by rhythmic counting. Instruction should be given on the way to push-off and on keeping the foot facing straight forward.

FOOT DEFORMITIES

Another complication is the presence or development of foot deformities. As has already been seen, *clawing of the toes* is a possible and a crippling deformity. Two factors may bring this about. As the plaster is applied round the foot it may lift the heads of the first and fifth metatarsals so that the heads of the second, third and fourth are lower and the 'anterior transverse arch' is lost. This hampers the action of the lumbricals and interossei. Lack of exercise of these muscles will lead to atrophy. In walking, the lumbricals should contract at the same time as the long flexor and extensor muscles of the toes (during the transference of the foot forward and the push-off), in order to counteract the tendency of the flexors to curl the toes and the extensors to hyperextend the metatarsophalangeal joints. If they do not do so, clawing of the toes results, a proper thrust off cannot be obtained, undue pressure comes on the metatarsal heads and pain results.

Another possible deformity is that of *flat foot*. This may occur because muscle weakness leads to the use of the foot in the position of weakness. This leads to abnormal strain on the medial ligament of the ankle joint and on the 'spring' ligament. These ligaments gradually yield and, as they do so, the calcaneus falls into eversion, the space between the sustentaculum tali and the navicular widens and the talus is displaced, pushing the navicular and cuneiforms forwards and laterally. If uncorrected, structural changes will occur in the foot. These complications should be prevented by adequate exercise within the plaster and progressive strengthening exercises when the plaster is removed. A very careful watch should be kept on the placing of the foot in standing and walking.

OEDEMA

Occasionally a further complication in the form of persistent oedema, arises as soon as the plaster is removed. This oedema is the result of loss of tone in all the structures of the leg. Normally the blood vessels are supported by the dense deep fascia, the tone of the muscles, and the condition of the vascular walls. Enclosing the limb within a rigid support takes away the need of support while at the same time resulting in diminution in the bulk and tone of fascia and muscular tissue. Consequently, when the plaster is removed, there is insufficient support for the blood vessels. These dilate, congestion occurs and there is increased filtration of fluid. The tissues become 'water-logged' and there is greater difficulty in moving the joints. Vigorous exercise within the plaster does much to minimize this complication, but the best way of preventing it is the substitution of a firm but not rigid bandage in the form of a Viscopaste or Cellanband immediately the plaster is removed, and the constant practise of exercises which are rapidly progressed in strength. These should be given with the leg elevated at first.

INABILITY TO RUN AND JUMP

Because of the weakness of the calf muscles, though a normal gait may be obtained, the patient may fail to re-acquire the power to run and jump and climb stairs. Thus intensive physiotherapy should be applied to these muscles as soon as the plaster is removed. Strong exercises are essential. At first these may be done in half lying against manual, weight and spring resistances in the available range. Progression should rapidly be made to standing. In this position the calf muscles have to lift the weight of the body and this can be made more difficult by standing with the toes on a raised bar or the narrow side of a form and by holding weights in the hands. Going upstairs, spring upwards preparatory to jumping, climbing the ribs, and running, all help in the development of the calf muscles. The calf muscles can be considered sufficiently strong when the patient can stand and balance on the toes of the injured limb.

Therefore, when the plaster is removed, physiotherapy consists mainly of graded exercises, measures to increase range in joints, and re-education in walking, climbing stairs, running and jumping.

Chapter XXII

INJURIES ROUND
THE ANKLE AND FOOT

S prains of the ankle, rupture of tendo-calcaneus, fractures and fracture-dislocations around the joint, and fractures of the calcaneus are some of the most frequent injuries seen in the physiotherapy department. To understand their treatment a sound knowledge of the anatomy of the region is essential. A few of the most important features will, therefore, be stressed.

The ankle joint is contructed in such a way as to give it the necessary strength and stability for weight-bearing while at the same time permitting dorsiflexion and plantarflexion, both of which are essential for normal gait and activities.

Strength and Stability

The talus is firmly fitted into a socket formed by the lower ends of the tibia and fibula, the interosseous and inferior transverse tibio-fibular ligaments and the medial and lateral ligaments of the ankle. The fact that the socket is a jointed one gives it elasticity and therefore strength. But because it is jointed the two bones are held together by particularly strong ligaments—transverse and interosseous, and if these should be torn the stability of the joint would be lost since the bones would separate and the foot would be upward and laterally displaced.

The line of gravity of the body passes in front of the ankle joint. There is therefore a natural tendency for the leg bones to ride forward on the talus. To ensure stability and prevent this the socket is narrower behind than in front. It is also deeper behind, the greater depth being gained by the downward projection of the posterior surface of the tibia, and the presence of the transverse tibio-fibular ligament, which lies below the level of the tibia. If this ligament is torn or the posterior flange fractured then forward dislocation of the leg bones can occur.

To prevent unwanted side to side or tilting movements of the talus, which would result in instability and weakness of the foot, the leg bones project down by means of the malleoli on either side of the talus. Stability is further enhanced by powerful ligaments which stretch from the malleoli not only to the talus, but also to the calcaneus and, in the case of the medial ligament, to the navicular. Complete rupture of either of these ligaments would mean that on inversion or eversion of the foot the talus would tilt. This would make walking on sloping, rough or moving surfaces difficult and uncomfortable, and would seriously weaken the foot.

Dorsiflexion and Plantarflexion

These movements at the ankle are permitted since the socket is 'open' in front and behind. The anterior and posterior ligaments are weak. There is no downward projection in front and only a small flange behind. The normal person's toes clear the ground by about one inch in walking, and to do this the foot must be capable of dorsiflexing to approximately 90°. Greater dorsiflexion is required for normal step climbing. The average range of dorsiflexion is about 25° beyond the right angle, but this range can be increased by movements at the tarsal joints.

Plantarflexion is necessary for the normal transference of the body weight forward and upward. The average range is greater than dorsiflexion about 35°, and it too is increased by movements at the tarsus.

Limitation in either movement is serious since they are both essential for the normal heel-toe gait and stiffness is rarely sufficiently compensated for by increased movements at the tarsal joints since these also are often involved in injuries round the ankle joint.

The function of the foot itself is twofold

It acts as a means of balance when supporting and transmitting the body weight, and as an organ of propulsion in walking, climbing, running and jumping.

The foot is required to act as a *balancing agent* because it forms a very small base for the body. When standing on one foot the body tends to sway and the line of gravity quickly falls outside this base. To prevent loss of balance there is continuous interplay between the invertors and evertors making minor adjustments at the talo-calcaneal, talo-calcaneo-navicular and calcaneo-cuboid joints. This keeps the body weight within the base. If these joints become stiff, adjustments are impossible and maintenance of balance becomes difficult.

Organ of Propulsion. To propel the body forward with minimum energy the foot must work as a second order lever. Thus the *fulcrum* provided by the first metatarsal head is strong. The head of the first metatarsal is large and beneath it are two sesamoid bones. If faulty use of the foot following injuries throws the strain of the 'push-off' on to the heads of the second, third and fourth metatarsals then trouble results since they are small and not equipped with sesamoids. The *power arm* is longer than the weight arm since the calcaneus projects well back behind the ankle joint—a feature peculiar to man—while the weight is transmitted in front of the joint. The power is very skilfully applied because it is provided by the gastrocnemius and soleus inserting into the posterior surface of the calcaneus. Soleus is a penniform muscle and so provides the power to overcome the inertia in lifting the body weight, while gastrocnemius is long and fusiform and gives the speed and range and so the 'spring' of the movement. If these muscles are weakened they cannot lift the body weight and the heel-toe gait and ability to run and jump are impaired.

Arched formation of foot

In order to overcome the shock in weight transmission the foot is constructed in the form of an arch, but unlike many architectural arches it is capable of changing its shape, permanent flattening being prevented by ligaments, aponeurosis, muscles and tendons. This means that the lever is segmented and a segmented lever can only work if it is capable of being converted into a rigid arched lever. Each time the calf muscles lift the heel the muscles which stretch from one end of the arch to the other contract and convert the segmented lever into a rigid arch. These muscles are the flexor hallucis longus, flexor digitorum longus et brevis and the abductor hallucis. If these muscles are weakened by disuse or injury their function is impaired and the gait is affected. Usually walking then produces pain in the sole of the foot. In the same way if the joints are stiffened this conversion and alteration in the height of the arch is impossible.

The Toes

The toes are extremely important because they give a larger surface for weight-bearing when the 'push off' occurs and so reduce the strain on the metatarso-phalangeal joints, and because they grip the ground and so prevent the foot slipping back as the thrust occurs. They are kept flat on the ground by the combined action of the long and short flexors and the lumbricals. The greatest danger in foot injuries is that they will become clawed and no longer able to fulfil these functions. Clawing develops if the intrinsic foot muscles are allowed to atrophy because then the long extensors extend the metatarso-phalangeal joints and the long flexors flex the interphalangeal joints without the synergic action of the lumbricals and the flexor digitorum brevis.

The intrinsic foot muscles are important not only to prevent clawing, but also to support the arched formation of the foot and restore it to its normal height after it has been depressed by weight.

Clearly all foot and ankle injuries, therefore, require special attention to the intrinsic foot muscles since if, as is so often the case, rigid immobilization is required, intrinsic action is very much reduced and trouble is likely to arise when the plaster is removed and unsupported weight-bearing permitted.

It will be realized that considerable trouble can arise following fractures, dislocations and sprains in this region. The *stability* of the ankle joint is dependent on its bony configuration and its ligaments rather than on its muscles and rupture of the ligaments allowing partial or complete dislocation may lead to permanent disability.

Stiffness of the joints leads to impairment of balance and shock-absorbing powers as well as to faulty gait, while *atrophy* of muscle means loss of the normal spring in activities, lack of support to the arch as the heel is lifted, and the danger of clawed toes.

PHYSIOTHERAPY IN FOOT AND ANKLE INJURIES

Strength of Muscles

In all cases in which the foot is immobilized there will be diminished function of the leg and foot muscles. The powerful calf muscles can no longer lift the heel, this action being simulated by the forward rock on the convex sole of the boot worn over the plaster. Since there is no heel lift the long and short flexors of the toes do not act to brace the arch and since it is difficult to press the toes against the sole of the boot the intrinsic muscles are often not brought into action. All these groups will, therefore, atrophy and when the plaster is removed their weakness will impair functional activities and may well lead to the development of foot deformities. Attempts must therefore, be made to lessen the atrophy during the period of immobilization and to restore the muscles to normal strength when the plaster is removed. During immobilization the repeated practice of vigorous toe flexion and extension, which the patient can perform against his own resistance, will help to maintain the condition of the anterior and posterior tibial groups of muscles, by working the long flexors and extensors concentrically and tibialis anterior and posterior synergically.

In half lying attempted plantarflexion within the plaster will produce contraction of the gastrocnemius and soleus lessening atrophy if it is done vigorously and often enough. If the tendo-calcaneus has been ruptured it is, however, wiser to omit this exercise.

To exercise the intrinsic muscles of the foot the patient should try to spread the toes out and press them against a board held beneath them; he should attempt to brace the arch of the foot and should be trained to flex the metatarso-phalangeal joints with the inter-phalangeal joints extended. This is not an easy exercise to do and always requires teaching on the un-injured foot first. One method which often proves successful is to slip the finger underneath the foot from the medial side so that it presses against the heads of the second and third metatarsals. A finger of the other hand is placed lightly over the dorsum of the toes to help to keep them straight. The patient is then asked to try to lift up from the underneath finger keeping the toes and the heads of the first and fifth metatarsals down. This is repeated and repeated until the help of the fingers is no longer required. It is then tried on the injured foot with a firm support beneath the toes. It is not easy since help cannot easily be given beneath the heads of the metatarsals. An explanation of the importance of this and all the other exercises must be given.

Walking in the plaster, if permitted, will produce some contraction of the muscles, particularly if the patient tries to think of the normal pattern of walking and to press the toes against the boot.

When the plaster is removed more strengthening exercises can be added as a range of movement in the foot and ankle is now possible. Strengthening exercises for the calf will progress as in the treatment of fractures of the tibia and fibula (see p. 418).

The intrinsic muscles can be developed by exercises in sitting, pressing the toes against the ground, shortening the foot and lumbrical action. Progression is made to standing and then the patient is taught to use these muscles in walking, contracting the lumbricals as the heel is lifted so that the toes are kept flat against the ground.

To exercise the long flexors and so support the segmented lever as the heel is raised, the patient is taught in sitting to lift the heel and at the same time brace the arch. He can then progress to the same exercise in standing As soon as he can manage, exercises and walking on his toes are valuable provided there is no clawing of the toes or pain beneath the metatarsal heads. The dorsiflexors do not as a rule show as marked weakness, but they should also be exercised.

Mobility of Joints

Following most injuries in this region, especially if lengthy immobiliza-tion has been required, there is limitation of range in the joints. Rupture of tendo-calcaneus, fractures and fracture-dislocation of the ankle, particu-larly affect the ankle joint though all joints of the foot may be involved;

fractures of the calcaneus usually result in great limitation in the joints of inversion and eversion. In the latter case the foot is often not immobilized and there is great swelling. Elevation of the leg and early active movements will lessen the danger of organization of the exudates and adhesions. Usually in this case the surgeon will permit movements almost at once while the foot is being rested and particular attention must be paid to inversion and eversion.

In the event of injuries round the ankle in which a below-knee plaster is worn attempts must be made to stimulate the absorption of exudate by vigorous toe exercises, rhythmic muscular contractions and hip and knee exercises, all of which will stimulate the circulation and aid drainage.

Stiffness is not usually a trouble following sprains of the ankle or foot, but if the medial or lateral ligament have been stretched or partially torn they may become adherent to the bone over which they pass and movement may then be painful and limited. Early movement with the ligament protected by strapping and sometimes transverse frictions over the ligament should prevent the adherence.

When any form of immobilization is discarded, general mobilizing exercises are begun often preceded by wax, hot-water baths, or short-wave therapy to soften and relax the tissues. Passive mobilization of the small joints of the foot is valuable though any forcing is best avoided. The manipulations advocated by the late Dr. Mennell are particularly useful. Balance exercises are essential to help to increase the mobility both of the ankle and the foot, standing on the injured foot, walking along a line, walking on the narrow side of a form are all useful for this purpose.

Re-education of functional activities

If the patient is wearing strapping, as for a sprained ankle or a below-knee plaster for a fracture, he usually requires instruction in correct walking and managing stairs. Usually no crutches or sticks are needed, but if there is much pain and the patient cannot be encouraged to walk well, it is better to use crutches for a few days than to develop faulty habits. The simplest way to teach the patient is to let him stand between parallel bars or two steady chairs with a mirror in front and practise, getting his weight evenly distributed between the two feet. At first he will almost always put all his weight on the uninjured limb. This can often be corrected by using rhythmic stabilization, pushing him gently towards the sound side while telling him to resist this ('don't let me push you'). When he can take weight evenly on both legs then he is ready to try to take weight on the injured limb only. He is first taught to feel this on the uninjured leg by lifting the injured one off the ground; he then tries this on the injured side. When he can stand on the injured leg and flex and adduct the other hip he is ready to begin step taking. He brings the injured leg through a short distance, taking care to keep the foot pointing straight forward, and puts it on the ground; he then transfers his weight on to it and brings the other leg forward an equal distance. When he can do this without hurrying the good leg through he next learns to transfer his weight on to this foot by rocking forward on the convex sole of the boot. He is then progressed to walking with some support by the parallel bars and then with no support. Many patients can manage this in one treatment session, others require several. When the patient can walk without a limp then he is taught to climb stairs so that he is independent at home and can get on and off a bus or train.

When strapping is removed the patient usually experiences no difficulty in walking normally, but if a plaster has been worn there is stiffness of joints, weakness of muscles, sometimes pain in the foot, and fear to be contended with and training has to start again. It can be carried out in the same way, but this time he has to learn to transfer weight from the injured foot by raising the heel instead of rocking on the sole, and as he swings the leg through to dorsiflex the foot and put the heel down first. Patients vary in their ability to walk correctly quickly depending very largely on their temperament and again if they cannot master it quickly it is better to supply crutches for a short time than to allow a limp.

The patient now has to be taken much further in the exercises and he cannot be considered to be ready for discharge if he has a heavy job or one demanding use of ladders and scaffolding until he can manage these with perfect confidence. Therefore when he can walk without a limp he has to be progressed to running and jumping, to climbing stairs and then ladders and to moving about well above ground level.

The extent of the progression in the treatment depends upon the job to which the patient has to return and some of the day should be spent if possible in a workshop or occupational therapy department where he is doing work which either helps his particular disability or encourages him to forget it.

SPRAINS OF THE ANKLE

The ankle is usually sprained by a sudden unexpected twist of the foot such as might occur when walking on uneven ground, slipping off the edge of the kerb or twisting on a stone. Occasionally it is sprained as a result of a fall with the foot beneath the body, though in this case the great violence often results in a fracture-dislocation.

Most commonly it is the anterior and middle fasciculi of the lateral ligament of the ankle which are stretched, but the lateral talo-calcaneal ligament and dorsal ligaments of the lateral tarsal and tarso-metatarsal joints may all be involved. Conversely the ligaments on the medial side of the foot may be stretched if the twist is in the opposite direction.

The actual *injury* varies from a stretching of the ligament followed by sero-fibrinous exudate, to a tear of a few fibres or in severe injuries an avulsion of the ligament from the malleolus sometimes tearing off with it a flake of bone. In each injury there will be damage to the soft tissues around, with bleeding and considerable inflammatory exudate. There may also be teno-synovitis of the tendons on whichever side of the joint is involved. On examination bruising and swelling will be found around the injured region. In severe injuries this will spread up the leg and down on to the dorsum of the foot and toes. Walking is painful and there is localized tenderness, the exact spot depending on which part of the ligament is damaged. If the lateral ligament is sprained it is the anterior and middle fibres which are usually affected and the tenderness is, therefore, just in front and just below the lateral malleolus. Dorsiflexion and plantarflexion are relatively free and painless though the extreme of plantarflexion, stretching the anterior fibres, is painful. Inversion will be limited and painful.

TREATMENT

Treatment depends on the severity of the injury. *If the ligament is stretched and a few fibres only torn* there will be no loss of stability of the joint, and the main object is to get healing of the ligament without organization of the exudate, thickening of the ankle and adherence of the ligament. To attain this object the ligament must be protected from further damage and the exudate rapidly absorbed. One of the most usual ways of carrying this out is to strap the ankle with firm adhesive strapping. This gives support to the ligament and prevents sudden strains. Usually a 'stirrup' is applied from beneath the heel up either side of the ankle to the level of the tubercle of the tibia. Strips of strapping are then applied in the form of a figure of eight. While the strapping is applied the foot should be held plantargrade. To obtain quick absorption, exercise should begin at once, consequently the patient is instructed to walk in the strapping. The contraction of the muscles against the elastic resistance of the strapping has a compressing and then relaxing effect on the blood vessels, so stimulating venous and lymphatic drainage. With this method of treatment no physiotherapy is required unless the patient fails to walk correctly when encouragement and instruction will help. The strapping is removed when it begins to get loose about the tenth day and in most cases no further treatment is required. If there is residual swelling and limitation of extremes of movement, deep massage, including transverse frictions to the ligament and vigorous movements to restore full range, together with strengthening exercises to the peronei or invertors, should be used.

It will be realized that in common with most recent injuries the methods of treatment vary very greatly from one hospital to another. In some clinics the ankle is firmly bandaged instead of strapped and the patient sent to the physiotherapy department. Treatment then may be massage and active exercises or ultrasonic therapy. Massage is applied with the leg elevated to disperse the oedema and prevent adherence of the ligament. Slow deep effleurage is given to the foot and leg starting above the oedematous area and gradually encroaching on it and below. Gentle active exercises are then tried. Dorsiflexion and plantarflexion are usually free and comparatively pain free, but inversion or eversion, according to the injury, will be painful. The free movement is encouraged and the movement in the opposite direction performed within the limit of pain. The ankle is then re-bandaged and walking carefully supervised. It is better for the patient to walk slowly a short distance, with sticks or crutches if necessary, with a normal heel-toe gait, than to walk quickly unsupported, but with a stiff foot and a limp.

The day after the injury transverse frictions are applied over the damaged ligament. Kneading may also be used on the dorsum of the foot, affected side of the ankle and leg. Massage should be followed by active toe and ankle movements and inversion and eversion within the limit of pain. Gentle passive movements within the limit of pain are necessary for the small joints not voluntarily controlled; in the case of sprain of the lateral side of the foot these movements should include the calcaneo-cuboid and cubo-metatarsal joints. Treatment is not usually needed for longer than a week by which time the swelling should have subsided, movements should be full and walking normal.

If the ligament is completely torn the previous treatment will not be successful because the ligament will not heal in ten days, and if the ankle is not to lose its stability permanently the ligament must be healed. Should the ligament be completely torn, the talus is no longer held to the malleolus and every time the foot is twisted it tilts away from the bone and a gap occurs between the side of the talus and the malleolus. When the patient walks on an uneven surface momentary subluxation with pain on that side of the joint occurs and there is complaint of the ankle 'giving way' and of thickening in that region. The treatment in this type of injury is either to repair the ligament surgically or to immobilize the ankle in a weight-bearing below-knee plaster for ten weeks. Subsequent treatment will follow the lines indicated on page 428.

Chronic Sprain

If the damaged ligament heals, but with adherence to the bone, the patient will complain of puffiness of the ankle, and aching and swelling following prolonged walking or vigorous activities. On examination it is usually found that, while movements appear full, the extremes of plantarflexion and inversion are painful and limited. The treatment of choice then is deep, transverse friction to the adherent part of the ligament followed by passive mobilization and vigorous active exercises.

Recurrent Sprain

Occasionally, after a severe sprain, the patient complains of repeated 'turning over' of the ankle and inability to walk over rough ground and run and play games with any degree of confidence. This may well indicate that there has been an undetected complete tear of the ligament. If surgery is not then indicated a broadening out of the heel on the lateral side of the shoe will give greater stability and attempts should be made to hypertrophy the peroneal muscles by strong exercises. To do this the muscles must be worked against maximum resistance using springs or weights and by use of proprioceptive neuromuscular facilitation techniques. The second method is probably the more effective when the patient attends the department, but the first must be taught so that the patient can use this method at home.

RUPTURE OF TENDO-CALCANEUS

Rupture of Tendo-Calcaneus most often occurs at the narrowest point about $1\frac{1}{2}$ inches above its insertion. The fibrous sheath may remain intact and the proximal end of the tendon is retracted by spasm of the calf muscles. The sheath quickly becomes filled with blood and there is extensive swelling round the ankle from blood and inflammatory exudate.

The patient gives a history of sudden pain and a sensation of a blow on the back of the ankle during some activity. Walking is painful and there is an obvious limp. On examination there will be very weak plantarflexion produced by the long flexors of the toes, tibialis posterior and peroneus longus, but the patient is quite unable to stand on the foot and lift the heel. The prominence formed by the calf muscles lies at a higher level on the injured side and if bleeding is not too great a gap may be palpable between the separated ends of the tendon.

TREATMENT

To avoid repair of the tendon by fibrous tissue with consequent lengthening and permanent weakness, suture is essential. Relaxation of the calf muscles to relieve the strain on the suture line is necessary therefore the leg is immobilized in an above-knee plaster with the knee flexed and the foot plantarflexed for three weeks. During this period the patient uses crutches and no weight is taken on the leg. At the end of this period the plaster is changed to a weight-bearing plaster with the foot at a right angle. This is worn for three to five weeks; the plaster is then removed and the patient walks with the heel of the shoe raised to lessen the work of the calf muscles.

PHYSIOTHERAPY

During the period of immobilization physiotherapy aims at lessening the organization of the oedema, thus exercise of joints not immobilized is very important. Supervision of walking is also undertaken.

When the plaster is removed it is usual to find considerable atrophy and weakness of the calf muscles, limitation of ankle movements due to fibrous tissue formation and a limp which is the result mainly of calf weakness. Attention is concentrated on building up the strength of the calf muscles (see p. 419) and training the patient to walk with a heel-toe gait. As in all tendon ruptures movement in the opposite direction, in this case dorsi-flexion, is limited and active exercises will be needed to regain the range; passive work should not be given and attempts to stretch tendo-calcaneus are dangerous because they may result in lengthening of the fibrous repair and permanent weakening of the calf muscles.

PARTIAL RUPTURE OF THE CALF MUSCLES

Less severe trauma may cause a rupture of a few fibres of one of the bellies of gastrocnemius. This is accompanied by quite considerable bleed-ing and oedema. Plantarflexion is possible, but weak; walking is painful, and there is a limp.

TREATMENT

The injury is treated by firm strapping to limit the bleeding together with immediate use of the muscle. With the foot plantarflexed a few strips of strapping are applied around the calf and the leg is then strapped from the toes to the knee. The heel of the shoe is raised. This method of treat-ment ensures that there is little atrophy and minimum formation of scar tissue. As the muscle contracts against the strapping, fluid is squeezed out of the muscle. At the same time the muscle cannot contract fully because the heel is raised and pain on walking is, therefore, reduced.

When the strapping is removed physiotherapy is given to disperse any residual oedema, to soften and stretch out fibrous tissue in the muscle and to restore full power in the muscles and confidence in the leg. If the patient is placed in prone lying, heat and deep massage can be given to the muscle and the thickened areas on either side of tendo-calcaneus. Deep transverse frictions will stretch the fibrous tissue in the muscle. Progressive strengthening exercises and re-education of functional activities are also necessary. In the athlete it is particularly important that this injury should be treated with care. To prevent the patient losing confidence he should be encouraged to carry on with his training, with the leg strapped, but competitive sport should be forbidden until the muscle is back to normal.

Some authorities prefer to remove the strapping daily for ultrasonic therapy, but heat and massage should be avoided for the first few days because they are likely to increase the bleeding.

FRACTURES AND FRACTURE-DISLOCATION OF THE ANKLE JOINT

There are a wide variety of fractures in this region and many attempts at classification have been made. Percival Pott, in 1769, described a fracture round the ankle though it is not clear which type of fracture he was describing. For convenience all the different varieties have been included in the term Pott's fracture and according to their severity divided into three degrees. The first degree covered those injuries in which dislocation was not present, the second those in which medial or lateral displacement of the joint occurred, and the third in which separation of the inferior tibiofibular joint with lateral and upward dislocation of the foot was present. These terms are now less commonly used and classification is made according to the stress which causes the injury as well as the extent of the injury.

Sir Reginald Watson-Jones classified these injuries into five different groups and this classification is used here.

Avulsion of the ligaments without fracture is the result of inversion or eversion strains of the foot and they are treated by immobilization in a weight-bearing below-knee plaster for eight to ten weeks.

Avulsion of the ligaments with malleolar fracture is a common injury. As the ligament is ruptured it takes with it a bit of the malleolus. Often there is little or no displacement and no difference in treatment is required. If there is much displacement internal fixation by means of a nail or screw may be necessary (see Plate XXIX). This is followed by immobilization in exactly the same way as before.

Malleolar fractures without avulsion of ligaments are the result of the thrust of the talus against the malleolus. Which malleolus is fractured depends upon the direction of the thrust. If the foot is fixed and the patient twists towards the opposite side as he falls the talus is thrust against the lateral malleolus and an oblique fracture occurs. If the patient falls without twisting to the same side an abduction force is applied, producing a transverse fracture of the fibula, while if he falls to the opposite side a transverse fracture of the medial malleolus results, but if he twists as he falls to this side a spiral fracture occurs. Provided that the ligaments are not torn the stability of the ankle joint is not affected and treatment by strapping or a crepe bandage with immediate walking is all that is strictly necessary. But these fractures are painful and a below-knee weight-bearing plaster will relieve pain and give confidence with the result that the patient walks better. This is, therefore, usually applied for five or six weeks.

Fractures with lateral or postero-lateral displacement of the joint mean that there is a complete rupture of the medial ligament and, if postero-lateral, a fracture of the posterior margin of the lower end of the tibia also. The injury is produced by a violent lateral twist of the foot or a severe abduction strain. In the former injury the fracture is an oblique break of the lateral malleolus, in the latter the fibula breaks obliquely somewhere in the lower third of the shaft though it can be higher. In this injury the interosseus tibio-fibular ligament will also be torn and the lower ends of the tibia and fibula separated so that the foot is laterally and often upwardly displaced. In both cases if the patient falls forward at the same time the talus thrusts against the back of the tibia which, therefore, breaks allowing the leg bones to slide forward.

These fractures require careful reduction and prolonged immobilization to ensure healing of the ligaments and a stable ankle joint. The usual method of treatment is to apply a padded plaster cast from toes to knee, with the foot plantargrade, for ten days to three weeks according to the severity of the injury. At the end of this time the plaster is changed for an unpadded cast in which the patient can walk. This is retained for eight to ten weeks. If there has been tearing of the tibio-fibular ligaments weight-bearing is delayed for eight to ten weeks when a further three or four weeks in a weight-bearing plaster is usually necessary. This is because serious disability will be inevitable if the ligaments do not heal since the foot will gradually dislocate upwards and laterally as weight is borne. Some surgeons prefer to screw the tibia and fibula together before applying the plaster in order to lessen the danger of this occurring. Instead of immobilizing the leg for so lengthy a period, the plaster may be removed at the end of six or eight weeks and an outside iron with inside T-strap are used for another six weeks; this prevents abduction of the foot at the ankle.

Fractures with medial or postero-medial dislocation are the result of the exactly opposite injury of the previous group. The medial malleolus is fractured and the lateral ligament avulsed, often the lateral malleolus being torn off with the ligament. The posterior margin of the tibia may also be fractured. Treatment will be on exactly the same lines as the preceding group, a padded plaster cast being applied for the first three weeks, followed by an unpadded plaster, in which the patient walks, for a subsequent six or seven weeks. In this case an inside iron with outside T-strap may be substituted after six to eight weeks.

Fractures with forward displacement. These are less common injuries usually resulting from a fall on to the heels forcing the foot forwards and fracturing the anterior margin of the tibia. These fractures may require internal fixation and all are immobilized in a plaster for ten weeks. Weight-bearing is usually postponed for several weeks.

It will be noted, therefore, that in spite of the variety of injuries treatment from the physiotherapists' angle is much the same. Practically all patients are immobilized in a below-knee plaster for a varying length of time according to the nature of the injury. If the patient is allowed to bear weight he will be fitted with a boot or an iron and T-strap. When the latter is worn it can be removed for non-weight-bearing exercises, but must be worn for walking. Physiotherapy follows the points discussed at the beginning of the chapter, but particular attention should be paid to the use of the foot in standing and walking, especially when the plaster or iron and T-strap are removed. The foot is temporarily weakened by damage to ligaments and atrophy of muscles and there is, therefore, a great tendency to stand and walk with the foot turned out, which will, if allowed to persist, lead to the development of a flat foot as well as strain on the joints of the whole of the lower extremity.

FRACTURES OF THE CALCANEUS

A fall from a height on to the feet is the most common cause of fractures of the calcaneus. The severity of the injury varies from an isolated fracture of the tuberosity or sustentaculum tali without displacement to a serious compression fracture in which the tuberosity is driven up and the articular surface of the talo-calcaneal joint is crushed and comminuted and fragments driven into the body of the bone.

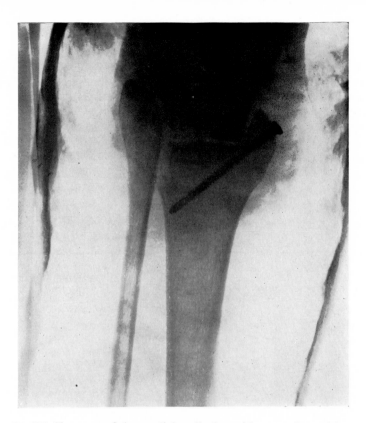

XXIX. Fracture of the medial malleolus with screw in position
(see p. 436)

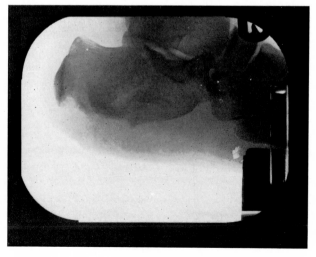

XXX. X-ray showing fracture of the os calcaneus
(see p. 439)

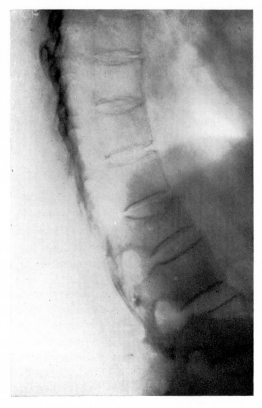

XXXI. Crush fracture of a dorsal vertebra
(*see* p. 443)

Rupture of Tendo-Calcaneus

Isolated injuries rarely cause trouble and are most often treated by protection in a weight-bearing below-knee plaster retained for six weeks and followed by a crepe bandage for a subsequent two weeks. *Compression fractures* however present certain very special problems and there is a good deal of divergence of opinion as to how they should be treated. Crushing of the bone results in broadening and shortening of the heel and this may well lead to difficulty in wearing a normal shoe. Comminution of the articular surface almost always means loss of the smooth contour and difficulty in inversion and eversion. Later there may be arthritis and sometimes peroneal spasm and flat foot. The extensive exudate which always results from these lesions to infiltrate the fibro-fatty material covering the heel and the scarring which results from its organization leads to pain and tenderness beneath the heel, making walking difficult. This is further complicated if bony irregularities form calcaneal spurs (see Plate XXX).

If the patient is young and it is possible to correct the deformity this is usually attempted and may involve the use of traction or of pins to depress the posterior fragment or elevate the central portion of the bone, This is usually followed by non-weight bearing plaster for six or eight weeks or even longer. Some surgeons apply a plaster shoe in which the pin is incorporated for four weeks. This allows early active movements. At the end of four weeks the patient is allowed to be up on crutches, but weight is not taken until union is satisfactory in eight to twelve weeks.

For older patients it is usually considered wisest to accept displacement and concentrate on preventing intra-articular adhesions, pain, and stiffness by early movements. The patient is treated in recumbency with the foot elevated and a crepe bandage applied from the toes to the knee. Massage may be given to disperse the oedema and lessen organization and active exercises are started at once. Ankle movements are usually fairly free, but inversion and eversion are very limited and special attention must be paid to these movements. If the patient cannot actively invert and evert the foot, these movements should be done very gently passively. Toe movements are valuable because they stimulate the circulation and lessen joint stiffness. When the swelling has subsided the patient is allowed up wearing a crepe or elastic bandage to prevent gravitational oedema. At first no weight is taken but after a few days he may try partial weight-bearing, progression being made according to the reaction—if there is any increase in pain, heat or swelling, the patient should not bear any weight for another one to two weeks. By this method it is hoped that moulding of the comminuted articular surface will occur and adhesion formation reduced. Results are usually good and the patient will probably be back at work in five to six months from the time of injury.

Complications

These may be dealt with in various ways. *Stiffness* of the tarsal joints has to be dealt with by repeated active exercises preceded by some form of heat. *Pain and tenderness* under the heel are often relieved by fitting into the heel of the shoe a sorbo pad into which a depression has been cut to be beneath the tender area to relieve pressure. Galvanism and massage sometimes prove helpful to soften the scar tissue which is the source of trouble. *Slackness* of the calf muscles can be overcome in the course of time by repeated exercise progressing from free and resisted exercises in half lying to heel lifting in sitting and, when the patient can take his weight, in standing. Gradually the muscles shorten and eventually the patient should be able to stand on the toes of the injured foot.

FRACTURES OF THE METATARSALS

A sudden violent inversion of the foot when the peronei are actively contracting may result in an avulsion of the tubercle at the base of the fifth metatarsal. The fracture will heal easily, but walking is painful and to avoid a limp the foot is strapped or a below-knee weight-bearing plaster is applied for three weeks.

Direct injury, such as a heavy weight falling on the foot, is liable to fracture the shaft or neck of the metatarsals. If the necks are fractured the heads may be displaced downwards and if not replaced will make walking painful. This fracture is, therefore, reduced and immobilized in a below-knee weight-bearing plaster which usually includes the toes. The plaster is retained for four weeks.

It is possible for the shaft or neck of the second or third metatarsal to be fractured spontaneously. There is no history of injury, but complaint of the sudden onset of pain in the foot. It is thought that the fracture may be due to long-continued stress such as might occur on prolonged walking if the patient is not accustomed to it. It seems particularly liable to occur if the second metatarsal is longer than the first and so takes greater strain in each 'thrust-off' in walking. The fracture heals readily and immobilization is not necessary, but to relieve pain and permit better walking the foot is strapped or immobilized in a below-knee plaster for three or four weeks.

In each case physiotherapy follows the usual plan, exercises and training of walking in the plaster or strapping and again when these are removed. When the foot is free particular attention should be paid to those muscles which support the transverse arch of the foot, the interossei and lumbricals, the adductors and flexor brevis hallucis.

Chapter XXIII

FRACTURES OF THE VERTEBRAE AND RIBS

FRACTURES OF THE SPINE

Before considering these fractures and their effects, it would be advisable to recall the parts of a single vertebra and their functions. Each vertebra consists of an anterior solid part, the body and a posterior part, the arch. The body serves to support the weight of the head and trunk. Each body is separated from its fellow by a disc of fibro-cartilage, consisting of an outer zone of concentric rings of fibrous tissue and fibro-cartilage and a central area of very elastic pulpy substance which serves to spread pressure over the whole surface of the disc. The arch is made up of four bars of bone, the two pedicles and the two laminae, which together with the posterior surface of the body, form a complete bony ring. When the vertebrae are articulated, the rings form a continuous canal which contains and protects the spinal cord and its membranes, the cauda equina and the beginning of the spinal nerves. Each arch supports seven processes, four of which are articular, while the other three are long and act as levers in movement. The spinous process acts as a lever for extension and rotation while the transverse processes provide leverage for side flexion and rotation.

If the spine is fractured, any part of the vertebra may be broken. In some fractures there will be no danger of damage to nervous tissue; in others the risk will be considerable.

Fractures of the vertebrae can be classified into two main groups; those of the vertebral body, and those of the processes.

FRACTURES OF THE PROCESSES

These involve the transverse processes more often than the spines. One or more transverse process may be torn off as a result of muscular pull.

441

Thus a patient may fall to one side and try to save himself by violent contraction of the quadratus lumborum. In so doing the lumbar processes may be simply cracked or may be wrenched off. The actual bony injury is relatively unimportant, but it is a severe, soft tissue injury because many muscle fibres will be torn, areolar tissue will be stretched, blood vessels will be ruptured and sensory nerve endings irritated. Therefore, much scar tissue is likely to form. Pain, muscle spasm, bruising and swelling will be the outstanding features.

If this injury involves only a crack without displacement, it is not treated as a fracture but as a soft tissue injury. To relieve pain and spasm and prevent further damage to soft tissues, the patient is usually confined to bed for a few days and often the lumbar region is firmly strapped for a period of three to four weeks. After a few days rest the usual principles of treatment of soft tissue injuries will be followed. *Promotion of absorption* will be aided by muscular contractions. *Prevention of muscle atrophy and loss of joint range* will be carried out by active exercises within the limit of pain. In a few weeks the condition of the tissues should be normal. If rest is not given and vigorous active work is undertaken too soon, more exudate will be caused and spinal movements will be limited and much incapacity will follow.

If the violence has been more severe and displacement of the bony fragments has occurred, then there will have been much tearing of muscle, and so a longer period of immobilization is required. A plaster jacket, extending from the buttocks to the inferior angles of the scapula, is sometimes used. As soon as the plaster is dry the patient is encouraged to resume normal activity, and physiotherapy will be carried out on lines similar to those used in fractures of the body of the vertebra which are treated in plaster (see page 444). Some surgeons prefer not to apply a plaster jacket but treat on the same lines as crack fractures without displacement.

In many fractures of the transverse processes, whether displaced or not, there may be an interference with autonomic function, presumably due to the fracture haematoma producing pressure on the sympathetic nerves. This appears as a paralytic ileus, with a feeling of fullness, distension and absent bowel sounds. In the great majority of cases it will respond to conservative treatment of gastric suction and intravenous fluids.

A similar lesion may occur in fractures involving the vertebral bodies.

FRACTURES OF THE BODY

These fractures are nearly always the result of forcible flexion of the spine, though very occasionally hyperextension produces the injury. The site is usually at the junction of a mobile segment with a relatively immobile one, hence at lumbo-dorsal or cervico-dorsal junctions. Most common of all are fractures of the body of the twelfth dorsal and first lumbar vertebrae. If an individual falls from a height on to the buttocks or feet, the spine will be slightly flexed and the vertical compression force will compress the bodies of several vertebrae. The bodies will become wedge-shaped by the elastic disc will remain unharmed (see Plate XXXI). Little, if any, damage of ligaments occurs and the fracture is stable with no danger of displacement or dislocation. A different type of injury is produced in cases in which the spine is suddenly and acutely flexed. This often occurs when a miner, working in a stoop position, sustains a heavy fall of coal on to his back from the roof. Sharp angulation occurs and the vertebra, at the maximum point of angulation, is comminuted. The anterior part of the lower margin of the vertebra above is driven into the upper surface of the comminuted vertebral body below. In this case the intervertebral disc must be damaged and permanent thinning of the disc space will result. There will also be momentary dislocation of the articular facets with considerable damage to the ligaments so that this fracture is not a stable one.

In a third group of cases the force falling on the flexed spine is moving forward and so drives one segment of the vertebral column forward on the one below. In this case dislocation will occur, either the laminae or the pedicles being fractured, or the articular processes being dislocated. These dislocations are liable to be complicated by damage to the spinal cord or cauda equina. Such damage may also occur if the vertebral body is comminuted in acute flexion and a fragment of bone is displaced back into the vertebral canal.

Treatment of these fractures depends on whether they are wedge compression fractures and therefore stable, comminuted and unstable, or fracture-dislocations.

In most cases, reduction of the fracture is obtained by hyperextending the spine, because this exerts a stretch on the anterior longitudinal ligament which is firmly attached to the margins of the vertebral bodies and to the intervertebral discs. As the ligament is stretched, it, working on the pivot provided by the articular processes, pulls out the bodies and corrects the compression and wedging. If there is fracture or dislocation of the articular processes, this would be dangerous because the pivot is no longer available and open reduction may be necessary.

COMPRESSION FRACTURES

These are not usually immobilized. The patient is kept in bed for a month, lying flat on a firm mattress over fracture boards. At the end of this period he is usually allowed to sit up and walk and he should be able to return to work by twelve weeks after the injury.

Physiotherapy during the period of recumbency aims at maintaining the strength of the spinal muscles. For the first two weeks the exercises are done in the lying position and include such work as back arching, head pressing back, rhomboid, abdominal and gluteal contractions, foot and breathing exercises. At the end of a fortnight it is usual to allow the patient to roll into the prone-lying position and in this position back and hip extension exercises can be progressed.

When the patient begins to get up, extension exercises are progressed and stress is now laid on correct sitting and standing postures and relieving strain on the back by training the patient in correct lifting.

Usually at six to eight weeks easy side flexion, rotation and flexion exercises are begun, though some surgeons do not permit flexion exercises.

COMMINUTED FRACTURES

These fractures are usually immobilized in a plaster jacket applied with the patient in hyperextension. Its extent depends upon the level of the lesion. If the first lumbar or the twelfth dorsal vertebra is fractured, the jacket will extend, on the anterior aspect from symphysis pubis to supra-sternal notch and on the posterior aspects from the cleft of the buttocks to the inferior angles of the scapulae. If the injury is a fracture in the upper part of the vertebral column, it may be necessary to carry the plaster up to the neck and over the top of the head and in front up to the chin. An alternative method is to arthrodese two or three vertebrae. In this case the patient is treated on a plaster bed for two to three months and this is followed by a light plaster corset and later by a back-brace. The aims of physiotherapy if the patient is treated in a plaster jacket are similar to those for any fracture immobilized in plaster.

If the spine is immobilized for some months, the *spinal muscles will be liable to atrophy*. It is, therefore, essential to exercise the back and abdominal muscles throughout the period of fixation. This can be done by rhythmic contractions and attempts to perform movements pressing against the plaster. Both groups of muscles may also be exercised statically by active exercises of the head and hips, the former, provided that the fracture is not a high one, necessitating plaster extending over the head. Some of the positions which can be used are lying and crook lying, prone lying and knee sitting, stoop sitting and standing. Quite heavy exercise may be obtained by weight lifting while the jacket is being worn. It is particularly important that the spinal muscles should be maintained in good condition as they have to support the spine when the plaster is removed. In cases in which immobilization is not used, spinal exercises will still be necessary, as bed rest is usual for several weeks, and full function of back and abdominal muscles will not therefore be obtained. It is particularly important, if a plaster is not worn, that spinal muscles should be strong.

Owing to the extent of the plaster, respiration may be impaired. It is therefore very *important to encourage as full movements of the thorax* as possible. The patient should be taught to gain maximum expansion and recoil by pressing out against the plaster and withdrawing the walls of the thorax from it. Deeper respiration can be encouraged by the use of light activities and games which can be adequately performed in plaster jackets.

In the very early days, if a plaster jacket is worn, the patient may find balance and walking difficult, owing to the hyperextended position, and *sitting and walking will need help and teaching.*

Reasonable *mobility* will be maintained by the use of static contractions within the plaster and full range movement of the joints which are not enclosed. The more games and activities which can be used the better, as they will stimulate general circulation. In those cases which are not immobilized, spinal exercises are gradually progressed and mobility maintained. Extension exercises are usually given first in lying and prone lying. When the patient is allowed to sit up, trunk side-flexion and rotation exercises are gradually introduced.

When a plaster is removed there will be found to be some atrophy of spinal muscles and some limited movement of the spine. The patient has acquired the habit of bending the trunk by flexion at the hips, and it will be a habit difficult to break now that the spine can be used. Hence an important principle is to encourage the *restoration of normal spinal movements* and restore the correct method of movement. This can be carried out by the use of active exercises, both strengthening and mobilizing, particularly concentrating on those which obtain movement in the affected region of the spine. Games are of great value in the later stages; swimming, football and netball are all of value. Patients who will be returning to heavy work should go on to outdoor activities; digging, sawing and mowing can all be used. If a really good course of treatment is followed, the patient should be able to return to work within two to three months of the removal of the plaster.

FRACTURE-DISLOCATIONS WITHOUT DAMAGE TO THE SPINAL CORD OR CAUDA EQUINA

These fractures are usually treated by open reduction followed by plaster immobilization for four months, and physiotherapy resembles that of the preceding group.

FRACTURE DISLOCATIONS WITH SPINAL CORD OR CAUDA EQUINA LESIONS

These are one of two types. Either conductivity is temporarily impaired as a result of shock, contusion or stretching without destruction of nerve cells or fibres; or there is laceration of nerve tissue with much permanent loss of function. The final result depends on the type of injury and the level at which it has occurred. If the injury has not destroyed nerve tissue, then fairly rapid recovery, beginning in two to three weeks, is most probable. If the damage is destructive, then recovery depends upon whether the cord or the nerves have been involved. If the cord has been damaged, no recovery of destroyed tissue will occur, since nerve cells and nerve fibres without a neurilemma cannot recover. If nerves outside the cord have been lacerated recovery should occur, as they have a nuerillemma and their cells are intact. The recovery may not, however, be complete.

The level of injury makes quite a considerable difference. In the upper dorsal region the spinal cord almost completely fills the vertebral canal. Forward displacement of the body of the vertebra, therefore, will result in crushing of the cord between the lamina of the vertebra above and the upper border of the body of the vertebra below. Serious and generally irreparable damage usually results. In the upper lumbar region the vertebral canal is larger and the cord consequently has more room to move, hence less damage is likely to result. Below the level of the first lumbar vertebra the nerves of the cauda equina occupy the vertebral canal. These nerves form a less solid structure and are more mobile, and so, though they may be contused or stretched, the whole cauda equina is rarely transected.

Injury to nervous tissue may therefore be severe or slight, permanent or only very temporary. The immediate result of damage, however slight or severe, is cessation of function due to shock. Below the level of injury there will be complete flaccid paralysis, loss of all forms of sensation, retention of urine, loss of reflexes and disturbance of circulation. At the level of the injury there may be hyperaesthesia. If the cord has been contused only, gradual recovery beginning in the first few weeks will be seen and full recovery is to be expected. If some destruction of cells and fibres has taken place, full recovery is not to be expected. There will then be mild residual paralysis and sensory loss.

In cases in which the cord has been completely crushed or divided, recovery of function is impossible. After a varying period, often about three weeks, the area of spinal cord below the level of the lesion will recover from spinal shock and begin to function again, although it cannot receive any message from any part of the brain. The result of this return to function, uncontrolled by higher centres, is the restoration of reflex movements and the onset of flexor and adductor spasticity, with the continued absence of voluntary movement and all forms of sensation. With the onset of flexor and adductor spasticity and the loss of voluntary movement, adaptive shortening of the fibro-elastic elements of the flexor and adductor muscles tends to take place. This results in irritation of muscle and tendon sensory end organs and flexor spasms become still more frequent. If great care is not taken, deformities develop which will make impossible the wearing of splints and consequently debar the patient from ever walking again. Profound atrophy of muscles inevitably occurs as voluntary movement is impossible and joints rapidly become stiff, if suitable steps are not taken to prevent this from occurring. The extensive disturbance of circulation, so characteristic of the first few weeks, gradually lessens as subsidiary spinal vasomotor centres become established and the development of pressure sores is not now so likely. Incontinence of urine and faeces will be present since these become purely reflex.

Contusion of the cauda equina is usually followed by rapid recovery. More severe injuries will have caused damage to some of the nerve fibres forming the cauda equina. The lower the level of the lesion the less damage will have occurred, since many fibres will have already left the vertebral canal. In such lesions, therefore, the iliopsoas, adductors and quadriceps muscles may easily have escaped paralysis. Muscles supplied by damaged nerves will remain flaccidly paralysed and cutaneous sensibility will be lost, but recovery is possible as, with nerve cells intact, growth of the proximal segment of the fibres will take place. A long time may elapse between the start of growth and the stage of recovery as there will be a considerable distance to span. As much as two years may elapse. Consequently perfect recovery is unlikely since during this time, degeneration and atrophy of all structures supplied by the nerves is liable to occur. In rare cases the cauda equina is irreparably damaged and a permanent flaccid paraplegia results.

If the spinal cord or cauda equina are damaged, immobilization in a plaster jacket or on a plaster bed is unsafe. This is because in the first few weeks vaso-motor control is lost and pressure sores can, therefore, develop very rapidly. Once developed, the fluid and protein loss from the open wound leads to serious deterioration in the patient's general condition. The patient is nursed on a sorbo mattress in the supine and side-lying positions, great care being taken to avoid bad positions and pressure on bony points. In the supine position a single pillow is used beneath the head, a pillow under the back maintains the spine in hyperextension and a firm pillow at the feet maintains dorsiflexion. In side-lying the under leg is protected by a pillow and one or two pillows are placed between the legs. The prone position is not used unless sores are already present when prone-lying, side-lying and lying on specially prepared and placed packs are used.

The patient is turned every two hours by a specially trained team of four. They stand on the same side, one supporting the head, one the shoulders, one the pelvis, and the fourth the legs. They lift together so that no movement of the spine occurs.

Very great care of the skin, bladder and bowels is necessary. These are at first dealt with by the nursing staff, but later the patient is taught how to help himself.

The physiotherapist forms part of the team of experts helping to train the patient to regain independence. Certain special objects can be fulfilled by passive movements and exercises.

Contractures and deformities must be prevented, circulation in the paralysed limbs must be maintained, vaso-motor control must be re-established and unaffected muscles must be hypertrophied to compensate for those paralysed. In addition the patient must be taught how to carry out the ordinary daily activities such as feeding, dressing, attending to toilet needs, moving from bed to chair and chair to car, standing and, in most cases, walking.

Prevention of contractures and deformities. Within a day or two of the accident passive movements of all joints of the paralysed limbs are begun. These are carried out slowly and carefully two or three times in full range, twice daily. Not only do these movements prevent contractures and stiff joints but they also stimulate the circulation and lessen the tendency to flexor spasm.

Vaso-motor control. Control of the blood vessels is temporarily lost and the effect is particularly noticeable in high thoracic lesions since the great splanchnic vascular area can no longer be constricted when the patient moves from the horizontal to the vertical position. For this reason when the patient is first allowed to sit and stand he is liable to faint. Hobson points out that this can be overcome by developing other vascular reflexes. This is done by constant changes of posture, deep breathing exercises and, where possible, by abdominal contractions. When the patient is allowed to sit up at eight to ten weeks, constant changes from lying to sitting and swinging exercises with the pelvis and legs suspended are most valuable.

Hypertrophy of unaffected muscles. If the lesion is above the sixth thoracic segment the spine, pelvis and legs will have to be moved by means of the latissimus dorsi, trapezius and shoulder girdle muscles. The latissimus dorsi is particularly important because it is innervated from the lower cervical segments while it is attached as low as the pelvis and lower vertebrae. A strong triceps is also necessary to prevent the elbows 'buckling' when the body and legs are lifted by the arms.

A few days after the injury, therefore, these muscles are exercised by drawing the arms down against the resistance of springs. The movements are bilateral so that an equal pull is exerted on the spine and movement of the vertebral column does not occur.

When the patient is allowed to sit up stronger exercises are given, one of the most effective being swinging and holding with the pelvis and legs suspended.

Balance in sitting. To begin with patients find it very difficult to sit, partly because of the paralysis of the muscles which normally control the spine and pelvis and partly because of the loss of all forms of sensation below the level of the lesion. Gradually the patient can learn to balance by making fuller use of the sensory messages, received from latissimus dorsi or any other intact spinal muscles.

Training begins by teaching the patient to see his position in the mirror, gradually he learns to feel it by keeping his eyes shut. By degrees balance no longer has to be thought of as he is trained to do simple movements in sitting, progressing until he can move the head, arms and trunk freely without losing his balance.

Balance in standing. The patient is taught to get up from the chair between parallel bars and stand with the shoulders well back and the hips extended. At first he requires assistance to steady his feet and keep his hips extended but gradually he can manage without. He will wear back splints or calipers and use a mirror in his practice. Balance is gradually gained in the same way as in sitting and when he can stand and balance with only finger-tip support he is ready to start walking.

Treatment is not complete until the patient is able to do all that is possible according to the level of the lesion. Many patients are able, when trained, to get in and out of the wheeled chair, manage their toilet needs, get in and out of a car and go up and down steps. Eventually as the paraplegic improves he can join in games and activities and learn a suitable occupation so that many patients are able to pursue a remunerative job.

FRACTURE OF THE RIBS

Fracture of one or more ribs may be the result of direct violence such as a fall on or against a hard object. The rib is then fractured at the site of the application of force. Alternatively it may be the result of a violent crushing force, such as when a patient is pinned against a wall by a heavy vehicle. In this case several ribs may be broken and they usually fracture at their point of maximum convexity near the angle of the rib. Very occasionally muscular violence, as in a sudden attack of coughing, may fracture a rib.

There is usually little displacement, though occasionally one fragment may be driven inwards to perforate the pleura and the lung.

Fixation is not, as a rule, required, since adequate immobilization is obtained by the intercostal muscles, but, as respiration produces movement and therefore pain at the fracture site, either Novocain may be injected to relieve the pain or strapping may be applied while the chest is in the position of expiration. This will be retained for seven to ten days.

Physiotherapy is not essential, but, sometimes when the strapping is removed, full use of the chest is not recovered and the patient complains of neuralgic pain. This can be relieved by a course of breathing exercises which aim at teaching the patient lateral costal breathing. They should be continued until the patient has full control of the thorax and neuralgic pain is no longer present.

CRANIOCEREBRAL INJURIES

These injuries have been discussed in Chapter XI (see p. 212).

Chapter XXIV

AMPUTATIONS

The majority of amputations are carried out in cases of peripheral vascular disorder, most of these in elderly patients. Amputation may also be necessary if a limb has been so badly damaged that it is impossible to save it, or if life may be endangered by its continued presence. Such damage might be caused by a severe accident or by gunshot or blast wounds. Malignant growths in the limbs usually need amputation. Amputation may also be necessary in some cases of acute infection which have not responded to treatment, particularly in the case of gas gangrene which, if the condition spreads, would endanger life.

With the exception of amputation of the leg for vascular disorders, if the uninjured limb is healthy, progress should be rapid, and the patient, using an artificial limb, should soon be ambulant.

If it is necessary to amputate a limb because of peripheral vascular disease certain special problems arise. The other limb would almost certainly be affected and will require treatment to improve its blood supply and delay the time at which amputation may be necessary. It does sometimes happen, however, that when one limb has to be amputated the circulation and condition of the other improves. Since the patients are elderly and circulation impaired it is vital that they are encouraged to be active as soon as possible after the operation, but these patients are less able to undertake vigorous exercise and this has to be borne in mind when post-operative physiotherapy is planned.

SITE OF AMPUTATION

If it is possible to choose the site at which amputation will be carried out the surgeon selects a position which will give a stump long enough to take an artificial limb and use it satisfactorily and yet one which is not too long, since there is often trouble with the circulation of a long stump. While modern prostheses can be made to fit almost any length of stump, a reasonable length is necessary to provide a lever to use the appliance, and for this reason the surgeon will plan to leave ten to twelve inches of femur

451

or five to six inches of tibia and four to five inches of fibula. In the upper limb eight inches of humerus and seven to eight inches of the radius and ulna, measured from the tip of the olecranon will give a most satisfactory stump. In some lower limbs a trans-knee amputation is carried out. This is particularly suitable for elderly patients since disarticulation takes only about half an hour and is therefore accompanied by much less surgical shock than if the amputation is done through the femur. In addition since the femur and its cartilages are intact the proprioceptive sense will be normal and the patient will know where his foot is in space. Alternately the amputation is carried out just proximal to the condyles. The periosteum is detached two inches distal to the site of amputation of the femur and then sewn over the end of the bone. Flexors and extensors, and adductors and fascia lata are sutured to each other thus avoiding the danger of contractures. The patella is incorporated so that weight is taken on it. Thus has the advantage of a less bulky stump, but the disadvantage of taking longer to carry out with more shock and giving a smaller weight-bearing surface.

PYLONS AND ARTIFICIAL LIMBS

In many lower-limb amputations a pylon is fitted about six weeks after the operation and this is worn until the stump has finished shrinking. The patient is then measured for an artificial limb which is supplied eight to ten weeks later. If the amputation is bilateral, short rocker pylons are worn for some months and often when artificial limbs are fitted they are made so that final height of the patient is three inches less than before the amputation. This depends on the condition of the cardiovascular system since the use of long legs is a greater strain and can affect the blood pressure.

A different approach is sometimes made in order to speed up rehabilitation. Immediately after the operation a plaster socket is applied. This has a metal junction to which an adjustable pylon tube with a foot can be attached. As soon as the surgeon permits, often twenty-four hours after the operation, the temporary pylon tube and foot is fitted to the socket and the patient is trained to stand, balance and walk with elbow crutches. At about twelve to fourteen days the plaster socket is removed and the patient is fitted with a leg having a metal socket and pelvic band suspension.

When an arm has to be amputated an artificial limb is fitted as early as possible, but while the patient is waiting for this he is trained to use the stump. Various pieces of equipment can be attached to it by plaster, strapping or leather gauntlets. By this means he gets accustomed to finding the stump useful and will then make better progress when the artificial limb is supplied.

Amputations

POST-OPERATIVE CARE

In lower limb amputations the patient is nursed lying supine on a firm mattress over fracture boards, with the stump flat on the bed. If a plaster socket has been fitted discomfort may be felt at the upper posterior border of the plaster. A small pillow is then placed under the buttock but it must not extend beneath the plaster. There is a tendency for both above- and below-knee stumps to flex. This is prevented in the former case by a roller towel and sandbags and in the latter by a posterior splint. In the above-knee amputation the patient should be prone several times each day to prevent flexion contracture.

Patients who have not been fitted with a plaster socket usually get up when the sutures have been removed. During the period in bed and before the pylon is fitted measures are taken to prepare the patient for the wearing of the pylon and later of the artificial limb. Very great care is given to the development of a stump which is ideal for the wearing and use of the artificial limb. The ideal stump is one which is rounded in shape, the skin should be free from folds and the end of the stump firm. The wound must be soundly healed, mobile and painless. The circulation should be well established.

Before the artificial limb is supplied shrinkage of the stump should be complete. This is aided by a system of bandaging or by the immediate fitting of a plaster socket. If a plaster socket is fitted bandaging will only be necessary at night or if the temporary pylon has to be removed during the day, but in this case, to prevent the stump becoming oedematous and the wound breaking down, care must be taken when the patient is moved to push the socket gently but firmly upwards.

Good condition of the skin is achieved by teaching the patient how to care for it. He is taught to wash the stump regularly and if there is any scaling at the end to massage in a few drops of vegetable oil.

For good use of the limb, there should be full range of movement at the proximal joints and no contractures should have developed. Certain muscle groups must be particularly strong. In an above-knee amputation the extensors and adductors are particularly important and the quadriceps if the amputation is below or through the knee. Exercises are therefore begun immediately after the operation.

In all cases the unaffected limb must be kept in good condition and trunk and arm muscles must be developed.

When the pylon is fitted the patient has to be taught to stand, balance, walk, fall and get up from the floor, get in and out of the bath, walk on uneven and inclined surfaces, manage stairs and take off and put on the pylon. Eventually he has to be taught to use the artificial limb.

Amputations

PART PLAYED BY THE PHYSIOTHERAPIST

Physiotherapy has the following aims: to assist in the shrinkage of the stump; to help in the prevention of contractures; to ensure full range of movement in the proximal joints; to strengthen muscles acting on the stump; to help to improve the patient's physical fitness and strengthen the unaffected limbs and trunk muscles. In addition she will train the patient in everyday activities and teach him how to care for the stump and use the pylon and artificial limb.

Shrinkage of the Stump. The stump must fit the socket firmly if the patient is to use the limb well and the socket must not rapidly become loose. Immediately after the operation it is often bulky and oedematous, though the size will decrease as traumatic oedema subsides and the muscular tissue atrophies. Rapid reduction in size and increased firmness is achieved by bandaging, since this reduces oedema and aids venous return. Two six-inch crepe bandages are required for an above-knee amputation (two four-inch ones for a below-knee and above-elbow and two three-inch ones for a below-elbow amputation). These should be firmly sewn together and rolled into one. The bandage is put on with the patient lying flat. The first turn begins in the groin, is taken down the front of the stump, over the centre of the end, up the back to the gluteal fold where both this end and the first are held by the patient's fingers and thumb. It is then carried down the back over the medial side of the end, up the front to the groin where it is grasped by the patient, then down the front to the lateral side of the end and up the back to be fixed again. It is now taken round the top of the thigh, not too tightly, to secure the previous turns. It is then brought obliquely down the back of the thigh to the lowest part of the lateral side of the stump. A figure-of-eight is then made up the thigh and around the waist (see Fig. 45). The same method is used for a below-knee stump, two four-inch bandages being used.

In applying this bandage, it is essential that certain rules should be followed. Briefly they comprise the following points: the bandage must be taken right up to the groin so that a roll of flesh does not form above it, which would later hang over the socket of the artificial limb; it must be taken round the waist so that it is anchored and does not slip down, but it must not hold the stump flexed; care should be taken to place the crossings of the figure-of-eight turns towards the lateral side of the thigh and so prevent pulling the stump into flexion; the bandage must be applied so as to exert pressure on the end and sides of the stump and the soft tissues should be compressed upwards and laterally; care must be taken to exert even pressure so that one particularly tight turn of bandage does not obstruct venous and lymphatic return causing oedema distally and the development of a 'waist' in the stump. Pressure should be greatest at the lower end of the stump and very gradually decrease as the turns of bandage reach the groin. Bandaging should be started as soon as the wound is healed, though it may be some days before maximum tension can be obtained. The bandage should be reapplied four times a day and must be worn until the pylon is fitted and then it must be applied at night or any time in the day when for some reason the pylon or artificial limb is removed.

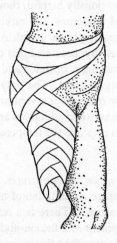

FIG. 45. STUMP BANDAGE

Even if the patient has worn an artificial limb for many years, if he is unable for some reason to wear it for even a very short time, the stump will increase in size, as much as two inches, if it is not bandaged and it will take six to eight weeks to get it back to its original size. It is usually necessary to teach a relative how to apply the bandage.

Certain affections of the stump are liable to occur, though some of these can be avoided if care is taken. One difficulty is the tendency for boils and sore areas to occur in the groin. The best way to avoid these is to keep the skin scrupulously clean. Sometimes the circulation of the stump is defective and stump exercises are probably the best way of dealing with this. Massage should be avoided as it never appears to be helpful and it sometimes seems to irritate. Short wave treatment to the stump may prove of value.

Tenderness and pain in the stump may be a very troublesome feature and may be localized owing to a tender neuroma, or generalized when its origin is unknown. Each of the nerves will develop a terminal enlargement known as a neuroma. These are tender on pressure for some weeks after the amputation, but they gradually lose their sensitiveness. Occasionally a neuroma will become sensitive again if the skin is adherent to the underlying soft tissues when the artificial limb is worn. Massage of an adherent scar may help to free it, and although it is always difficult to loosen, the special manipulations advocated for loosening scar tissue should be used. It has been found that vibrations applied to the end of the stump with the mechanical vibrator are occasionally helpful, though it is not clear in what way they help. Generalized tenderness can rarely be successfully treated, though ultra sound occasionally proves useful. Another method is hypnosis. The patient is taught self-hypnosis and this often results not in totally relieving the pain, but in making it bearable and ensuring that it does not prevent the patient sleeping at night. The only really successful way to deal with the problem is by means of a myoplastic operation in which the flexors and extensors, abductors and adductors are sutured over the end of the stump. This appears to improve the temperature of the stump and its circulation.

Mobility of joints and prevention of contractures. An artificial limb cannot easily be fitted or worn if there is limitation of movement in the proximal joint, or if there are contractures. There is a tendency in an above-knee amputation for the development of a flexion-abduction deformity. This is due to the fact that the majority of the flexors and abductors have not been cut at the operation, whereas both the extensors and adductors have been grossly affected. The flexors also are much stronger than the extensors. This deformity must be prevented. Exercises are started as soon as the surgeon permits, often within a few days of the operation. Some surgeons prefer only passive movements of the hip to be given for the first five days on the grounds that there is a large painful wound and the patient will be unwilling to move the stump actively. In an above-knee amputation the patient should to asked to turn into the prone position for extension of the hip which should be practised in this position many times a day. The position will help check the tendency to flexion deformity. This position may not be possible in cases of arterio-sclerosis with high blood pressure, and side-lying with the head and shoulders raised should then be used. Progression may be made when the wound is healed by adding resistance to extension and adduction and by changing the starting position to standing. A careful watch should be kept that the movement is really taking place in the hip joint and not occurring by tilting of the pelvis.

In a below-knee amputation a flexion deformity tends to develop; progressive exercises should be given to strengthen the quadriceps muscle.

A full range of shoulder joint and shoulder girdle is particularly important if the amputation is above the elbow. An adduction-medial rotation deformity is liable to occur. Exercises should begin at once to maintain range and strengthen the abductors and lateral rotators. If the amputation is below the elbow both flexion and extension are necessary and these movements should be practised.

Strengthening of stump muscles. All the stump muscles must be strong and resisted work should begin as soon as the wound is healed. In the above-knee amputation the extensors and adductors must be particularly strong because they are essential to help in the correct use of the artificial limb. When the patient brings the limb forward, the strong abductors tend to swing it into abduction. He has therefore to adduct the stump strongly in the socket to prevent this. If the limb has a knee joint, in order to lock it in extension, the patient presses the heel against the ground at the end of the forward swing and then strongly extends the stump against the socket. Thus the extensors must be particularly strong. To hypertrophy these muscles, progressive resisted work is used and both movements can be carried out by work against springs or weights. Great care is again necessary when extending against weights to prevent the movement being performed by a forward tilting of the pelvis. In the below-knee amputation special attention is given to the extensors. In the upper limb—according to the level of amputation—the abductors and medial rotators of the shoulder or the flexors and extensors of the elbow are progressively strengthened.

Sensation. When the patient begins to use a pylon he finds difficulty in balance, because he is used to knowing his position as a result of sensations from the soles of his feet and the joints of the lower extremity. He has now to train himself to recognize his position by the position of the stump in the socket. Before the limb is worn, there is not a great deal which can be done, except by teaching him to think of the position of the stump and to feel objects with it; but when the limb is fitted, he is taught to sense the position of the stump in the socket in various positions of the leg and must not, therefore, be allowed to look down at the leg even when he first gets on his feet.

Balance. If a limb, probably weighing about twenty-eight pounds, is removed, it must inevitably upset the balance of the body. When the patient first sits up, the stump tends to flex and leave the support and the

457

patient tends to fall back. He must be taught therefore to sit slightly forward and press the thigh against the bed or chair. When he can do this he can progress to simple exercises in sitting.

At about the tenth to twelfth day he is often allowed to stand. He is taught to stand holding on to the bed-end or the back of a steady chair and to try to stand up straight and adjust his weight over the remaining leg. He then has to try to balance without support for an increasing length of time, provided that the remaining leg is fit enough to allow this. When he has mastered this stage, he can try arm exercises in standing. If he can stand unsupported, he will master crutch-walking without fear. Balance will always be better if the general musculature is good and, provided that the physical condition of the patient is suitable, exercises are therefore given to strengthen the back and abdominal muscles.

Co-ordination. In order to avoid the mental discarding of the stump, the repugnance of it and therefore the inability to use the artificial limb properly, the term 'stump' should be avoided in talking to the patient and the words 'right' and 'left' arm or leg should be used. All exercises should include the remaining limb where possible, so that, with the exception of the special resisted work, exercises should be alternate, reciprocal or bilateral. Reciprocal movements are particularly important and stress should be laid on the use of this method in home exercises and care should be taken to see that the patient understands the reason.

The remaining limbs. If a leg has to be amputated and the other leg is not in a good condition, or if it is affected by vascular disease, and if the arms are not strong or their circulation is impaired, appropriate measures should be taken. Treatment given prior to amputation for impoverished circulation should continue as soon as the patient is fit enough. Thus Buerger's exercise may be recommenced after two to three weeks. If the leg is in very poor condition, crutch walking may impose too great a strain on its circulation and the patient will not then be able to walk. The treatment of the trunk and arms then becomes most important, as the patient must be as independent as possible. If the arm, shoulder girdle and trunk muscles are strengthened, he will be able to move himself about from bed to wheeled chair. A careful note must of course be made as to the condition of the heart and blood pressure, as occasionally strong work of any sort cannot be undertaken.

Walking. The patient usually gets up when the wound is healed or at about seven days. If a plaster socket has been applied immediately he may be allowed up as early as twenty-four hours later. In the former case training follows the usual routine, first training balance between the parallel rails, then progressing to taking steps. When he can walk with crutches he is taught how to sit down and stand up, manage stairs, walk on uneven surfaces and get up from the floor. When the pylon is fitted training starts again first in between the rails then with one rail and one stick, then two sticks in the rails, then two sticks and out of the rails. It is important at this point to teach the patient to bring the pylon only up to the toe of the good leg instead of, as he tends to do, taking a longer stride with the pylon. This ensures that his weight is taken over the dead centre of the top of the pylon so that the balance is correct. Gradually as his confidence increases the stride can be lengthened.

If a temporary pylon tube and foot are used the patient is assisted out of bed as soon as the surgeon permits. While this is being done the prosthesis is supported and gently pressed upwards, otherwise the socket does not remain in firm contact and the stump becomes oedematous and the wound may break down. The patient is encouraged to stand taking as much weight as possible but supported by a nurse and a physiotherapist. The pylon foot is slightly behind the other leg so that the weight is taken through the ischial tuberosity. On the first day the patient should stand for about five minutes and this may be repeated three times. As soon as the patient can stand with elbow crutches he is taught to transfer weight from one leg to the other, and by three to four days he should be taking a few steps. When the pylon with metal socket and pelvic suspension is fitted the same method is followed. Once the patient can walk with elbow crutches treatment is progressed as in the former method—training walking on uneven surfaces, on an incline, up and down stairs, getting up from the floor and all activities of daily living.

SPECIAL POINTS IN RELATION TO OTHER AMPUTATIONS

In below-knee amputations the principles of physical treatment are the same. The tendency to a flexor contracture has to be watched, since this would make it difficult to wear a limb. As the position of rest is with the knee slightly flexed, it is important to see that the knee is kept straight after the amputation, and, if necessary, a back splint should be worn for a few days. As soon as exercises are permitted, active extension must be encouraged. The muscle which particularly requires strengthening is the quadriceps, because the knee will flex by gravity, but the quadriceps will be required to extend it. Thus progressive strengthening exercises are essential.

In an above-elbow amputation the essential feature is to obtain a full range of movement in the shoulder joint and joints of the shoulder girdle, as, without this, the artificial limb cannot be fully used. Great care must be taken, therefore, to keep these joints mobile. Exercises are usually begun rather earlier than in the leg, often twenty-four hours after the operation. An adduction-medial rotation deformity is liable to occur and the abductor and lateral rotator muscles require attention.

If the amputation is below the elbow, both flexion and extension are necessary and these movements should be developed, beginning when the sutures are out.

Arm amputees can usually be fitted with the limb early. This is valuable, because the longer the patient remains with one arm only, the better will he manage to be independent and the less co-operative will he be in learning to use an artificial limb, which is always a difficult procedure. For this reason, these patients are usually sent to residential limb-fitting centres and it is rare for the physiotherapist to be required to train the patient in the use of an upper limb prosthesis.

BIBLIOGRAPHY

AMPUTATION

Amputation and Artificial Limbs, by R. D. Langdale Kelham and George Perkins (Oxford University Press).
The Rehabilitation of Amputees (Her Majesty's Stationery Office).
Rehabilitation of the Lower Limb Amputee, by W. Humm (Baillière, Tindall and Cassell).

ANATOMY

Anatomy, Regional and Applied, by R. J. Last (J. and A. Churchill).
Cunningham's Text Book of Anatomy, edited by J. C. Brash (Oxford Medical Publications).
A Method of Anatomy, by J. C. Boileau Grant (Baillière, Tindall and Cassell).
Principles of Anatomy as seen in the Hand, by F. Wood-Jones (Baillière, Tindall and Cassell).

BURNS

A New Approach to the Treatment of Burns and Scalds, by L. Colebrook (Fine Technical Publications).
Burns and their Treatment, by I. F. K. Muir and T. L. Barclay (Lloyd-Luke).
Physical Methods in Plastic Surgery, by Joseph P. Reidy (Actinic Press).

DISEASES OF THE CHEST AND THORACIC SURGERY

A Clinical Introduction to Heart Disease, by C. Bramwell (Oxford University Press).
An Introduction to Congenital Heart Disease, by L. Schamroth and F. Segal (Blackwell).
An Introduction to Surgery, by Geoffrey Flavell (Oxford University Press).
'Extra-corporeal circulation', by P. E. Ghadiali, Brompton Hospital—Physiotherapy for Medical and Surgical Thoracic Conditions, 19.
'Surgical Treatment of Tetralogy of Fallot', by H. H. Bentall, from *Recent Advances in Surgery* (Churchill).

Bibliography

'The Surgery of the Aortic Valve' by W. P. Cleland, from *Recent Advances in Surgery* (Churchill)

Thoracic Surgery for Physiotherapists, by G. M. Storey (Faber).

DISEASES OF THE EAR, NOSE AND THROAT

Diseases of the Ear, Nose and Throat, by H. Ludman (Pitman Medical and Scientific Publishing Co. Ltd.).

Diseases of the Nose, Throat and Ear, by I. S. Hall (Livingstone).

DISEASES OF THE NERVOUS SYSTEM AND NEUROSURGERY

Anatomy of the Human Body, by R. D. Lockhart, G. F. Hamilton and F. W. Fyfe (Faber).

An Introduction to Neurosurgery, by W. Bryan Jennett (Heinemann).

Applied Physiology, by Samson Wright (Oxford University Press).

Diseases of the Nervous System, by Lord Brain (Oxford University Press).

Essentials of Clinical Neuroanatomy and Neurophysiology, by John T. Manter and Arthur Gatz, (F. A. Davies).

Gray's Anatomy (Longmans, Green and Co.).

Injuries of the Brain and Spinal Cord and their Coverings, by Samuel Brock (Cassell).

Peripheral Nerve Injuries, by Ruth E. M. Bowden (H. K. Lewis).

Principles of Neurological Surgery, by Loyal Davis and Richard Davis (Kimpton).

Rehabilitation of the Hand, by C. B. Wynn Parry (Butterworths).

The Ciba Collection of illustrations, Vol. 1.

Various papers published by members of the unit staff.

FRACTURES AND SOFT TISSUE LESIONS

Fractures and Dislocations, by G. Perkins (Oxford University Press).

Fractures and Joint Injuries, by Sir R. Watson-Jones (Livingstone).

Fractures and Orthopaedic Surgery for Nurses and Physiotherapists, by A. Naylor (Livingstone).

Fractures and Soft Tissue Lesions, by P. D. London (Livingstone).

Injuries of the Knee Joint, by I. S. Smillie (Livingstone)

'The Mechanism, Reduction Technique and Results in Fractures of the Os Calcis', by Peter Essex-Lopreste. *British Journal of Surgery*, Vol. XXXIX, No. 157, March 1952.

'Progress in the Treatment of Fractures', by G. Perkins. *Physiotherapy*, December 1955.

'Re-education of the Injured Shoulder', by R. Barrie Brookes (unpublished).

Bibliography

'The Regeneration of Bone after Fracture', by T. T. Stamm. Report of Annual General Congress of the Chartered Society of Physiotherapy. *Physiotherapy*, October 1945.

Short Practice of Surgery, by A. J. Harding Rains and W. Melville Capper (H. K. Lewis).

'Some remarks on the Repair of Flexor Tendons in the Hand, with special reference to the Technique of Free Grafting', by A. B. Watson (Reprinted from the *British Journal of Surgery*, Vol. XLIII, No. 177, July 1955).

Sports Injuries. Their Prevention and Treatment, by Donald F. Featherstone (John Wright and Sons).

'Tenosynovitis and Tenovaginitis', by D. H. Griffiths. *British Medical Journal*, 22 March 1952.

GENERAL AND GYNAECOLOGICAL SURGERY

Modern Gynaecology with Obstetrics for Nurses, by Winifred Hector and G. Bourne (Heinemann).

Principles and Practice of Surgical Nursing, by D. F. Ellison Nash (Edward Arnold).

A Short Practice of Surgery, by Bailey and Love (H. K. Lewis).

Surgery for Nurses (Bailey and Love). Edited by McNeill Love and A. Clain (H. K. Lewis).

Surgery for Nurses, by J. Moroney (Livingstone).

Textbook of Operative Surgery, by E. L. Farquharson (Livingstone).

ORTHOPAEDICS

Essentials of Orthopaedics, by Philip Wiles (Churchill).

Orthopaedics for Nurses, by M. C. Wilkinson and G. R. Fisk (Faber)

PATHOLOGY

Pathology, by J. H. Dible and Thomas B. Davie (Churchill).

Textbook of Pathology, by William Boyd (Kimpton).

PHYSICAL TREATMENT

Ambulation, by Dening, Deyoe and Ellison (Funk and Wagnalls Company).

Physical Medicine and Rehabilitation, edited by Basil Kiernander (Blackwell).

Textbook of Medical Conditions for Physiotherapists, by J. E. Cash (Faber and Faber).

Ultrasonic Therapy, by W. Summer and Margaret K. Patrick (Elsevier Publishing Co.).

INDEX

Index

Index

Index

Index

Index